NOURISHING *FATS*

Other Books by Sally Fallon Morell

Nourishing Broth: An Old-Fashioned Remedy for the Modern World

Nourishing Traditions: The Cookbook That Challenges Politically Correct Nutrition and the Diet Dictocrats (with Mary G. Enig, PhD)

The Nourishing Traditions Book of Baby & Child Care (with Thomas S. Cowan, MD)

The Nourishing Traditions Cookbook for Children (with Suzanne Gross)

Eat Fat Lose Fat (with Mary G. Enig, PhD)

NOURISHING *FATS*

Why We Need ANIMAL FATS *for* HEALTH *and* HAPPINESS

SALLY FALLON MORELL

Foreword by Nina Teicholz

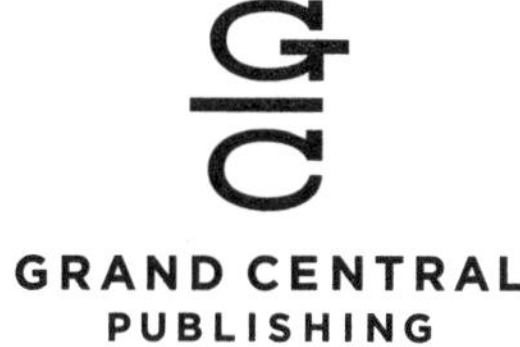

GRAND CENTRAL PUBLISHING

New York Boston

Grand Central Publishing
Hachette Book Group
1290 Avenue of the Americas, New York, NY 10104
grandcentralpublishing.com
twitter.com/grandcentralpub

First edition: January 2017

Image credits: page 4 *Good Housekeeping* magazine; page 13 and 63 *Journal of the American Medical Association;* page 53 The American Heart Association; page 100 *Life* magazine.

Grand Central Publishing is a division of Hachette Book Group, Inc. The Grand Central Publishing name and logo is a trademark of Hachette Book Group, Inc.

The publisher is not responsible for websites (or their content) that are not owned by the publisher.

The Hachette Speakers Bureau provides a wide range of authors for speaking events. To find out more, go to www.hachettespeakersbureau.com or call (866) 376-6591.

Library of Congress Cataloging-in-Publication Data

Names: Fallon, Sally, author.
Title: Nourishing fats : why we need animal fats for health and happiness / Sally Fallon Morell ; foreword by Nina Teicholz.
Description: New York : Grand Central Life & Style, [2017] | Includes bibliographical references and index.
Identifiers: LCCN 2016040436| ISBN 9781455592555 (trade pbk.) | ISBN 9781455592562 (ebook)
Subjects: LCSH: Lipids in nutrition. | Lipids—Metabolism. | Lipids—Physiological effect. | Fat—Health aspects.
Classification: LCC QP751 .F35 2017 | DDC 612.3/97—dc23
LC record available at https://lccn.loc.gov/2016040436

ISBNs: 978-1-4555-9255-5 (trade paperback), 978-1-4555-9256-2 (ebook)

Printed in the United States of America

LSC-C

Printing 5, 2022

To the memory of Mary G. Enig, PhD

Contents

Foreword

Lately there's been a growing chorus of voices challenging the conventional wisdom on dietary fat. Long-standing ideas have been upended—about which fats are bad and which are good, as well as the general notion that fat overall is a major driver of chronic disease. A large number of rigorous studies now show that you can eat plenty of fat and be slim and healthy—or health*ier*, even. Indeed, in 2015, after thirty-five years of recommending the low-fat diet to Americans, the U.S. government decided to lift its caps on total fat, albeit in such a quiet and confusing way that the public seems hardly to know.

People are even less aware of the origins of this shift—what we might call the Great Fat Reconsideration. With the recent proliferation of bloggers and book writers riding a wave of burgeoning enthusiasm about the surprising virtues of butter, eggs, whole milk, and so on, most people don't realize that many of these ideas trace directly back to the Weston A. Price Foundation, and especially to the work of Sally Fallon Morell together with her late, close colleague Mary G. Enig, PhD.

The partnership between Fallon Morell and Dr. Enig was a central force in propelling forward the rethinking of fats over the last twenty years. In 2006, for instance, they co-authored *Eat Fat, Lose Fat*, which detailed how higher-fat diets helped people maintain good health. This idea dates back a century at least, but its current renaissance has only unfolded over the past five years or so, putting these two women squarely ahead of the curve.

Taking on the scientific orthodoxy like this was second nature to Dr. Enig, who occupied a singular space in the academic world of "lipidology" (fats). A leading expert who published in academic journals, she simply lacked the fear *not* to challenge the prevailing dogma. For this she weathered a storm of criticism from her all-male colleagues who called her "nutso" and a "zealot," yet Dr. Enig fiercely stood her ground.

In the 1970s, she was one of the earliest researchers to signal the alarm about the dangers of *trans* fats—it took mainstream scientists another two decades to catch up—and also she spoke out, more generally, about the politics and health problems of vegetable oils. It was Dr. Enig, in fact, who lured me into studying this subject. With her seemingly unbelievable stories about how executives from the vegetable oil industry had repeatedly tried to shut down her work, I knew that Dr. Enig, hardly a kook, was truly a pioneer.

Fallon Morell, meanwhile, skillfully fused the science—Dr. Enig's charts of carbon-chain atoms and carboxyl groups—with the larger cultural and historical context. Put another way, she performed the crucial job of translating nutrition into *food*. She did this, in part, by writing *Nourishing Traditions*, a best-selling cookbook that combined recipes derived from ancient traditions, along with riveting, surprising stories about the origins of those traditions. Yes, ancient peoples prized organ meats above all other cuts and let bacteria run amok in their dairy products. For the average American, these were mind-bending revelations.

In this way, Sally Fallon Morell has carried forward the work of Dr. Price, the dentist whose stunning photos of healthy "primitive" peoples, along with accounts of their diets, provides a historical, anthropological record of how humans ate before the onset of chronic diseases. Modern nutrition science ignores all this history at its peril—which is why her work in preserving and furthering this crucial knowledge is such a profound contribution to the many researchers and laypeople now trying to rediscover our lost food culture.

Another important part of Dr. Price's legacy that Fallon Morell has skillfully charted into present day is a focus on nutrients, especially those needed for women and children. Nutrition scientists in the 1920s and '30s used to ask the question, so crucial to any animal, namely, what is the best diet for promoting healthy growth and reproduction? What must a pregnant woman eat to ensure a healthy baby and then feed that baby to ensure its healthy development? Attention to these issues vanished in the 1950s, when nutrition scientists swung around to focus instead on the growing epidemic of heart disease, which afflicted middle-aged men. The needs of women and children were thus subsumed to those of men. And this remains true today—such that the U.S. government's recommended diets are actually deficient in quite a few key nutrients, and consequently, lunches fed to our children in schools cannot support healthy growth, according to the government's own standards. Getting information about how to provide adequate nutrition to children is now nigh-well impossible.

Except for the Weston A. Price Foundation. Through the work of Fallon Morell, this group has become a beacon for parents in the United States and throughout the world on how to buy and cook food that will result in truly healthy children. Hopefully this focus on nutrients will catch on among the new crop of leaders embracing higher-fat diets. Thus far, however, it's been the the singular, brave work of Sally Fallon Morell and her foundation that has kept this vitally important information alive. Through her, so many women, including myself, have learned how to bring up healthy children, and for that, she rightly deserves a medal.

Now Sally Fallon Morell has written a new book, focusing on different kinds of dietary fats. Full of fascinating stories as well as the underlying science, the book carries on the spirit of her partnership with Dr. Enig. It also explains how fats play an interlocking role with crucial nutrients. In short, it combines the many strands of Fallon Morell's work to date. Plus, some of her excellent recipes.

NINA TEICHOLZ
Author of *New York Times* bestseller *The Big Fat Surprise*

NOURISHING
FATS

CHAPTER 1

The Greatest Villains

In 1911, William Procter and James Gamble, makers of soap and candles, introduced a revolutionary new product. They called their product Crisco.

Crisco's main ingredient was—and still is—cottonseed oil,* but cottonseed oil subjected to a special process to make it hard at room temperature. Developed by Procter and Gamble with the help of German chemist E. C. Kayser, the process of partial hydrogenation rearranges the hydrogen atoms in fat molecules. The resulting fat—now bleached, emulsified and deodorized—resembled lard.

P&G initially used this new industrially hardened fat to replace expensive lard and tallow in their candles and soap. But electricity had arrived, the market for candles fell precipitously, and the company needed new markets. Since the new product resembled lard, why not sell it as a food?

Marketing began in 1912. An ad appearing in the February 1912 *Home Directory* stressed the product's "vegetable" origin: "Great interest centers in the effort to establish the correct proportion of vegetable and animal products in the daily diet. Every important test made lately has confirmed the popular idea that all other things being equal, a vegetable product is more desirable than an animal one, and there can be no question of the desirability of replacing a greasy animal fat with a flaky vegetable product." The copy urged housewives to use Crisco for frying, as shortening, and for "general cooking" and praised its clean, fresh odor. "Better than Butter for Cooking," it promised. Readers learned that "Crisco is being placed in the grocery stores as rapidly as possible."

Procter & Gamble's next step was pure marketing genius—they published and gave away a cookbook touting the joys of cooking with their new magic fat. *The Story of Crisco* featured two hundred fifty recipes, everything from lobster bisque to pound cake, all made with Crisco.

The Story of Crisco's long introduction mixes pseudoscience with subtle persuasion. Considered a classic in marketing strategy, its language appealed to housewives of the emerging middle class, eager for modernization.[1]

* A waste product of the cotton industry.

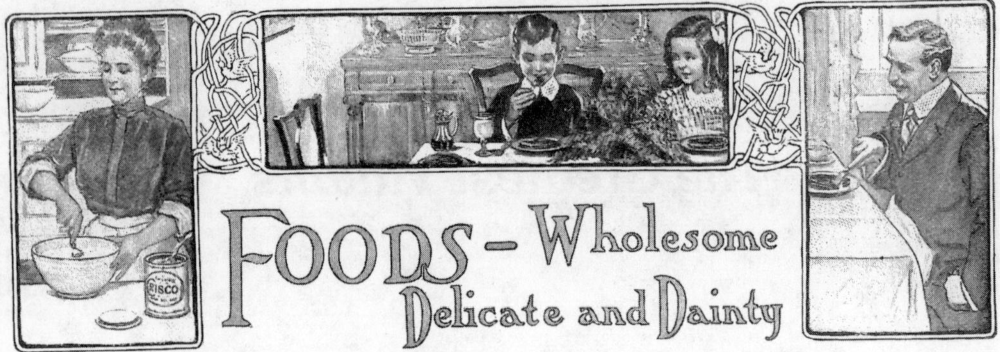

Their Intelligent Preparation

THERE is nothing more important to the American housewife than the preparation of wholesome, delicate and dainty foods for her family. More and more people now realize that by intelligent eating, not only can they avoid such common ills as headache and indigestion, but can do much to make good health their normal condition.

Great interest centers in the effort to establish the correct proportion of vegetable and animal products in the daily diet. Every important test made lately has confirmed the popular idea that all other things being equal, a vegetable product is more desirable than an animal one, and there can be no question of the desirability of replacing a greasy animal fat with a flaky vegetable product.

Crisco, the new product for frying, for shortening and for general cooking, is purely vege-

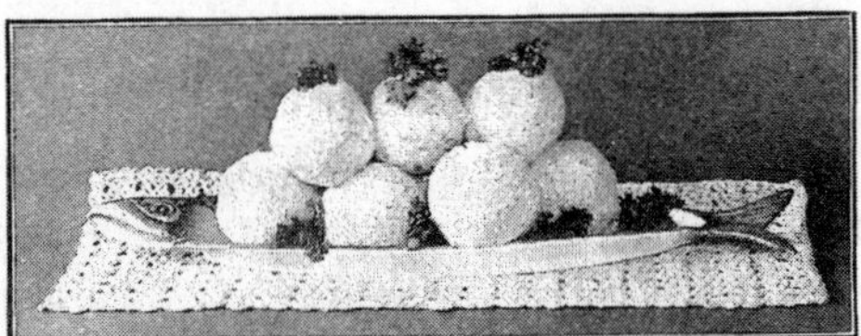

In Crisco, Fish Balls Fry in *One* Minute

table and should be used for cooking where you now use fats of animal origin, such as butter or lard. It is in no sense a compound or mixture of oils and fats. There is absolutely no animal matter in it.

Exquisitely Clean

CRISCO is absolutely clean and pure in origin and manufacture. It never gets strong, it stays sweet and fresh. It is put up in immaculate packages protected from dust and store odors. No hands ever touch it, no unsanitary paddles, boats or tubs. As soon as you see Crisco, you will be impressed with its purity. It is a delicious cream white, pleasing and appetizing in appearance. The color, flavor and odor are natural, there is nothing artificial about it.

Notice its Delicate Aroma

CRISCO has the fresh, pleasant odor of a vegetable product. It has *none* of the disagreeable features so characteristic of compounds or mixtures of oils and fats. Its use is not attended by even the slightest odor in the kitchen, nor do Crisco fried foods or pastries have any suggestion of the offensive odor or flavor which accompanies the use of cottonseed oil or lard compounds. Test it in hot biscuits. Open a Crisco biscuit when it is very hot and notice the delightful biscuit aroma. This is one of the most pleasing qualities of Crisco, for the strong odor of the ordinary fats in common use has made them thoroughly objectionable.

Purchase a package of Crisco today. Use it throughout your cooking and see how wholesome, delicate and dainty it makes your food.

On request, we shall mail a fully illustrated booklet, showing many other advantages of Crisco, the new and heretofore unknown, strictly vegetable product for frying, for shortening and for general cooking.

Packages 25c, 50c, and $1.00 except in the Far West

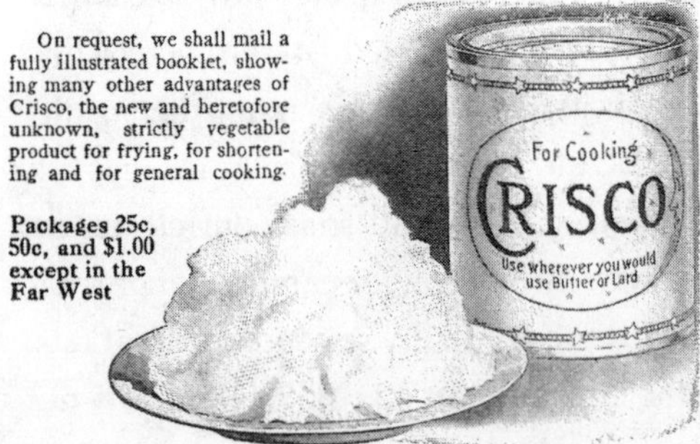

Crisco is Purely Vegetable.

CRISCO — Better than Butter for Cooking

Crisco is being placed in the grocery stores as rapidly as possible. If your own grocer does not keep it, you probably will find it in one of the other stores in your neighborhood; if not, on receipt of 25c in stamps or coin, we will send you by mail or express, charges prepaid, a regular 25c package. If you order from us, write plainly your name and address, and also let us have the name of your grocer. Not more than one package will be sent direct from us to any one customer.

THE PROCTER & GAMBLE CO., Dept. H, Cincinnati, Ohio.

The cookbook presents Crisco as healthier, more digestible, cleaner, more economical, more enlightened and more modern than lard; it portrays women who use Crisco as good wives and mothers, their houses are free of strong cooking odors and—every mother's dream—their children grow up with good character.* "Domestic scientists," employed by Procter & Gamble, taught the use of Crisco at cooking schools and at free demonstrations held in theaters and public facilities. One specific target: high school girls enrolled in home economics classes.

P&G also had the brilliant idea of presenting Crisco to the Jewish housewife as a kosher food, one that behaved like butter but could be used with meats. Because it made kosher cooking easier, Jews adopted Crisco and margarine—imitation lard and imitation butter—more quickly than other groups, with unforeseen consequences.

Procter & Gamble's strategy was obvious: demonize the competition, but do it in a way that would appeal to the thrifty turn-of-the century housewife, eager to be modern and clean.†

Crisco was not the first manufactured fat presented as suitable for human consumption. In 1869, Emperor Napoleon III of France offered a prize to anyone who could make a satisfactory alternative for butter, "suitable for use by the armed forces and the lower classes." French chemist Hippolyte Mège-Mouriès invented a substance he called oleomargarine, later shortened to "margarine." The principal raw material in the original formulation was beef fat, but in 1871, Henry W. Bradley of Binghamton, New York, patented a process for creating margarine that combined vegetable oils (primarily cottonseed oil) with animal fats. With cheaper ingredients, the margarine business promised great profits.

In *Life on the Mississippi*, published in 1883, Mark Twain recalls a conversation he overhears between a New Orleans cottonseed oil purveyor and a Cincinnati margarine drummer. New Orleans boasts of selling deodorized cottonseed oil as olive oil in bottles with European labels. "We turn out the whole thing—clean from the word go—in our factory in New Orleans...We are doing a ripping trade, too." Cincinnati reports that his factories are turning out oleomargarine by the thousands of tons, an imitation that "you can't tell from butter." He gloats at the thought of market domination. "You are going to see the day, pretty soon, when you won't find an ounce of butter to bless yourself with, in any hotel in the Mississippi and Ohio Valleys, outside of the biggest cities...And we can sell it so dirt cheap that the whole country has got to take it...butter don't stand any show—there ain't any chance for competition. Butter's had its day—and from this out, butter goes to the wall. There's more money in oleomargarine than—why, you can't imagine the business we do."[2]

Early ads for margarine had little copy and made no claims; instead, pictures of healthy babies and pretty girls conveyed wholesome goodness. The best they could do was imply equivalence at a lower price. And there was

* We now know that *trans* fats in products like Crisco interfere with the production of sex hormones, like testosterone and estrogen (more on that later in the book). Crisco *was* likely to make the children of these mothers less interested in sex.

† Besides all the health risks of partially hydrogenated oils, modern Crisco contains residues of strong defoliating chemicals.[a]

much resistance. People still preferred butter—in part because they could make it in their kitchens. Butter consumption in 1900 was about eighteen pounds per person per year,[3] or about five teaspoons per day, and probably a lot higher among farm families. Early visitors to America, such as de Tocqueville, noted that Americans were a butter-eating nation, that they put butter in or on everything including soups, sauces, meat, vegetables, porridge and puddings.[4] Early cookbooks included recipes for salad dressing based on melted butter.[5] People cooked in lard, bacon fat and beef dripping because that was what they had.

In the early 1900s, the chief medical concern was poor health in children—infectious disease, rickets, anemia and growth problems—problems rightly attributed to poor nutrition. On the basis of research carried out in the 1920s and 1930s, the British Medical Association recommended that all British people consume 80 percent more milk, 55 percent more eggs, 40 percent more butter and 30 percent more meat. The British government introduced free school milk—that would be full-fat milk—and encouraged the consumption of more animal foods, especially eggs.

Following this policy, childhood deaths from diphtheria, measles, scarlet fever and whooping cough fell dramatically—well before the advent of antibiotics and vaccinations.

I Can't Believe It's Butter

U.S. Per Capita Consumption in Pounds

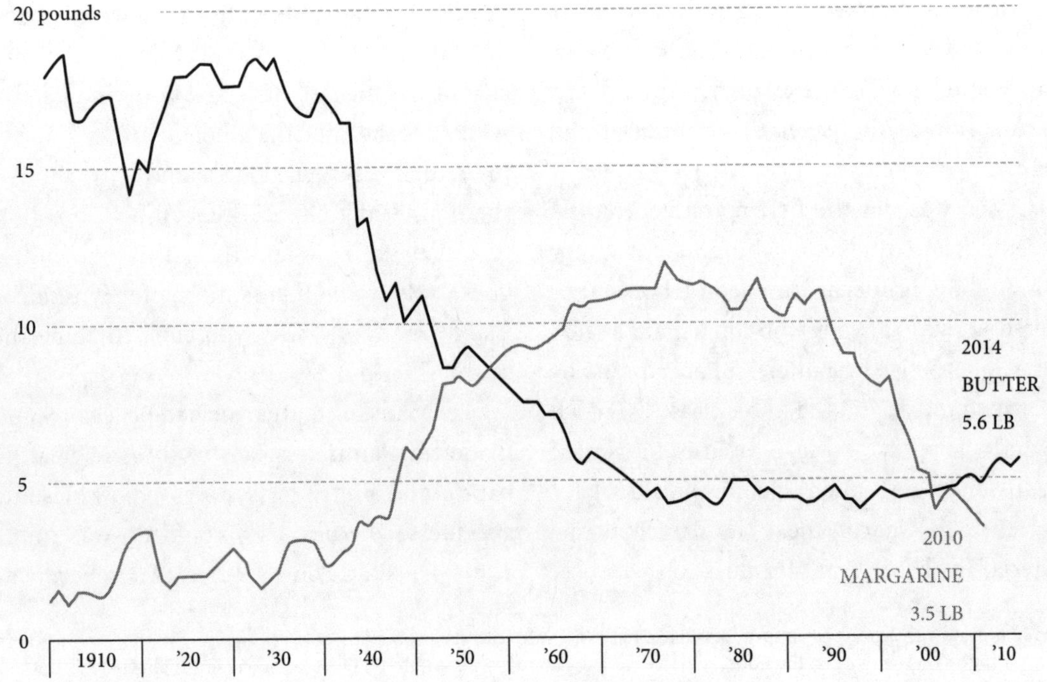

Note: Last margarine data is from 2010.
Source: U.S. Department of Agriculture; U.S. Census Bureau/*The Wall Street Journal*

Rickets and other childhood afflictions became rare. These recommendations continued into the Second World War, when all British children received a ration of eggs, cod liver oil and orange juice. During these years, the life expectancy in England climbed to sixty years in 1930 and seventy years in 1960.[6]

In America as well, most American doctors recognized the value of milk, eggs, butter, liver, cod liver oil and meat in the diet. Doctors told mothers to prepare liver once a week in order to prevent anemia, and housewives judged the quality of milk by the amount of cream it contained. *The American and His Food*, published in 1940, listed milk, cheese, eggs, liver, fatty fish, green vegetables, raw fruits, butter and cod liver oil as "highly protective foods" and legumes, cereals, bread, nuts, sugar, jam, honey, margarine, olive oil and other vegetable oils as "nonprotective foods."[7]

The Story of Crisco notwithstanding, advertisers found it difficult to make claims based on science or health benefits in this climate of common sense. They relied on price as the deciding factor. And then an innocent molecule called cholesterol entered the public consciousness. Cholesterol conveniently occurs only in animal foods, especially in saturated animal fats like lard and butter.

THE THEORY THAT CHOLESTEROL CAUSES heart disease dates from 1779 when Caleb Parry, an English physician, published his discovery that obstructed coronary arteries caused angina pectoris or chest pain.[8] In 1910 the German chemist Adolf Windaus reported that these lesions contained six times as much cholesterol as a normal arterial wall.[9]*

In 1912, just as Crisco was coming to market, Nikolai N. Anichkov, a Russian scientist, induced atherosclerosis—obstructions in the arteries—by feeding foods like egg yolks and purified cholesterol to vegetarian rabbits. One year later he announced the discovery that cholesterol was "the primary factor" in initiating atherosclerosis.[10] (One minor detail: Anichkov fed his rabbits cholesterol dissolved in vegetable oil, not saturated animal fats. Subsequently researchers routinely used vegetable oils as a base for cholesterol to induce atherosclerosis in animals.[11])

But the fabulous marketing opportunity that awaited the makers of margarine, shortening and industrial vegetable oils did not materialize until after the Second World War. In the 1950s, a new health problem emerged—not rickets or other obvious manifestations of malnutrition—but heart disease, especially sudden death from myocardial infarction or heart attack.

While turn-of-the-century mortality statistics are unreliable, they consistently indicate the fact that heart disease caused no more than 10 percent of all deaths, considerably less than infectious diseases such as pneumonia and tuberculosis. Heart disease in 1900 usually manifested as gradual heart failure after a serious case of typhoid fever, not as sudden death by heart attack. The first recorded U.S. case of myocardial infarction (MI)—the scientific term for heart attack—occurred in 1920[12]; three thousand deaths from MI occurred in

---

* Windaus won a Nobel Prize in Chemistry in 1928 for his work on sterols and their relation to vitamins. The main focus of his work involved the transformation of cholesterol through several steps to vitamin D_3 (cholecalciferol). He gave his patents to Merck and Bayer, which in 1927 brought out Vigantol, a vitamin D_3 supplement still in use today.[a]

1930. By 1960, coronary heart disease (CHD) was the leading source of mortality in the United States, causing more than three hundred thousand deaths annually. The greatest increase came under the rubric of myocardial infarction.[13] What was causing this new epidemic?*

In 1950 an American doctor, John Gofman, later known for his work on the dangers of x-rays and atomic radiation, resurrected the hypothesis that blood cholesterol was to blame. He noted, "For reasons still unknown, coronary heart disease suddenly took off during the 1920s throughout the industrialised world. By the 1940s it was becoming the major cause of premature death. And nobody knew why."[14]

Nobody knew why, but it was easy to theorize. One explanation was the decrease in infectious disease following the decline of the horse as a means of transport and the removal of horse manure from city streets, the installation of more sanitary water supplies, and the advent of better housing. These measures allowed more people to live to adulthood and thus made them more likely to experience a heart attack.

The other theory focused on a dietary change. Since the early part of the century, when the Department of Agriculture began tracking food "disappearance" data—or the amount of various foods going into the food supply—a number of researchers had noticed a change in the kind of fats Americans were eating. Butter consumption was declining while the use of vegetable oils, especially oils hardened to resemble butter or lard, was increasing—dramatically increasing. By 1950 butter consumption had dropped from eighteen pounds per person per year to just over ten. Margarine filled in the gap, rising from about two pounds per person at the turn of the century to about eight. Lard consumption plummeted from fifteen pounds per person per year to about three. Consumption of vegetable shortening—used in the home and in crackers and baked goods—remained relatively steady at about twelve pounds per person per year (up from zero in 1912), but consumption of liquid vegetable oil more than tripled—from just under three pounds per person per year to more than ten.[15] Sugar consumption was up as well, from less than ten pounds per year in 1820 to almost eighty pounds in 1950.[16] The statistics pointed to one obvious conclusion—to combat the rise in heart attacks, Americans should return to eating the traditional foods that nourished their ancestors, including meat, eggs, butter and cheese, and avoid the newfangled foods based on industrial oils (and sugar) that were flooding the grocers' shelves.

Even as the evidence pointed to the dietary shift toward oils and sugar as a cause, researchers continued to align themselves behind the idea that cholesterol was to blame for the epidemic. In 1954 a young researcher from Russia named David Kritchevsky repeated Anichkov's rabbit experiment. Kritchevsky agreed with the original findings: cholesterol added to vegetarian rabbit chow caused the formation of atheromas. In the same year,

* The rate of deaths from heart disease has declined since the 1960s, but even today, heart disease is still the leading cause of death in the United States, with over six hundred thousand per year according to some sources, costing more than one hundred billion dollars annually.[a]

Kritchevsky published a paper describing the beneficial effects of cholesterol-free polyunsaturated fatty acids—found in liquid vegetable oils—for lowering cholesterol.[17]

Another early researcher was Dr. Edward H. Ahrens. For decades, Ahrens conducted research on blood cholesterol levels to determine whether a dietary change could prevent atherosclerosis. His research showed that the substitution of liquid vegetable oils for solid animal fats could reduce levels of the villainous cholesterol molecule, at least for the duration of short-term human experiments. The discovery did *not* show that liquid oils could lower the rate of heart disease, but many used it as justification for urging a switch from saturated animal fats to liquid polyunsaturated oils.*

Much credit for popularizing the cholesterol theory of heart disease goes to the persuasive and strong-willed Ancel Keys, a University of Minnesota researcher. His various epidemiological studies made him the most famous scientist in the nutrition world as he championed the idea that saturated fats raise cholesterol and therefore cause heart attacks. It was Keys, more than any other, who promoted the idea of the Mediterranean diet as low in fat and cholesterol, and rich in vegetables and beans. These conclusions came from dietary surveys carried out in Italy, Greece and middle Europe in the early 1950s, when these populations were still recovering from the wartime shortages—and they were carried out during Lent![18] The idea that the Italian diet—rich in cured pork products, cheese and meat—is low in saturated fat contradicts all the evidence. Keys fancied himself a gourmet but does not seem to have enjoyed linguine Alfredo or pepperoni pizza during frequent sojourns in Italy.†

Another member of this rogue's gallery was Jeremiah Stamler, MD, the doctor credited with introducing the term "risk factors" into the field of cardiology. Listed as an author on over four hundred papers, starting in 1948 with a study entitled, "The effect of a low fat diet on the spontaneously occurring arteriosclerosis of the chicken,"[19] and continuing to 2015, Stamler insists even today that dietary cholesterol raises serum cholesterol, a premise that has faded with overwhelming findings to the contrary. Even during the heyday of cholesterol research, Stamler was highly selective in the studies he cited to justify his assertions. In a 1988 paper Stamler maintained that dietary cholesterol "has a substantial impact on blood cholesterol." As proof, he cited seven studies, and ignored many others. Two of these were irrelevant liquid diet studies and

---

* Getting human subjects to consume the right amounts of various fats—including bizarre diets that contained large amounts of pure saturated or polyunsaturated fatty acids—to determine their effect on blood cholesterol levels is not an easy task. "We had an awful time at first," said Dr. Ahrens in a 1984 interview. "It was boring as the devil for the patients, who had to eat the same diet every day for weeks. It was hard on the dietitians, and we didn't have precise enough control of the dietary mix." At the suggestion of a pediatrician at Rockefeller, who advised him to "feed them like babies," he put his patients on a diet of formula, becoming one of the first researchers to use this now-common technique. One is justified in asking what relevance studies on bottle-fed inmates have for normal people living in the real world and eating real food.[a]

† I lived with a French family in Montpelier, France, in 1968—a location as Mediterranean as Mediterranean can be. We ate ham, pâté, cheese, butter, eggs and meat every day. We ate fruits and vegetables occasionally—strawberries (with cream) in the late spring and sometimes a green salad—but never beans. Bread, of course, came with every meal. When journalist Nina Teicholz asked a Keys associate why the eminent scientist never included France in his surveys, she learned that "Keys did not like to travel in France."[a]

the remaining five indicated trivial effects of dietary cholesterol.[20] When the International Atherosclerosis Project found no relationship between diet and degree of arterial obstruction or proneness to heart disease, he continued to insist that "a highly significant correlation was found between intake of fat and severe atherosclerosis at autopsy."[21] In 1963, sponsored by Mazola Corn Oil and Mazola Margarine, Stamler coauthored a booklet called *Your Heart Has Nine Lives*, urging people to substitute vegetable oils for butter and other "artery-clogging" saturated fats.[22]

Dr. Frederick Stare, head of Harvard University's Nutrition Department for over forty years, added to the confusion surrounding cholesterol and saturated fat. He wrote a popular syndicated column that promoted the consumption of polyunsaturated oils and urged readers to reduce consumption of saturated fat and dietary cholesterol by avoiding eggs, meat and butter. In one 1969 column he stated, "To my knowledge, I've never heard of too much polyunsaturated fat for man."

He knew how to play fast and loose with the science: in a promotional piece specifically for Procter & Gamble's Puritan Oil, he cited two experiment and one clinical trial as showing that high blood cholesterol is associated with coronary heart disease (CHD).[23] However, neither experiments had anything to do with CHD, and the clinical trial did not find that reducing blood cholesterol had any effect on CHD events. Nor was he bothered by any conscience for consistency. In 1986, he published a letter to the editor in *FDA Consumer* claiming, "far too much emphasis to the hazards of saturated fat and dietary cholesterol and not enough to the hazard of too many calories is given by the magazine." In a 1989 letter to the editor of the *Journal of the American Medical Association* he asserted that "The [blood] cholesterol factor is of minor importance as a risk factor in cardiovascular disease."*[24]

Irving Page served as president of the American Heart Association (1956–57) and in 1961 coauthored—with Ancel Keys, Jeremiah Stamler and Frederick Stare—the American Heart Association's revised dietary guidelines. The new guidelines recommended that Americans reduce the consumption of total fats and cholesterol and increase the amount of polyunsaturated fats, this despite the fact that Page and Stare had previously published papers showing that the increase in coronary heart disease mirrored the rise in consumption of vegetable oils.[25] Only a few years earlier, Keys had proposed the theory that the increasing use of hydrogenated vegetable oils might actually be the underlying cause of heart disease.[26]

The 1968 AHA statement went further and quantified just how much fat and cholesterol people should be eating, with recommendations to limit cholesterol to 300 milligrams per day (typical diets contain 600–800 milligrams per day) and total fat to 30–35 percent of calories, comprised equally of saturated,

* Both Ancel Keys and Fred Stare received substantial funding from the sugar industry, and both vigorously objected to the premise that excess sugar consumption might be harmful, thus deflecting attention from sugar to animal fats as a cause of heart disease.[a] In a 1971 paper, Keys cherry-picked data in order to attack John Yudkin, a British researcher who argued that sugar consumption was a major culprit. "The public is grossly misled by repetitions in print of the claim that victims of CHD tend to be persons who habitually consume more sugar than the average for the population."[b] He objected to Yudkin's use of statistical associations, a practice at which Keys was a master.

polyunsaturated and monounsaturated fatty acids (typical diets contain 40–80 percent of calories as fat). These recommendations remain even to the present, enshrined in the USDA Dietary Guidelines.

It was these early researchers who formulated the "diet-heart theory" (that dietary choices can affect cholesterol levels in the blood) and the "lipid hypothesis" (that blood cholesterol levels determine proneness to heart disease). The appeal to the industrial oil industry was obvious—seed oils, as opposed to animal fats like butter, tallow and lard—contain no cholesterol and very little saturated fat. If feeding polyunsaturated oils from vegetable sources lowered serum cholesterol in humans, at least temporarily, and feeding vegetarian animals cholesterol caused plaque buildup in their arteries—oils were the clear solution! Using this shaky science, researchers put forward the idea that Americans could avoid heart disease by reducing animal products in their diet and lowering their cholesterol by substituting polyunsaturated oils. And this line of argument *just happened* to prove a boon to those who produced products that could substitute for butter, cream, eggs and lard.

Procter & Gamble was the first in the industry to capitalize on this opportunity brought forth by this new theory of heart disease prevention. In 1948, P&G made the American Heart Association (AHA) the beneficiary of their popular "Walking Man" radio contest, which the company sponsored. The show raised almost two million dollars for the organization and transformed it (according to the AHA's official history) from a small, underfunded professional society into the powerhouse it remains today.[27] Originally founded in 1924 to study the effects of diseases like rheumatic fever on the heart, the organization morphed into the most influential advocate for a diet low in cholesterol and saturated fat. Their advice, even today, is unwaveringly fat-phobic: avoid butter, cream, ice cream, egg yolks and whole milk in favor of industrial seed oils, soft margarines, skinless chicken breasts, lean meat, egg whites and low-fat salad dressings.[28] The AHA remains the main force in the war on animal fats—with no concern about the consequences.

IN THE YEARS THAT FOLLOWED, a number of population studies demonstrated that the animal model—especially one derived from vegetarian animals like rabbits—was not a valid approach for studying the problem of heart disease in human omnivores. As early as 1936, pathologists K. E. Lande and W. M. Sperry at Harvard University looked at cholesterol levels and degree of coronary artery occlusion in individuals who had died a sudden death. They found no correlation; there were individuals with low cholesterol and a high degree of occlusion and individuals with high cholesterol and a low degree of occlusion.[29]

A much publicized 1955 report on artery plaques in American soldiers killed during the Korean War showed high levels of atherosclerosis, but another report—one that did not make it to the front page of the *New York Times*—found that Japanese natives had almost as much pathogenic plaque—65 percent versus 75 percent—even though the Japanese diet at the time was lower in animal products and fat.[30] A 1957 study of the largely vegetarian Bantu found that they had as much atheroma as other races from South

Africa who ate more meat.[31] A 1958 report noted that Jamaican blacks showed a degree of atherosclerosis comparable to that found in the United States, although they suffered from lower rates of heart disease.[32] A 1960 report noted that the severity of atherosclerotic lesions in Japan approached that of the United States.[33] The 1968 International Atherosclerosis Project, in which over twenty-two thousand corpses in fourteen nations were cut open and examined for plaques in the arteries, showed the same degree of atheroma in all parts of the world—in populations that consumed large amounts of fatty animal products and those that were largely vegetarian, and in populations that suffered from a great deal of heart disease and in populations that had very little or none at all.[34] These studies pointed to the likelihood that the thickening of the arterial walls is a natural, unavoidable process. The diet-heart theory and the lipid hypothesis put forward by American researchers did not hold up to these population studies, nor did it explain the tendency to fatal clots associated with myocardial infarction.

But the lipid hypothesis had already gained enough momentum to keep it rolling, in spite of the contradictory studies that were showing up in the scientific literature. In 1957, Dr. Norman Jolliffe, director of the Nutrition Bureau of the New York Health Department, initiated the Anti-Coronary Club, in which a group of businessmen, ranging in age from forty to fifty-nine years, were placed on the Prudent Diet. Club members used corn oil and margarine instead of butter, cold breakfast cereals instead of eggs, and chicken and fish instead of beef. A control group of men the same age ate eggs for breakfast and had meat three times a day. Jolliffe, an overweight diabetic confined to a wheelchair, was confident that the Prudent Diet would save lives, including his own.

That same year, 1957, the food industry initiated advertising campaigns that touted the health benefits of products low in fat or made with vegetable oils. A typical ad read: "Wheaties may help you live longer." Wesson recommended its cooking oil "for your heart's sake," and a *Journal of the American Medical Association* ad described Wesson oil as a "cholesterol depressant." Mazola advertisements assured the public that "science finds corn oil important to your health." Medical journal ads recommended Fleischmann's Unsalted Margarine for patients with high blood pressure. Such advertising continued unabated through the 1960s and 1970s. A 1970 ad for Fleischmann's "Golden Corn Oil" Margarine, appearing in the *Journal of the American Medical Association*, showed a heart wrapped in a Fleischmann's Margarine wrapper with the headline, "Eat to your heart's content." The text sauntered along in the same jaunty, pseudoscientific style as *The Story of Crisco*. "According to latest medical opinion, a low-saturated-fat, low-cholesterol diet is still one of the best ways to a man's heart. Such diets invariably include a vegetable oil margarine—like Fleischmann's."

The vegetable oil industry soon discovered a foolproof advertising technique: get the guys in white coats to do your advertising for you. Dr. Frederick Stare, head of Harvard University's Nutrition Department, came first, promoting vegetable oils in his syndicated column. Later, Dr. William Castelli, director of the Framingham Study, provided an endorsement for Procter & Gamble's Puritan Oil; Dr. Frederick Stare also promoted Puritan. Dr. Antonio Gotto, Jr., former president of the

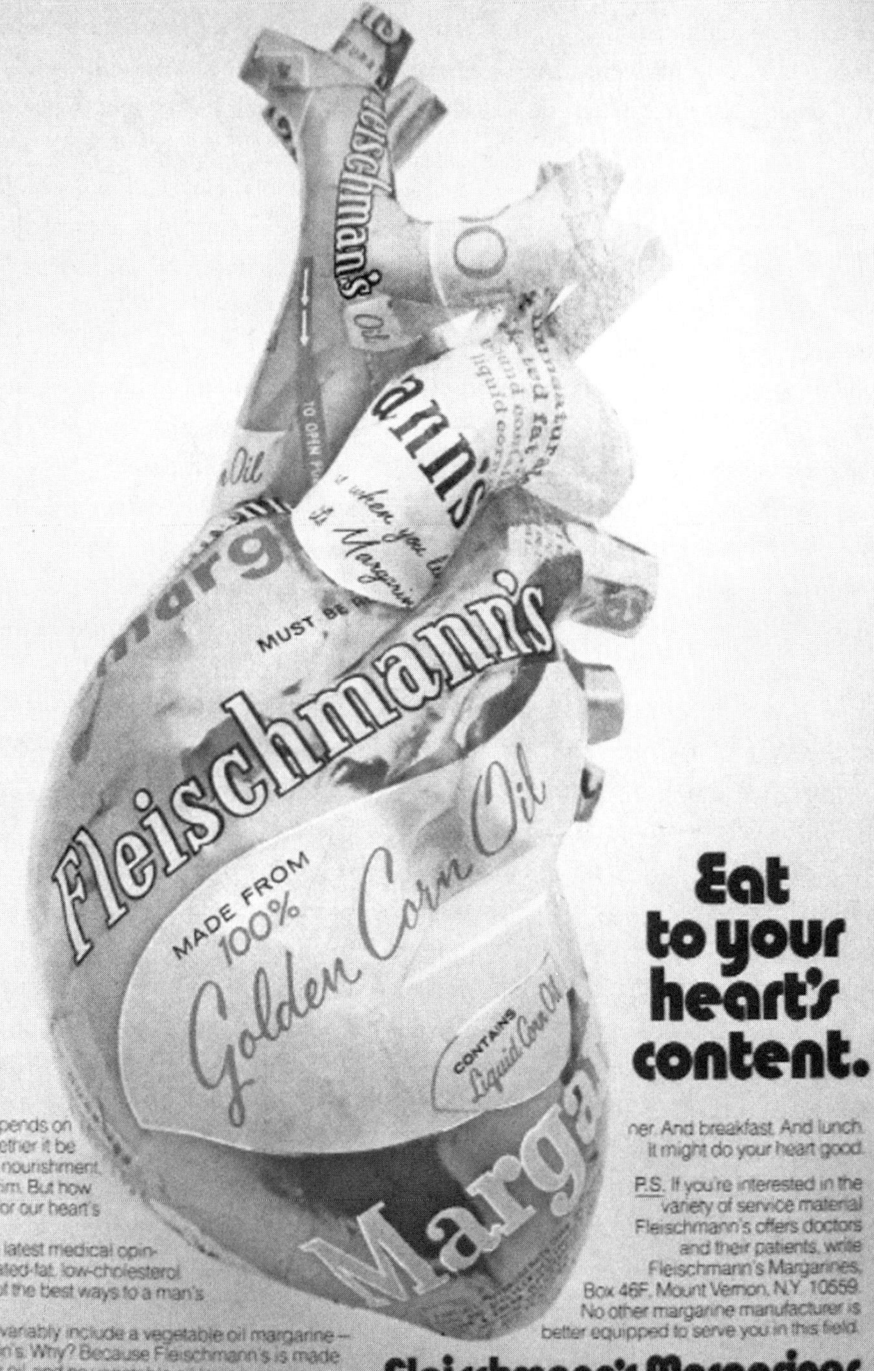
Fleischmann's
MUST BE
MADE FROM 100% Golden Corn Oil
CONTAINS Liquid Corn Oil
Eat to your heart's content.
What we eat depends on why we eat. Whether it be for pleasure, for nourishment, or just to keep trim. But how many of us eat for our heart's benefit?
According to latest medical opinion, a low-saturated-fat, low-cholesterol diet is still one of the best ways to a man's heart.
Such diets invariably include a vegetable oil margarine—like Fleischmann's. Why? Because Fleischmann's is made from 100% corn oil, and no vegetable oil lowers serum cholesterol better than corn oil. No margarine tastes better, either. Fleischmann's has that light, distinctive flavor that has helped make it America's favorite premium margarine.
Strike a blow for better diets. Invite Fleischmann's to dinner. And breakfast. And lunch. It might do your heart good.
P.S. If you're interested in the variety of service material Fleischmann's offers doctors and their patients, write Fleischmann's Margarines, Box 46F, Mount Vernon, N.Y. 10559. No other margarine manufacturer is better equipped to serve you in this field.
Fleischmann's Margarines
... made from 100% corn oil. Fleischmann's comes Lightly Salted, Unsalted, and Soft. And for half the calories, half the fat of regular margarines, try delicious Diet Fleischmann's.

American Heart Association, sent a letter promoting Puritan Oil to practicing physicians—printed on letterhead from the De Bakey Heart Center at Baylor College of Medicine.[35] The irony of Gotto's letter is that De Bakey, the famous heart surgeon, coauthored a 1964 study involving seventeen hundred patients, which also showed no definite correlation between serum cholesterol levels and the nature and extent of coronary artery disease.[36] In other words, those with low cholesterol levels were just as likely to have blocked arteries as those with high cholesterol levels. But while studies like De Bakey's moldered in the basements of university libraries, the vegetable oil campaign took on increased bravado and audacity.

The American Medical Association at first opposed the commercialization of the diet-heart theory and warned that "the anti-fat, anti-cholesterol fad is not just foolish and futile... it also carries some risk."[37] The American Heart Association (AHA), however, was committed.

Your Heart Has Nine Lives—a little self-help book by Stamler and sponsored by the makers of Mazola Corn Oil and Mazola Margarine—showed up in the 1960s, advocating the substitution of vegetable oils for butter and other so-called "artery clogging" saturated fats. Stamler did not believe that lack of evidence should deter Americans from changing their eating habits. The evidence, he stated, "was compelling enough to call for altering some habits even before the final proof is nailed down... the definitive proof that middle-aged men who reduce their blood cholesterol will actually have far fewer heart attacks waits upon diet studies now in progress." His version of the Prudent Diet called for substituting low-fat milk products such as skim milk and low-fat cheese for cream, butter and whole cheese, reducing egg consumption, and cutting the fat off red meats. Heart disease, he lectured, was a disease of rich countries, striking rich people who ate rich food, including "hard" fats like butter.[38]

It was in 1966 that the results of Dr. Jolliffe's Anti-Coronary Club experiment were published in the *Journal of the American Medical Association*.[39] Those on the Prudent Diet of corn oil, margarine, fish, chicken and cold cereal had an average serum cholesterol of 220 mg/dl, compared to 250 mg/dl in the meat-and-potatoes control group. Blood pressure also dropped and the Prudent Dieters lost weight. However, the study authors were obliged to note twenty-six deaths in the Prudent Diet group, including eight deaths from heart disease, versus only six deaths, none from heart disease, among those who ate meat three times a day. Dr. Jolliffe was dead by this time. He succumbed in 1961 to vascular thrombosis, although the obituaries listed the cause of death as complications from diabetes. The "compelling proof" that Stamler and others felt certain would vindicate wholesale tampering with American eating habits was not yet "nailed down."

According to insiders promoting the diet-heart theory and the lipid hypothesis, the numbers involved in the Anti-Coronary Club experiment were too small to provide meaningful results. Dr. Irving Page urged a national diet-heart study involving one million men, in which the results of the Prudent Diet could be compared on a large scale with those on a diet high in meat and fat. With great media attention, the National Heart, Lung, and Blood Institute organized the stocking of food warehouses in six major cities, where men on the Prudent Diet could get tasty polyunsaturated donuts and other fabricated food items free of charge. But a pilot study involving two thousand men resulted in exactly the same number of deaths in both the Prudent Diet and the control group. A brief report in *Circulation*, March 1968, stated that the study was a milestone "in mass environmental experimentation" that would have "an important effect on the food industry and the attitude of the public toward its eating habits."[40] But the million-man Diet-Heart Study was abandoned in utter silence "for reasons of cost." Its chairman, Dr. Irving Page, died of a heart attack.

ALTHOUGH THE AHA HAD COMMITTED itself to the lipid hypothesis and the unproven theory that liquid vegetable oils afforded protection against heart disease, concerns about partially hydrogenated (industrially hardened) vegetable oils were sufficiently great to warrant the inclusion of the following statement in the organization's 1968 statement on diet and heart disease: "Partial hydrogenation of polyunsaturated fats results in the formation of *trans* forms which are less effective than *cis, cis* [natural] forms in lowering cholesterol concentrations. It should be noted that many currently available shortening and margarines are partially hydrogenated and may contain little polyunsaturated fat of the natural *cis, cis* form." The AHA printed one hundred fifty thousand statements but never distributed them. The shortening industry strongly objected, and a researcher named Fred Mattson of Procter & Gamble convinced Campbell Moses, medical director of the AHA, to remove the statement.[41] The final AHA recommendations for the public contained three major points—restrict calories, substitute liquid oil for saturated fats like butter, and reduce cholesterol in the blood through diet.

Other organizations soon fell in behind the AHA in urging the replacement of animal fat with vegetable oils. By the early 1970s the National Heart, Lung, and Blood Institute (NHLBI), the American Medical Association (AMA), the American Dietetic Association (ADA) and the National Academy of Science (NAS) had all endorsed the lipid hypothesis, urging Americans in the "at risk" category to avoid animal fats.

Since Kritchevsky's early rabbit studies, many other trials had shown that serum cholesterol can be lowered by increasing ingestion of liquid polyunsaturated oil.* But proof that lowering serum cholesterol levels could stave off CHD remained elusive. That did not prevent the American Heart Association from calling for "modified and ordinary foods" to support a dietary shift toward newfangled oils and away from traditional fats. These foods, said the AHA literature, should be made available to the consumer, "reasonably priced and easily identified by appropriate labeling. Any existing legal and regulatory barriers to the marketing of such foods should be removed."[42]

* The physiological explanation goes like this: when excess polyunsaturates are built into the cell membranes, resulting in reduced structural integrity or "limpness," cholesterol is sequestered from the blood into the cell membranes to give them necessary "stiffness." This results in lower cholesterol levels in the blood, at least temporarily.

The man who made it possible to remove any "existing legal and regulatory barriers" was Peter Barton Hutt, a food lawyer for the prestigious Washington, DC law firm of Covington and Burling. Hutt once stated, "Food law is the most wonderful field of law that you can possibly enter."[43] After representing the edible oil industry at his law firm, he temporarily left to become the FDA's general counsel in 1971.

The regulatory barrier the AHA was referring to, and that Hutt would challenge, was the Food, Drug and Cosmetic Act of 1938, which stated that "there are certain traditional foods that everyone knows, such as bread, milk, and cheese, and that when consumers buy these foods, they should get the foods that they are expecting... [and] if a food resembles a standardized food but does not comply with the standard, that food must be labeled as an 'imitation.'"

The 1938 Food, Drug and Cosmetic Act became law partly in response to consumer concerns about the adulteration of ordinary foodstuffs. Chief among those needing protection were butter and olive oil—foods with a tradition of suffering competition from imitation products. As the FDA's general counsel, Hutt guided his agency through the legal and congressional hoops to establish a new "Imitation Policy" in 1973. This new policy attempted to provide for "advances in food technology" and give "manufacturers relief from the dilemma of either complying with an outdated standard or having to label their new products as 'imitation'... [since] such products are not necessarily inferior to the traditional foods for which they may be substituted."[44] Hutt considered the word "imitation" as oversimplified, inaccurate and "potentially misleading to consumers." The new regulations defined "inferiority" as "any reduction in content of an essential nutrient that is present at a level of two percent or more of the US Recommended Daily Allowance (RDA)." The new imitation policy meant that imitation sour cream, made with vegetable oil and fillers like guar gum and carrageenan, need not carry an imitation label as long as added minerals and artificial vitamins brought key nutrient levels up to the same amounts as those in real sour cream. Coffee creamers, imitation egg mixes, processed cheeses and imitation whipped cream no longer required the imitation label, but could be sold as real and beneficial foods, low in cholesterol and rich in polyunsaturated fatty acids.

These new regulations were adopted without the consent of Congress, continuing the trend, instituted under Nixon, of the White House using the FDA to promote certain social agendas through government food policies. This policy effectively increased the lobbying clout of special interest groups, such as the edible oil industry, and short-circuited public participation in the regulatory process. The FDA's new imitation language allowed food processing innovations that manufacturers regarded as "technological improvements" to enter the marketplace without the onus of oversight brought on by greater consumer awareness and congressional supervision. Along with "technological improvements" the FDA ushered in the era of ersatz foodstuffs—convenient counterfeit products that were weary, stale, flat and immensely profitable.

CONGRESS VOICED NO OBJECTION TO the FDA's usurpation of its powers, but entered the contest on the side of the lipid hypothesis. The Senate Select Committee on Nutrition and Human Needs, chaired by

George McGovern during the years 1973 to 1977, actively promoted the use of vegetable oils. "Dietary Goals for the United States," published by the committee, cited U.S. Department of Agriculture data on fat consumption, and stated categorically that "the overconsumption of fat, generally, and saturated fat in particular... have been related to six of the ten leading causes of death" in the United States. The report urged the American populace to reduce overall fat intake and to substitute polyunsaturated vegetable oils for saturated fat from animal sources—margarine and corn oil for butter, lard and tallow.[45] Opposing testimony included a moving letter by Dr. Fred Kummerow of the University of Illinois urging a return to traditional whole foods and warning against consumption of soft drinks. In the early 1970s, Kummerow had shown that *trans* fatty acids in partially hydrogenated vegetable oil caused increased rates of heart disease in pigs.[46] This was a direct challenge to the lipid hypothesis driving the country's food choices, but his letter remained buried in the voluminous report. A private endowment allowed him to continue his research as government funding agencies such as National Institutes of Health refused to give Kummerow further grants.

McGovern committee members were also aware of another damning unpublished study, this time on calves and cholesterol. While the study was not mentioned in the committee's final report, it compared calves fed saturated fat from tallow and lard with those fed unsaturated fat from soybean oil. The calves fed tallow and lard did indeed show higher plasma cholesterol levels than the calves fed soybean oil, and researchers found fat streaking in their aortas. But the calves fed soybean oil showed a decline in calcium and magnesium levels in the blood, possibly due to inefficient absorption. They utilized vitamins and minerals inefficiently, showed poor growth, poor bone development, and had abnormal hearts.* More cholesterol per unit of dry matter was found in the calves' aortas, livers, muscle, fat and coronary arteries. These findings led the investigators to an important conclusion: the lower blood cholesterol levels in the soybean-oil-fed calves may have been the result of cholesterol transfer from the blood to other tissues. The calves in the soybean oil group also collapsed when they were forced to move around, and they were unaware of their surroundings for short periods. They also had rickets and diarrhea.[47] These unfortunate side effects of a vegetable oil diet in calves should have served as a warning on the effects of the diet-heart theory applied to children, but no one on the committee was paying attention.

One person who was paying attention was Mary G. Enig, a graduate student in the lipids department at the University of Maryland. When she read the McGovern committee final report, she was puzzled. Enig was familiar with Kummerow's research, and she knew that the consumption of animal fats in America was not on the increase—quite the contrary, use of animal fats had declined steadily since the turn of the century. A report in the *Journal of American Oil Chemists*—which the McGovern committee did not use—showed that animal fat consumption had declined from 104 grams per person per day in 1909 to 97 grams

---

* Milk replacer given to calves today contains animal fat as the third ingredient. Human babies are not so lucky. They get polyunsaturated oils in their formula—no animal fats and no cholesterol for them!

per day in 1972, while vegetable fat intake had tripled from a mere 21 grams to almost 60.[48] Total per capita fat consumption had tripled over the period, but this increase was mostly due to an increase in unsaturated fats from vegetable oils—with 50 percent of the increase coming from liquid vegetable oils and about 41 percent from margarines and shortenings made from vegetable oils.

She also knew about a number of studies that directly contradicted the McGovern committee's conclusions that "there is . . . a strong correlation between dietary fat intake and the incidence of breast cancer and colon cancer," two of the most common cancers in America. All she had to do was look to other countries. Greece, for example, had less than one-fourth the rate of breast cancer compared to Israel, but the same dietary fat intake.[49] Spain had only one-third the breast cancer mortality of France and Italy, but the total dietary fat intake was slightly greater.[50] Puerto Rico, with a high animal fat intake, had very low rates of breast and colon cancer.[51] The Netherlands and Finland both used approximately 100 grams of animal fat per capita per day, but breast and colon cancer rates were almost twice as high in the Netherlands compared to Finland.[52] The Netherlands consumed 53 grams of vegetable fat per person compared to 13 in Finland. A study from Cali, Columbia, found a fourfold excess risk for colon cancer in the higher economic classes, which used less animal fat than the lower economic classes.[53] A study on Seventh-Day Adventist physicians, who avoid meat, especially red meat, found they had a significantly higher rate of colon cancer than non-Seventh-Day Adventist physicians.[54]

Enig analyzed the U.S. Department of Agriculture data that the McGovern committee had used and concluded that it showed a strong *positive correlation* between total fat and vegetable fat consumption to total cancer deaths, breast and colon cancer mortality, and breast and colon cancer incidence. The data also showed an essentially strong *negative correlation* or no correlation between animal fat consumption and total cancer deaths, breast and colon cancer mortality, and breast and colon cancer incidence. In other words, the data that the McGovern committee used showed that vegetable oils seemed to predispose someone to cancer while animal fats seemed to protect against cancer. She also noted that the analysts for the committee had manipulated the data in inappropriate ways—for example adding when they should have subtracted—in order to obtain mendacious results in favor of vegetable oils.

Enig submitted her findings to the *Journal of the Federation of American Societies for Experimental Biology* (FASEB), in May 1978, and her article was published in the FASEB's *Federation Proceedings*[55] in July of the same year—an unusually quick turnaround. The assistant editor, responsible for accepting the article, died of a heart attack shortly thereafter. Enig's paper noted that the correlations pointed a finger at the *trans* fatty acids and called for further investigation.

Enig's paper sent alarm bells through the edible oil industry. In early 1979, while still a graduate student, she received a visit from S. F. Reipma of the National Association of Margarine Manufacturers. Reipma was visibly annoyed. He explained that both his association and the Institute for Shortening and Edible Oils (ISEO) kept careful watch to prevent articles like Enig's from appearing in the scientific literature. He claimed that Enig's paper should never have been published. While he thought that ISEO was "watching out," he admitted, "we left the barn door open, and the horse got out." Reipma challenged Enig's use of the USDA data, claiming that it was in error. He knew it was in error, he said, "because we give it to them."

A few weeks later, Reipma paid Enig a second visit, this time in the company of Thomas Applewhite, an advisor to the ISEO and representative of Kraft Foods, Ronald Simpson with Central Soya, and an unnamed representative from Lever Brothers. They carried with them—in fact, waved them in the air in indignation—a two-inch stack of newspaper articles, including one that appeared in the *National Enquirer*, all reporting favorably on Enig's *Federation Proceedings* article. Applewhite's face flushed red with anger when Enig repeated Reipma's statement that "they had left the barn door open and the horse got out," and his admission that the margarine industry had sabotaged the Department of Agriculture food data.

In spite of Enig's efforts to right the wrongs of the McGovern committee, the Committee's recommendations bolstered dietary trends already in progress—the increased use of vegetable oils, especially in the form of partially hydrogenated margarines and shortenings. In 1976, the FDA established GRAS (Generally Recognized as Safe) status for hydrogenated soybean oil. A report prepared by the Life Sciences Research Office of the Federation of American Societies for Experimental Biology (LSRO-FASEB) concluded, "There is no evidence in the available information on hydrogenated soybean oil that demonstrates or suggests reasonable ground to suspect a hazard to the public when it is used as a direct or indirect food ingredient at levels that are now current or that might reasonably be expected in the future."[56] Armed with this assurance, the vegetable oil industry turned its attention to replacing animal fats with *trans* fats in the entire food supply.

WHILE THE U.S. GOVERNMENT ABANDONED its million-man diet-heart study "for reasons of cost," plenty of funding became available for other studies through the National Heart, Blood, and Lung Institute (NHBLI). These studies would form the justification that allowed the scientific and popular literature promote the diet-heart theory and the lipid hypothesis.

First was the Framingham Study, ongoing for forty years, which found virtually no difference in coronary heart disease "events" for individuals with cholesterol levels between 205 mg/dL and 294 mg/dL—the vast majority of the U.S. population. Even for those with extremely high cholesterol levels—up to almost 1200 mg/dL—the difference in CHD events compared to those in the normal range was trivial.[57] This did not prevent Dr. William Kannel, Framingham Study director in 1987, from making sweeping claims about the Framingham results. "Total plasma cholesterol," he said, "is a powerful predictor of death related to CHD."[58] It wasn't until more than a decade later that the real findings at Framingham were published—without fanfare—in the *Archives of Internal Medicine*, an obscure journal. "In Framingham, Massachusetts," admitted Dr. William Castelli, Kannel's successor, "the more saturated fat one ate, the more cholesterol one ate, the more calories one ate, the lower people's serum cholesterol... we found that the people who ate the most cholesterol, ate the most saturated fat, ate the most calories weighed the least and were the most physically active."[59] In other words, those eating butter and other animal fats had the lowest major risk factors for heart disease—low cholesterol levels, normal body weight and high physical activity.

NHLBI's Multiple Risk Factor Intervention Trial (MRFIT) also studied the relationship between heart disease and serum cholesterol levels, this time in three hundred sixty-two thousand men. Published in 1982, this trial found that annual deaths from CHD varied from slightly less than one per thousand at serum cholesterol levels below 140 mg/dL, to about two per thousand for serum cholesterol levels above 300 mg/dL, once again a trivial difference. Dr. John LaRosa of the American Heart Association claimed that the curve for CHD deaths began to "inflect" after 200 mg/dL, when in fact the "curve" was a very gradually sloping straight line that could not predict whether serum cholesterol above certain levels posed a significantly greater risk for heart disease. In addition, another key MRFIT finding—not reported in the media—was the unexpected fact that deaths from all causes (cancer, heart disease, accidents, infectious disease, kidney failure, etc.) were substantially greater for those men with cholesterol levels *below* 160 mg/dL.[60]

Considering the fact that orthodox medical agencies united together in their promotion of margarine and vegetable oils over animal foods containing cholesterol and saturated fat, it is surprising that researchers can cite only a handful of experiments indicating that dietary cholesterol has "a major role in determining blood cholesterol levels." One of these was a study involving seventy male prisoners directed by Fred Mattson[61]—the same Fred Mattson, formerly of Procter & Gamble, who pressured the American Heart Association into removing any reference to hydrogenated fats from their diet-heart statement a decade earlier. Funded in part by P&G, the research contained a number of serious flaws: selection of subjects for the four groups studied was not randomized; the experiment inexcusably eliminated "an equal number of subjects with the highest and lowest cholesterol values"; twelve additional subjects dropped out, leaving some of the groups too small to provide valid conclusions; and statistical manipulation of the results was shoddy. But the biggest flaw was the fact that the subjects receiving cholesterol did so in the form of reconstituted powder—an artificial diet. Mattson's discussion did not even address the possibility that the liquid formula diet he used might affect blood cholesterol levels differently than a diet of whole foods—even as other comparable studies indicated that this is the case. The culprit, in fact, in liquid protein diets appears to be oxidized cholesterol, formed during the high-temperature drying process. Oxidized cholesterol seems to initiate a buildup of plaque in the arteries.*[62] It was also purified, oxidized cholesterol (usually mixed with vegetable oil) that Kritchevsky and others used in their experiments on vegetarian rabbits.

The NHLBI had argued that a diet study using whole foods and involving large numbers of Americans would be too difficult to design

* Powdered milk containing oxidized cholesterol is often added (without labeling) to reduced-fat milk—to give it body—which the American public has accepted as a healthier choice than whole milk.

and too expensive to carry out, but the agency did have funds available to sponsor the massive Lipid Research Clinics Coronary Primary Prevention Trial (LRC-CPPT) in which all subjects were placed on a diet low in cholesterol and saturated fat. The researchers divided the subjects into two groups, one of which took a cholesterol-lowering drug and the other a placebo, but placed both groups on a low-cholesterol, low–saturated fat diet. Working behind the scenes, but playing a key role in both the design and implementation of the trials, was the same Dr. Fred Mattson.

An interesting feature of this particular study was the fact that a good part of the trial's one-hundred-and-fifty-million-dollar budget was devoted to sessions in which trained dietitians taught both groups of study participants how to choose "heart-friendly" foods—margarine, egg replacements, processed cheese, baked goods made with vegetable shortenings—in short, the vast array of manufactured foods awaiting consumer acceptance. As both groups received dietary indoctrination, study results could support no claims about the relation of diet to heart disease. Nevertheless, when the results were released, both the popular press and the medical journals portrayed the Lipid Research Clinics' trials as the long-sought proof that animal fats were the cause of heart disease. Rarely mentioned in the press reports was the ominous fact that the group taking the cholesterol-lowering drugs had an increase in deaths from cancer, stroke, violence and suicide.[63]

The Lipid Research Clinics' researchers claimed that the group taking the cholesterol-lowering drug had a 17 percent reduction in the rate of CHD, with an average cholesterol reduction of 8.5 percent. This allowed LRC trials director Basil Rifkind to claim that "for each 1 percent reduction in cholesterol, we can expect a 2 percent reduction in CHD events." The statement was widely circulated even though it represented a completely invalid representation of the data, especially in light of the fact that when the lipid group at the University of Maryland analyzed the LRC data, they found *no* difference in CHD events between the group taking the drug and those on the placebo.[64] Ironically, just three years later, the Framingham Study group published follow-up data on the original Framingham subjects. Their finding: for each 1 percent mg/dl drop of cholesterol there was an 11 percent *increase* in coronary and total mortality. In other words, the lower the cholesterol levels of the participants, the greater their risk of death.[65]

A number of clinicians and statisticians participating in a 1984 Lipid Research Clinics Conference workshop were highly critical of the manner in which the LRC researchers had tabulated and manipulated the results. The conference, in fact, went very badly for the NHLBI, with critics of the lipid hypothesis almost outnumbering supporters.

Dissenters were again invited to speak briefly at the NHLBI-sponsored National Cholesterol Consensus Conference held later that year, but their views were not included in the panel's report, for the simple reason that the NHLBI staff generated the report before the conference convened. University of Maryland researcher Dr. Beverly Teter discovered this fact when she picked up some papers by mistake just before the conference began, and found they contained the consensus report, already written, with just a few numbers left blank. Kritchevsky represented the lipid hypothesis camp with a humorous five-minute presentation, full of ditties. Edward

Ahrens, who pioneered earlier research to assess how dietary fats and cholesterol affected blood levels of cholesterol, nevertheless raised strenuous objections about the "consensus," only to have the conference organizers tell him that he had misinterpreted his own data, and that if he wanted a conference to come up with different conclusions, he should pay for it himself.

The 1984 Cholesterol Consensus Conference final report was a whitewash, containing no mention of the evidence that conflicted with the diet-heart theory and the lipid hypothesis. Dissenting attendees found their names listed as speakers, but with no record of what they said.

One of the blanks was filled with the number two hundred. The document defined all those with cholesterol levels above 200 mg/dL as "at risk" and called for mass cholesterol screening, even though the most ardent supporters of the lipid hypothesis had surmised in print that two hundred forty should be the magic cutoff point. Such screening would, in fact, be required on a massive scale as the federal medical bureaucracy, by picking the number two hundred, had declared a large portion of the American adult population as "at risk."* The report advocated the avoidance of saturated fat and cholesterol for all Americans now defined as "at risk," and specifically advised the replacement of butter with margarine.

The Consensus Conference also provided a launching pad for the nationwide National Cholesterol Education Program, which had the stated goal of "changing physicians' attitudes." NHLBI-funded surveys had determined that while the general population had bought into the diet-heart theory and the lipid hypothesis, and was dutifully using margarine and buying low-cholesterol foods, the medical profession remained skeptical. All doctors in America received a large "Physicians Kit," compiled in part by the American Pharmaceutical Association, whose representatives served on the NCEP coordinating committee. Doctors were taught the importance of cholesterol screening, the advantages of cholesterol-lowering drugs and the unique benefits of the Prudent Diet. Every doctor in America received a packet of NCEP materials, which recommended the use of margarine rather than butter. The men in white coats now served as hucksters for the vegetable oil industry.

IN NOVEMBER 1986, THE *JOURNAL of the American Medical Association* published a series on the Lipid Research Clinics' trials, including "Cholesterol and Coronary Heart Disease: A New Era," by longtime American Heart Association member Scott Grundy, MD, PhD.[66] The article is a disturbing combination of euphoria and agony—euphoria at the forward movement of the anti-cholesterol juggernaut, and agony over the elusive nature of real proof. "The recent consensus conference on cholesterol . . . implied that levels between 200 and 240 . . . carry at least a mild increase in risk, which they obviously do," wrote Grundy. This directly contradicted an earlier statement in which Grundy claimed that

* Mary G. Enig attended the conference and overheard an argument between cochairman Basil Rifkind and two other conference organizers, who protested strenuously the choice of two hundred as the risk point. Average cholesterol levels in America are two hundred forty, they argued, so how could someone with average cholesterol levels be characterized as "at risk"? But Rifkind cut them off. "No, no," he said, "at two hundred forty we wouldn't have enough people to test" (and by inference, to treat). Today any adult with a risk factor for heart disease, such as overweight or obesity, gets a prescription for a cholesterol-lowering drug, even if their cholesterol is already dangerously low.

the cause-and-effect connection was strong. Grundy called for "the simple step of measuring the plasma cholesterol level in all adults... those found to have elevated cholesterol levels can be designated as at high risk and thereby can *enter the medical care system... an enormous number of patients will be included* [italics added]." Who benefits from "the simple step" of measuring and monitoring cholesterol levels in all adults? Hospitals, laboratories, pharmaceutical companies, the vegetable oil industry, margarine manufacturers, food processors and, of course, medical doctors, just to name a few. "Many physicians will see the advantages of using drugs for cholesterol lowering," wrote Grundy, even though "a positive benefit/risk ratio for cholesterol-lowering drugs will be difficult to prove." In the thirty years since Grundy's prediction, sales of cholesterol-lowering drugs have reached fourteen billion dollars per year, even though a positive risk/benefit ratio for such treatment has never emerged from the studies. Physicians, however, have "seen the advantages of using drugs for cholesterol lowering" as a way of creating patients out of healthy people.

Grundy was equally inconsistent about the benefits of dietary modification. "Whether diet has a long term effect on cholesterol remains to be proved," he stated, but "public health advocates furthermore can play an important role by urging the food industry to provide palatable choices of foods that are low in cholesterol, saturated fatty acids, and total calories." Such foods, almost by definition, contain liquid or partially hydrogenated vegetable oils containing *trans* fatty acids. Grundy knew that the *trans* fats were a problem, that they raised serum cholesterol and contributed to many diseases—he knew because a year earlier, at his request, Mary G. Enig, PhD, then in private practice, had sent him a package of data detailing numerous studies that gave reason for concern, which he acknowledged in a signed letter as "an important contribution to the ongoing debate."[67]

Shortly thereafter, the *Surgeon General's Report on Nutrition and Health* emphasized the importance of making low-fat foods more widely available. Project LEAN (Low-Fat Eating for America Now), sponsored by the J. Kaiser Family Foundation and a host of establishment groups—such as the American Heart Association, the American Dietetic Association, the American Medical Association, the USDA, the National Cancer Institute, Centers for Disease Control and the National Heart, Lung, and Blood Institute—announced a publicity campaign to "aggressively promote foods low in saturated fat and cholesterol in order to reduce the risk of heart disease and cancer."[68]

Meanwhile, studies contradicting the diet-heart theory and the lipid hypothesis continued to accumulate. In 1988, the statistician Russell Smith, PhD, in consultation with Edward R. Pinckney, MD, published a summary of all the diet and cholesterol studies to date. *Diet, Blood Cholesterol and Coronary Heart Disease: A Critical Review of the Literature* catalogs the many papers that received no attention from the media, most of which refuted the cholesterol dogma or were inconclusive. In summary, Smith stated, "One need not go beyond the food consumption studies to know that the diet-CHD hypothesis is totally and unequivocally incorrect. These studies, combined with common knowledge, demonstrate clearly that the foods targeted by the NHLBI/AHA alliance as raising blood cholesterol and, therefore, indirectly causing atherosclerosis, decreased (animal fats) or remained constant (dietary cholesterol) during the 'epidemic.' The only trend which paralleled the recorded CHD mortality curve was that of vegetable fats...Attributing the 'epidemic' to animal fat consumption... is totally illogical and defies even the most elementary principles of scientific reasoning."[69]

Regarding the presentation of the cholesterol theory in the media, Smith was scathing: "Many hundreds and probably thousands of articles on diet and heart disease have been published in the last fifteen years in newspapers and magazines. Almost none of these articles have accurately reflected the known scientific facts, and many have given the public totally false or highly misleading information."[70]

For example, the press did not report on a multiyear British study involving several thousand men, published in 1983, half of whom were asked to reduce saturated fat and cholesterol in their diets, to stop smoking and to increase the amounts of unsaturated oils such as margarine and vegetable oils. After one year, those on the "good" diet had 100 percent more deaths than those on the "bad" diet, in spite of the fact that those men on the "bad" diet continued to smoke! But in describing the findings, the study's author ignored these results in favor of the politically correct conclusion: "The implication for public health policy in the U.K. is that a preventive programme such as we evaluated in this trial is probably effective."[71]

Numerous surveys of traditional populations have also yielded information that is an embarrassment to proponents of the diet-heart theory. For example, a study comparing Jews when they lived in Yemen and ate fats solely of animal origin to Yemenite Jews living in Israel, whose diets contained margarine and vegetable oils, revealed little heart disease or diabetes in the former group but high levels of both diseases in the latter.*[72] A comparison of populations in northern and southern India revealed a similar pattern. People in northern India consumed seventeen times more animal fat, but had an incidence of coronary heart disease seven times lower than people in southern India.[73] The Masai and kindred tribes of Africa subsist largely on milk, meat and blood. They are free from coronary heart disease and have low blood cholesterol levels.[74] Eskimos eat liberally of animal fats from fish and marine animals. On their native diet they are free of disease and exceptionally hardy.[75]

Colin Campbell, coauthor of the famous China Study, claims that his extensive study of diet and disease patterns in China found that those on plant-based diets suffered fewer health problems than those whose diets contained large amounts of animal foods. However, the researchers actually discovered that people living in the region in which the populace consumed large amounts of whole milk had half the rate of heart disease as several districts with low levels of animal consumption.[76] Several Mediterranean societies have low rates of heart disease even though fat—including highly saturated fat from lamb, sausage and goat cheese—comprises a large portion of their caloric intake. The inhabitants of Crete, for example, are remarkable for their good health and longevity.[77] A study of

* The study also noted that the Yemenite Jews consumed no sugar, but those in Israel consumed sugar in amounts equaling 25–30 percent of total carbohydrate intake.

Puerto Ricans revealed that, although they consumed large amounts of animal fat (mostly as lard), they had a very low incidence of colon and breast cancer.[78] A study of the long-lived inhabitants of Soviet Georgia revealed that those who ate the most fatty meat lived the longest.[79] In Okinawa, where the average life span for women is eighty-four years—longer than in the rest of Japan—the inhabitants eat generous amounts of pork and seafood and do all their cooking in lard.*[80] None of these studies appears in feature articles in the *New York Times.*

Researchers often attribute the relative good health of the Japanese, who have the longest life span of any nation in the world, to a low-fat diet. Although the Japanese eat few dairy fats, the notion that their diet is low in fat is a myth; rather, it contains moderate amounts of animal fats from eggs, pork (in popular foods like Spam), chicken, beef, seafood and organ meats. What they do not consume (or at least did not consume until recently) is a lot of vegetable oil, white flour or processed food (although they do eat white rice). The life span of the Japanese has increased since the Second World War with an increase in animal fat and protein in the diet.[81] Those who point to Japanese statistics to promote the low-fat diet fail to mention the fact that the Swiss live almost as long on one of the fattiest diets in the world. Tied for third in the longevity stakes are Austria and Greece—both with high-fat diets.[82]

As a final example, let us consider the French. Anyone who has eaten his way across France has observed that the French diet is loaded with saturated fats in the form of butter, eggs, cheese, cream, liver, meats and rich pâtés. Yet the French have a lower rate of coronary heart disease than many other Western countries. In the United States, over three hundred of every hundred thousand middle-aged men die of heart attacks each year; in France the rate is half of that, at one hundred forty-five per hundred thousand. In the Gascony region, where goose and duck liver form a staple of the diet, this rate is remarkably low: eighty per hundred thousand.[83] This phenomenon has gained international attention as "The French Paradox." But other European countries show paradoxical patterns as well. The highest rates of saturated fat consumption in Europe occur in France, followed by Switzerland, the Netherlands, Iceland, Belgium, Finland and Austria. Yet these same countries have the lowest rates of death from heart disease in Europe, while the countries with low rates of saturated fat consumption have higher rates of CHD.[84]

In spite of these glaring facts, the campaign to promote vegetable oils had worked very well. By the 1990s, the promoters had succeeded, by slick manipulation of the press and of scientific research, in transforming America into a nation that was well and truly oiled. Consumption of butter had bottomed out at about 4 grams per person per year (about one teaspoon per day), down from almost 18 grams at the turn of the century. Use of lard and tallow was down by two-thirds. Margarine consumption had jumped from less than 2 grams per person

* The Okinawan diet, rich in lard, was described in a 1996 article appearing in *Health* magazine. Damage control soon followed with two books describing the Okinawan diet as low in animal fat—in the late 1990s, according to the authors, the Okinawans were dutifully cooking in canola oil. But the Okinawans who had made it to their eighties grew up long before canola oil ever existed. Like all peoples of Chinese extraction, they cooked in rendered pig fat.[a]

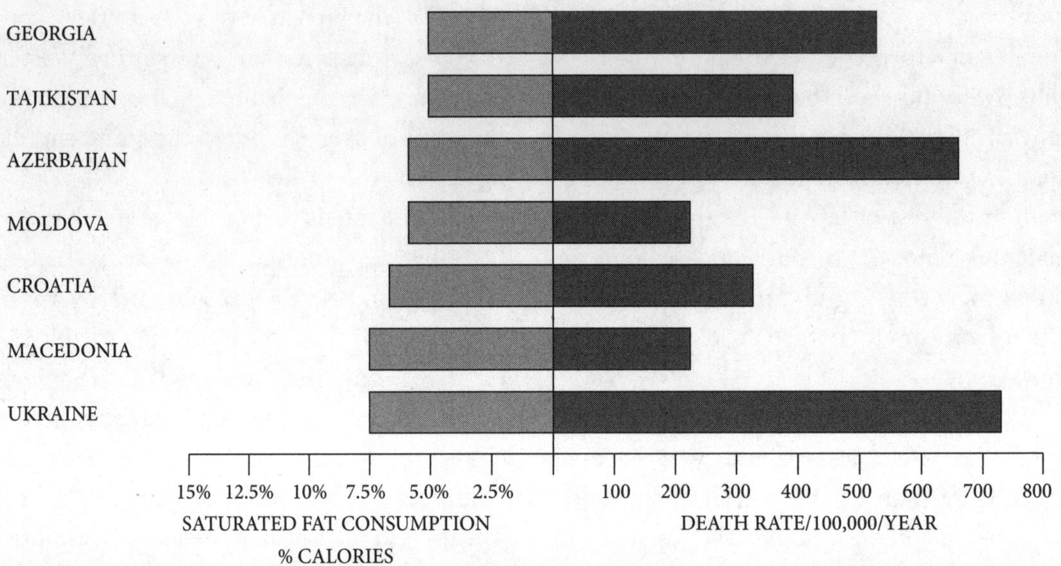

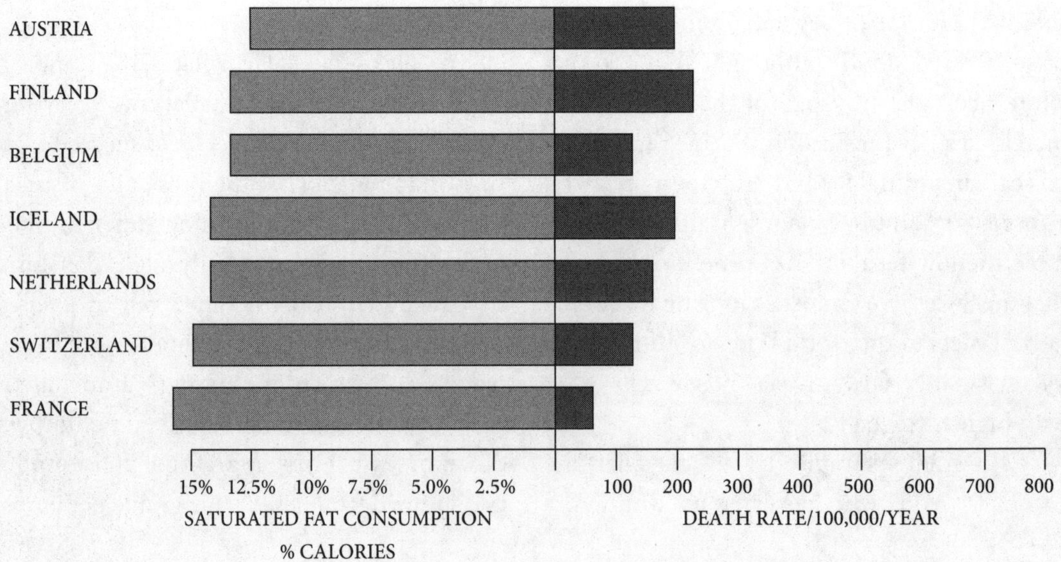

Source: European Cardiovascular Disease Statistics, 2005 Edition, www.heartstats.org/uploads/documents%5CPDF.pdf

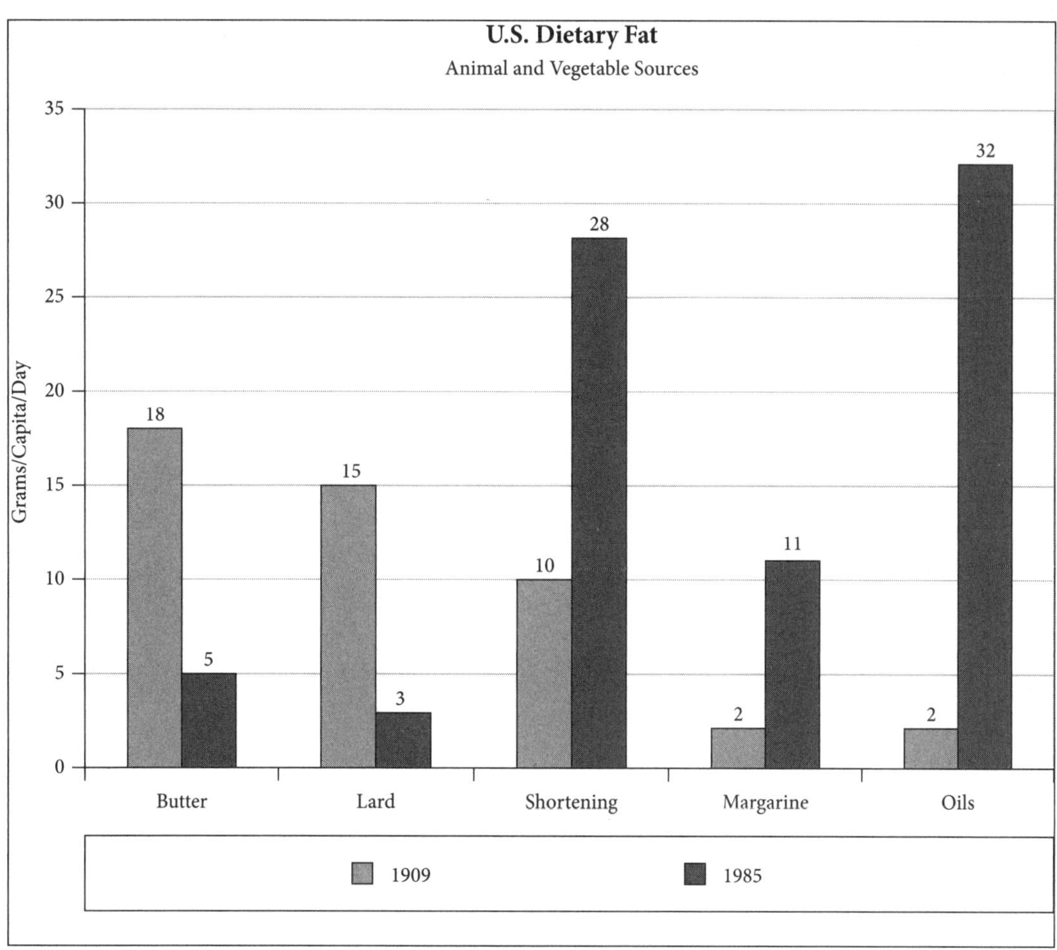

Source: U.S. Department of Agriculture

per day in 1909 to about 11 in 1960.[85] Since then margarine consumption figures have changed little, remaining at about 11 grams per person per day—perhaps because knowledge of margarine's dangers has been slowly seeping out to the public. However, for many years most of the *trans* fats in the American diet weren't from margarine alone, but from shortening used in fried and fabricated foods. American shortening consumption of 10 grams per person per day held steady until the 1960s, although the content of that shortening had changed from mostly lard, tallow or coconut oil—all natural fats—to partially hydrogenated soybean oil. Then shortening consumption shot up and by the 1990s had tripled to almost 30 grams per person per day.

But the most dramatic overall change in the American diet was the huge increase in the consumption of liquid vegetable oils, from slightly less than 2 grams per person per day in 1909 to over 30—a fifteenfold increase. Now that the dangers of hardened *trans* fats have become common knowledge, Americans are consuming more liquid vegetable oils than ever.

BY THE EARLY 1980s, ONLY one large source of saturated animal fat in American fast food remained—the tallow in fast-food fryers. McDonald's and other fast-food restaurants used beef or lamb tallow, and with good reason.* Highly saturated tallow is stable, can be reused many times, and gives a delicious, crispy final product. That was soon to change, thanks to the Center for Science in the Public Interest (CSPI).

One of America's most influential and vocal consumer-advocacy group, CSPI was founded in 1972, the year that Michael Jacobson, CSPI's executive director, published *Eaters' Digest*, a book filled with anti-saturated-fat rhetoric.

CSPI's 1988 publication, *Saturated Fat Attack*, condemned a long list of processed foods said to be made with coconut oil, palm oil, tallow, butter or lard. (Actually, processors used mostly partially hydrogenated oil for snack foods and baked goods, but often included a small amount of other fats and oils, which were, of course, listed on the label.) There were a few holdouts on the list, however: Hi Ho Crackers were made with coconut oil, Uneeda Biscuits were made with lard, Sara Lee Croissants were made with butter, and Pepperidge Farm used a blend that contained a lot of coconut oil.[86]

But it was the fast-food chains that received the brunt of Jacobson's wrath, because they used a blend of 91–95 percent beef fat or 100 percent palm oil for frying. Jacobson and CSPI orchestrated well-publicized demonstrations in front of McDonald's and a postcard campaign to the corporate offices of the fast-food chains to protest the use of these "artery-clogging" saturated fats for frying.

CSPI launched its campaign against "saturated" frying fats in 1984 and continued its efforts into 1986 when the organization added "tropical oils" to the list of supposed villains in the American diet. The campaign was successful; most fast-food restaurants soon switched to partially hydrogenated shortening. Movie theaters gave in very quickly as well—replacing the villainous coconut oil in their popcorn with shortening containing artificial butter flavor.†

While problems with *trans* fats in partially hydrogenated oil were well known at this time, CSPI continued to defend them throughout the decade. A 1987 article by Elaine Blume, published in CSPI's *Nutrition Action* newsletter, read like oil industry propaganda. Blume wrote: "From margarine to Tater Tots, partially hydrogenated vegetable oils play a major role in our food supply... In fact, hydrogenated oils don't pose a dire threat to health... Improving on Nature... Manufacturers hydrogenate... these vegetable oils so they won't become rancid while they sit on shelves, or during frying... it seems unlikely that hydrogenation contributes much to our burden of heart disease... The fact that hydrogenated oils appear to be relatively benign is cause for thanks, because these fats are everywhere."

Blume was at it again in March 1988 with another article, "The Truth About Trans." In it, she claimed: "Hydrogenated oils aren't guilty as charged... All told, the charges against *trans* fat just don't stand up. And by extension,

* Krispy Kreme doughnuts used lard.

† OSHA lists diacetyl, the artificial butter flavor used in movie theater and microwave popcorn as a toxic substance; the vapors can cause Popcorn Lung Disease (bronchiolitis obliterans), characterized by lung inflammation, hardening and scarring, and other serious symptoms. The disease is rare, but those who suffer from it often require lung transplants, as it is irreversible and can be life-threatening, ultimately obstructing the lungs.

hydrogenated oils seem relatively innocent... As for processed foods, you're better off choosing products made with hydrogenated soybean, corn, or cottonseed oil." This article was widely disseminated; Michael Jacobson provided it as a handout to members of the Maryland legislature during hearings when the University of Maryland lipids research group tried to introduce labeling of *trans* fatty acids in the state.

But by 1990, CSPI could no longer defend the indefensible. In October of that year, Bonnie Liebman, CSPI director of nutrition, published an article, "Trans in Trouble," which referred to recent studies by Dutch scientists showing that *trans* fats raised cholesterol. "That's not to say *trans* fatty acids are artery-cloggers," she wrote; "the fats in our foods may affect cholesterol differently than those used in the Dutch experiment... The Bottom Line... Trans, shmans. You should eat less fat... Don't switch back to butter... use a soft tub diet margarine."

On October 20, 1993, CSPI had the chutzpah to call a press conference in Washington, DC, and lambast the major fast-food chains for doing what CSPI coerced them into doing, namely, using partially hydrogenated vegetable oils in their deep-fat fryers. On that date, CSPI reversed its position after an onslaught of adverse medical reports linking *trans* fatty acids in these processed oils to coronary heart disease and cancer. Instead of accepting the blame, CSPI claimed that the fault lay with the major fast-food chains, including McDonald's, Burger King, Wendy's and Kentucky Fried Chicken, because they "falsely claim to use '100 percent vegetable oil' when they actually use hydrogenated shortening."*

According to the CSPI press release, "In 1984, CSPI organized the first national campaign to pressure fast-food restaurants and food companies to stop frying with beef fat and tropical oils, which are high in the cholesterol-raising saturated fats that increase the risk of heart disease. After six years of public pressure—including full-page newspaper ads placed by Nebraska millionaire and cholesterol-crusader Phil Sokolof—the industry finally relented in 1990. But instead of switching to vegetable oil for frying, CSPI's research shows, the companies opted for hydrogenated shortenings, which have a longer shelf life and can be used longer in deep-fat fryers."

In December 1992, Liebman wrote: "We've been crying 'foul' for some time now, as the margarine industry has tried to convince people that eating margarine was as good for their hearts as aerobic exercise... And we warned folks several years ago that *trans* fatty acids could be a problem... That's especially true now that we know that *trans* fatty acids are harmful, but we don't know how much *trans* are in different foods." Of course, CSPI had issued no such warning, but had defended *trans* fats for more than five years. And they offered no apology for falsely demonizing traditional fats. "Don't switch back from margarine to butter," wrote Liebman, "try diet or whipped margarine... use a liquid margarine."

CSPI's campaign was wildly successful. It is impossible to measure the suffering and grief that Liebman and Jacobson—as leaders of the major nutrition "activist" consumer

* Actually, a fat or oil or mixture of fats and/or oils is called a "liquid shortening" when it is used in baking and frying; similarly, when poured over lettuce and tomatoes, it is called a "salad dressing."

organization—have inflicted on many millions of an unknowing public. Thanks to CSPI, healthy traditional fats almost completely disappeared from the food supply, first replaced by manufactured *trans* fats known to cause many diseases, and then more recently, by dangerously rancid liquid oils. Jacobson was equally successful going after the popcorn in movie theaters so that this good dietary source of coconut oil—one of the supremely healthy fats on the planet—disappeared. "Today," bragged Jacobson, "'no tropical oils' is a badge of honor worn by many food packages."

Who benefits from the ongoing campaign against saturated fat? First and foremost, the soybean industry. Eighty percent of all oil, whether partially hydrogenated or liquid, used in processed foods in the United States comes from soybeans, as does 70 percent of all liquid oil sold in bottles to consumers. CSPI claims that its support comes from subscribers to its *Nutrition Action* newsletter, which continues even today to issue hysterical warnings against "artery-clogging" fats in steak, whole milk and fettuccine Alfredo. The one million subscribers provide more than 70 percent of CSPI's thirteen-million-dollar annual income, according to one report, but CSPI is extremely secretive about the value of its assets, the salaries it pays and the use of its revenues. If CSPI has large donors, they're not telling who they are, but in fact, in CSPI's January 1991 newsletter, Jacobson notes that "our effort was ultimately joined... by the American Soybean Association."[87]

Once the idea that saturated fats cause heart disease took hold, other modern diseases fell in line. The official organizations to combat stroke, Alzheimer's, cancer, diabetes, autoimmune disease, multiple sclerosis, obesity and even infertility found an easy scapegoat in saturated fats, using evidence that is even sketchier than that used to indict saturated fats for heart disease—anything to deflect attention away from the truly dangerous ingredients in the modern industrial diet.

ON APRIL 30, 1996, SENIOR researcher David Kritchevsky received the American Oil Chemists' Society's Research Award in recognition of his accomplishments as a "researcher on cancer and atherosclerosis as well as cholesterol metabolism." His accomplishments include coauthorship of more than three hundred seventy research papers, one of which appeared a month later in the *American Journal of Clinical Nutrition*.[88] This "Position paper on *trans* fatty acids" noted, "A controversy has arisen about the potential health hazards of *trans* unsaturated fatty acids in the American diet."

The controversy dates back to 1954. In the rabbit studies that launched Kritchevsky on his career, the researcher actually found that cholesterol dissolved in Wesson oil "markedly accelerated" the development of cholesterol-containing low-density lipoproteins; and cholesterol fed with shortening gave cholesterol levels twice as high as cholesterol fed alone.[89] The unavoidable conclusion: vegetable oils, and particularly partially hydrogenated vegetable oils, are bad news.

But Kritchevsky's "Position paper on *trans* fatty acids" took no position at all. Studies have given contradictory results, said the author, and the amount of *trans* in the average American diet is very difficult to determine. As for labeling, the study claimed, "There is no clear choice of how to include *trans* fatty acids on the nutrition label. The database is insufficient to establish a classification scheme for these fats." There may be problems with *trans*, said the senior researcher, but their use "helps to reduce the intake of dietary fats higher in saturated fatty acids. Also, vegetable fats are not a source of dietary cholesterol, unlike saturated animal fats." Kritchevsky and his coauthors concluded that physicians and nutritionists should "focus on a further decrease in total fat intake and especially the intake of saturated fat…A reduction in total fat intake simplifies the problem, because all fats in the diet decrease and choices are unnecessary…We may conclude," wrote Kritchevsky and his colleagues, "that consumption of liquid vegetable oils is preferable to solid fats."

Two years later, a symposium entitled "Evolution of Ideas about the Nutritional Value of Dietary Fat" reviewed the many flaws in the lipid hypothesis and highlighted a study in which mice fed purified diets died within twenty days, while whole milk kept the mice alive for several months.[90] One of the participants was David Kritchevsky, who noted that the use of low-fat diets and drugs in intervention trials "did not affect overall CHD mortality." Ever with a finger in the wind, this influential Founding Father of the lipid hypothesis concluded thus: "Research continues apace and, as new findings appear, it may be necessary to reevaluate our conclusions and preventive medicine policies."

Fast-forward to the present, when many scientists and writers have exposed the manipulation and fraud in heart disease research: the establishment is sticking to its story. Cholesterol and saturated fat, particularly saturated animal fat, remain public enemy number one, the greatest villains in the Western diet. *Trans* fats are largely gone, but liquid vegetable oils—possibly more dangerous—have taken their place, used in fried foods, processed foods and "healthy" soft spreads.

MUCH OF WHAT AMERICANS BELIEVE about nutrition and have put into practice comes from popular magazines, which for decades have derived a large portion of their advertising revenues from the industrial food industry—think back to advertisements for Crisco in the 1912 *Home Directory*. Today, the practice continues to shape American eating habits.

The American Council on Science and Health, which describes its mission as ensuring "that peer-reviewed mainstream science reaches the public, the media, and the decision-makers who determine public policy," tracks nutrition reporting in major magazines. In a 2001 report, fourteen out of twenty magazines received a rating as "excellent" or "good" sources of nutrition advice. (The three magazines rated excellent were *Parents*, *Cooking Light* and *Good Housekeeping*.) The report recorded as good news the fact that "for the first time since these surveys began, no magazine ranked as a poor source." What this means is that the food industry has control of all the major magazines, and not one of them can be expected to publish anything but the conventional dogma that saturated fat is bad for all ages, even babies and little children.[91]

At eatingwell.com you can read today about the daily diets of six "nutrition experts," as virtuous as virtuous nutrition experts can be. Lots and lots of low-fat foods in these diets—oyxmoronic low-fat sour cream and low-fat cheese—whole-grain foods like granola and whole wheat pasta, tofu, fish, 2 percent milk, and politically acceptable fast food like veggie burgers. Most of them admit to giving in to temptations like chocolate, ice cream, white bread, cake or pretzels. One "expert" drinks six diet sodas per day.

This advice is no different from what comes out of our universities, which are also recipients of food industry largesse. An August 2008 *Health and Nutrition Letter* from Tufts University, sent to students and dietitians, provides a list of thirty dietary suggestions, including lots of vegetables; lots of whole grains with just a very thin smear of spread on your bread; cooking in vegetable oils, no butter; less meat; more canned beans; less salt; and iced tea, black coffee or mineral water to drink. The article recommends eating from a small plate, never eating everything on your plate and never, ever eating seconds. The author does not provide any suggestions on what to do when the cravings hit just before bedtime, when the body tries to compensate for this virtuous starvation diet by making you eat a half-gallon of ice cream or a whole bag of potato chips.

Tufts nutrition professor Alice Lichtenstein has sided with the food processing industry throughout her career. As Americans make attempts to avoid processed foods, Lichtenstein declares that it is fine to reformulate real foods like meat and milk into low-fat versions "because you are focusing specifically on taking out saturated fat. But for other products such as cookies and brownies, it's not that useful." In other words, it's okay for consumers to consume lots of industrial fats and oils in baked goods, but not the natural fats in cheese and meat.[92]

What happens when you try to eat according to the current U.S. government guidelines? The *San Francisco Chronicle* reported on a group of four food and wine staffers from their offices who took the following mission upon themselves: "Spend two weeks following the US government's new [2010] dietary guidelines, glow smugly with the virtue and newfound health, then report on the findings." After fourteen days of chickpeas, skim milk, soy milk, rice cakes, kale and carrot sticks, the intrepid group discovered that they all felt "constrained and deprived." Blake Gray, one of the participants, summed it up: "I miss the pure pleasure of choosing the food that sounds most delicious and savoring each morsel without wondering what kind of oil it was cooked in. If I have to give some years off my life for this pleasure, I'm willing to do it—if only I knew in advance how many years I'm forfeiting." The group also found that following the guidelines was very difficult to do, requiring the help of calorie, fat and sodium lists to figure out whether they could have an additional piece of cheese or a cookie for dessert; and while the guidelines did steer them away from junk food, they found it difficult to reach their vegetable and grain quota. One participant observed that it was hard to "round people up for a nice meal of chick-pea stew," noting that she felt more isolated, with the world looking "a bit bleak." In short, hiding behind a pile of platitudes against processed foods, the guidelines offer a useless plan for real people living in the real world who want to eat real food.[93] With the vegetable oil industry pulling the strings in the background, the universities, the media, medical institutions and the government all sing the same sad song, making every effort to mislead a very confused public, which ricochets between virtuous, abstemious eating and indulgence in processed foods.

REDUCTIONIST TUNNEL VISION CAN LEAD to ludicrous conclusions, a prime example being the 2008 Overall Nutritional Quality Index (ONQI), developed by a "panel of twelve of the nation's foremost experts on nutrition" at Yale University's Griffin Prevention Research Center. The august experts rated commonly consumed foods on a scale of one to one hundred, with one hundred being the "healthiest," using a complex mathematical formula that looks at selected nutrients in a particular food, as well as the amount of fat, sugar, sodium, cholesterol, calories, glycemic load and other factors. The top-rated food under the ONQI system? Broccoli! All but one of the foods rated ninety and above are fruits and vegetables—radish gets a ninety-nine—the exception being nonfat milk with a ninety-one. Meats and seafood range from the twenties to the eighties in this system, with the lower numbers assigned to fatty cuts of meat such as baby back ribs and chicken wings. Obviously nonnutritious foods such as Popsicles, cheese puffs and sodas received ratings below twenty, but so do healthy traditional foods like fried eggs, salami and bacon.[94] Nutrient-dense foods—prized by traditional cultures as absolutely necessary for optimal health and normal reproduction—don't even show up in the ONQI list: butter, organ meats, fish eggs, cod liver oil and whole raw dairy products from grass-fed cows. It would be interesting to feed one group of laboratory rats a diet of high-rated foods such as broccoli, radishes and nonfat milk, and another group of rats a diet of low-rated foods such as fried eggs, salami and bacon, and compare the results. The scale system "will allow busy parents and others who care about nutrition a quick, at-a-glance way to see what food item is ultimately the healthiest without having to read every label."[95] An ominous statement! Can we expect to see the ONQI replace food labels sometime in the future?

A news item celebrating the eighty-fifth anniversary of Frigidaire's electric refrigerator recently listed the contents of the fridge, then and now. In 1918: a bottle of whole raw milk, eggs, lard, cream, churned butter, homemade lemonade, homemade cottage cheese, apple butter, homemade jelly, fresh meat. Today: one gallon reduced-fat ultrapasteurized and homogenized milk, eggs, fat-free margarine, flavored nondairy creamer, sports drinks, squeezable yogurt, colored ketchup, bagged salad, ice cream and frozen dinners. In other words, in 1918, Americans ate real food including plenty of animal fats; today Americans eat mostly processed food and the animal fats have largely disappeared—only eggs have survived the food Puritan finger wagging, probably because fake eggs are just too disgusting for words.

The biggest change during the last few decades is reflected in milk consumption patterns. In 1945, Americans consumed nearly forty-one gallons of whole milk per year, compared to only eight gallons per person today. Consumption of lower-fat milks was fifteen gallons in 2001, up from four gallons in 1945 and six gallons in 1970.[96] The change reflects more than thirty years of constant industry propaganda against animal fats as well as greatly increased intake of soft drinks and juice, which have largely replaced milk in children's diets. A 2002 study found that 51 percent of the average American child's daily liquid intake is made up of sweetened beverages, which is one of the likely reasons that obesity is steadily increasing.[97]

However, one recent and surprising trend is a rise in butter consumption over the last few years—not by leaps and bounds, but steadily upward—both in the United States and in Europe. This shift in consumption patterns may explain a resurgence of anti–saturated fat messages in the United States and overseas.

Britain's Food Standards Agency launched a "health" campaign in February 2009 costing over three million pounds to "raise awareness of the health risks of eating too much saturated fat," and lamenting the fact that "the UK is currently eating 20 percent more saturated fat than UK Government recommendations."

The highly coordinated campaign included a forty-second TV advertisement in which a "jug of saturated fat is poured down the sink, overloading and blocking a kitchen pipe to vividly bring to life the message that too much saturated fat is bad for your heart."* Print ads encouraged Britons to cut the fat off their meat, switch to lower-fat dairy products, and use vegetable oils instead of butter when cooking.[98] The campaign referred to a 2008 government report that claimed "more than 3,500 premature deaths could be avoided every year" if Britons consumed within the guideline daily amount of saturated fat.

In New Zealand, newspaper articles have urged the population to eat less bacon and sausage, avoid butter and pastries containing butter, and take children off full-fat milk after the age of two "to avoid clogging their arteries." One university professor has even called for a tax on "poison" butter.[99]

What modern dietary advice has done is whiplash most Americans between two extremes—between a puritanical low-fat diet and processed pornographic food, loaded with industrial fats and oils. A diet of skinless chicken breast, dry whole grains and unbuttered vegetables is bound to create cravings, which are most often met by indulging in junk food. Americans seesaw between virtuous eating and consuming a whole Sara Lee coffee cake alone in the evening hours when the body sends powerful messages signifying hunger even though the stomach is filled.

The only solution to such chaotic eating patterns is to return to a diet that provides our bodies with the nutrients they need, including saturated animal fats and the many nutrients they contain. The prescription for what ails the American eating dysfunction is butter, egg yolks, cream, whole milk, cheese, rich pâtés, fatty meats and chicken with succulent skin.

THE EXPERTS TELL US THAT saturated fat is bad because it raises cholesterol levels. But it seems that no matter what Americans are eating, experts say our cholesterol levels are too high. Hence the push for cholesterol-lowering statin drugs, the greatest boondoggle the pharmaceutical industry has ever enjoyed. Statin drugs bring many billions dollars per year on the premise that they save lives and have few side effects.[100] Are cholesterol-lowering drugs actually helping anyone other than the pharmaceutical companies?

In February 2015, the journal *Expert Reviews in Clinical Pharmacology* published a review article entitled, "How statistical

* The pipe comparison is wrong for many reasons, one of which is the fact that saturated fats are liquid in the tropics, where the temperature hovers above 80 degrees. At 98.6 degrees F, our bodies are warmer than tropical.

deception created the appearance that statins are safe and effective in primary and secondary prevention of cardiovascular disease." Authors David M. Diamond and Uffe Ravnskov conclude that although cholesterol-lowering statin drugs effectively reduce cholesterol levels, they fail to improve heart disease outcomes; they also describe how statin advocates have used deceptive statistical manipulations to create the false appearance that cholesterol reduction results in a reduction in heart disease.

According to Ravnskov and Diamond, statin advocates use a statistical method called relative risk reduction (RRR) to misuse and manipulate the data. This method amplifies any trivial way statin drugs could possibly benefit heart disease. The authors also describe how the directors of the clinical trials on statin drugs succeeded in hiding the drugs' significant, toxic side effects.

According to Ravnskov and Diamond, what has emerged, after thirty years of statin promotion, is the fact that these cholesterol-lowering drugs increase the risk of cancer, cataracts, dementia, diabetes and muscular-skeletal diseases—side effects that more than offset any possible, trivial benefits. In fact, in one of the most positive clinical trials on statins, researchers used statistical deceptions to transform a possible 1 percent heart benefit into a supposed 36 percent benefit through a meaningless relative risk reduction estimate. In the widely publicized JUPITER study, researchers misleadingly transformed a minuscule 1 percent benefit into a 54 percent benefit.[101] A second study, published in the same journal, indicates that statins may actually cause atherosclerosis and heart failure.[102]

Researcher David Evans has compiled the overall mortality of participants in the thirty-three statin trials to date (2015). The difference in the percentage of people alive at the end of the trials in the carefully selected treatment groups and in the control groups (which almost always have more smokers) in all the trials is trivial. When the total number of people in each trial is taken into account, the data reveal that 0.61 percent more people were alive who were taking statins at the end of the trials than the people taking a placebo.[103] The only sensible conclusion, after three decades of study, is that taking cholesterol-lowering medication will not prolong your life and may plague your later years with a number of painful and debilitating side effects.

Yet in what can only be described as nationwide insanity, statin pushers are now citing two studies as justification for putting people with "normal" cholesterol levels on statins. Millions more Americans now get prescriptions for cholesterol-lowering statin drugs because they also lower C-reactive protein (CRP), a marker for inflammation. One study is the above mentioned JUPITER study, in which the statin Crestor was said to "dramatically cut deaths, heart attacks and strokes in patients who had healthy cholesterol levels but high levels of a protein associated with heart disease."[104]

In reality, the actual differences in outcome in the JUPITER study were very small, with the difference in mortality between the statin and the control groups after nearly two years only 0.25 percent; and researchers stopped the trial early, just as the projected overall mortality of the statin group was about to surpass that of the placebo group. The selection process for trial participants was so rigorous that it screened out eight of ten senior citizens recruited, for conditions like inflammatory disease and for "unstated reasons." The stock of AstraZeneca, maker of Crestor, climbed 45 percent after JUPITER was halted.*

The second study doctors relied upon to justify statin prescriptions took place at UCLA. The study revealed that half of over one hundred thirty thousand hospital admissions for heart disease had normal levels of LDL-cholesterol—the so-called bad cholesterol. By the tortured logic of statin-numbed brains, this allowed researchers to claim that the ideal LDL level was set too high and the "majority of people would be recommended to take a statin."[105]

Meanwhile, research published in the *Proceedings of the National Academy of Sciences* suggests that cholesterol-reducing drugs may indeed reduce brain function. According to Yeon-Kyun Shin, a biophysics professor in the department of biochemistry, biophysics and molecular biology, studies indicate that the drugs may keep the brain from making cholesterol, thereby affecting the machinery that triggers the release of neurotransmitters. "Neurotransmitters affect the data-processing and memory functions," says Shin. "In other words, how smart you are and how well you remember things."[106] Another study found that obese men taking statins had a fifty percent *increase* in prostate cancer.[107] Statin promoter Professor Sir Richard Peto of Oxford University dismissed the findings as a "statistical fluke."

It is truly incredible the lengths to which scientists invested in the lipid hypothesis will go to explain away all the contradictions to their theory. They even have a creative explanation for the French paradox. According to Timo Strandberg from the University of Oulu, Finland, "Fewer coronary deaths during the 1970s and 1990s in France than in Britain (or in the US) were simply reflecting much lower saturated fat consumption and lower cholesterol levels in France during earlier decades. While saturated fat consumption started to increase in Britain from the late 19th century and reached a plateau during the 1930s, this increase did not happen in France, a Mediterranean country, until from the 1970s."[108] What are you smoking, dear Timo? Many Americans visited France in the 1970s and the 1990s and remember the pleasure of French full-cream cheeses, whipped cream, soufflés and plates swimming with butter. Even today, saturated fat consumption by the French is the highest in Europe, while rates of heart disease are the lowest.[109] According to Professor Strandberg, the low levels of heart disease in France today are due to the use of cholesterol-lowering statin drugs. "Eating lots of cream cheese and butter-rich croissants may not be so dangerous if you are on a statin," says the professor. What's really dangerous is advice from academics so blinded by their own dogma that they cannot distinguish fact from fiction, and who continue to promote the very low-fat or wrong-fat diets that are obviously killing us.

Doctors in the United States write over two hundred fifty million prescriptions for

* One very interesting fact emerged from the media discussions of the JUPITER trial—with JUPITER, cardiologists have finally acknowledged that cholesterol levels do not accurately reflect a tendency to heart disease. Dr. James Stein, MD, from the University of Wisconsin Medical School in Madison, praised the study for exposing the fact that current therapeutic LDL-cholesterol levels are not only arbitrary, but are in fact a poor indicator of cardiovascular risk. "Most patients with heart attacks have normal LDL-cholesterol values," he stated.[a]

cholesterol-lowering statin drugs per year, despite the long list of side effects: memory loss, cognitive decline, Parkinson's disease, muscle wasting, back pain, heart failure, weakness, impotence and fatigue.[110] Now another can be added to the list: diabetes. A study published in the *Archives of Internal Medicine,* which looked at data gleaned from the Women's Health Initiative, found a nearly 50 percent increase in diabetes among longtime statin users.[111] A 2011 analysis in the *Journal of the American Medical Association*[112] and a 2010 analysis in *The Lancet*[113] also found a higher risk of diabetes among those taking cholesterol-lowering drugs. Doctors may be hemming and hawing, but they continue to prescribe them. "I don't think there's any debate remaining, particularly in the higher doses, about whether statins slightly increase the risk of developing diabetes," says cardiologist Steven Nissen of the Cleveland Clinic. Yet he claims that statins are "among the best drugs we've got."[114] Even a spokesperson for the American Diabetes Association (ADA) urges the continuation of statins. "Every medication has risks and benefits," says Vivian Fonseca, president of the ADA, "but you don't want people to have heart attacks because they are so worried about getting diabetes."[115]

YOU CAN'T HELP BUT WONDER whether the folks involved in this tragic chain of events—from the eager beaver copywriter composing ads for Crisco, to the men in white coats who lied about the results of the Lipid Research Clinics' trials, to the dietitian-nuns foisting low-fat diets on growing children—you can't help but wonder whether they ever had a twinge of conscience, whether they ever heard the heart knocking softly on the back door of the brain. But as Upton Sinclair once said, "It is difficult to get a man to understand something when his salary depends on his not understanding it."

But achieving good health in this atmosphere of confusion *does* depend on understanding the fact that saturated fat and cholesterol are not dietary villains but vital factors in the human diet.

CHAPTER 2

A Short Lesson on the Biochemistry of Fats

"We're not worried about *trans* fats," a food industry executive once said to lipid researcher Mary G. Enig. "The chemistry of fats is complicated and the public will never understand."

The industry executive was wrong on both counts. *Trans* fats have become a buzzword for what's wrong with processed food, and the chemistry of fats and oils is not complicated.

Fortunately so, because a basic knowledge of how fats and oils are structured is necessary to understand just why *trans* fats are bad, why the recent industrial substitutes for *trans* fats are worse, and why saturated fat is not the villain the food industry and media have made it out to be.

Organic chemistry is the study of molecules found in life forms—molecules based on carbon, hydrogen and oxygen. An additional element, nitrogen, is an essential part of amino acids, the building blocks of protein. Carbohydrate molecules are complicated, protein molecules even more so, but the structure of fat molecules is simple and easy to understand.

Think of a carbon atom as a nucleus or center with four arms. These arms easily link with other carbon atoms, and also with hydrogen and oxygen. Fat molecules are chains of carbon atoms (from as few as four carbons to as many as twenty-six) that form a strong bond, carbon to carbon, with two of their arms. The other two arms mostly bond to hydrogen. At one end of the chain is another hydrogen (rather than another link with carbon), and at the other end is what is called a carboxyl group, where the final carbon is bonded with one arm to an oxygen-hydrogen compound and the other two arms are bonded to one oxygen molecule.

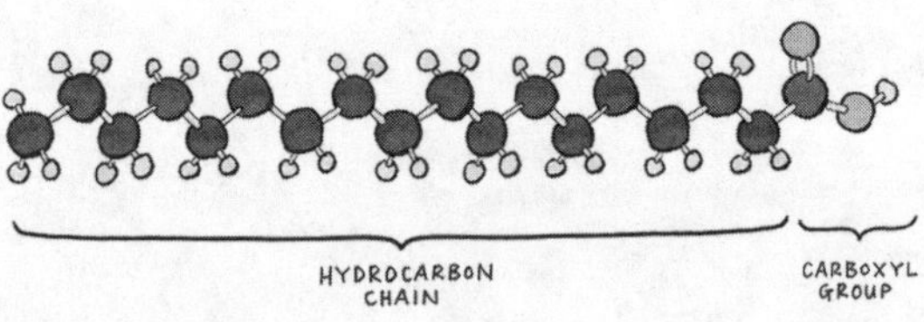

A fatty acid with a hydrocarbon chain and carboxyl group at one end.

The carboxyl group attached at the end technically makes the fat molecule an acid, so fat molecules are called fatty acids. The nomenclature is confusing because most acids, like vinegar or lactic acid, are water soluble. Fatty acids, however, do not dissolve in water.

Fatty acids are classified in two ways: by their degree of "saturation" and by their length.

A FATTY ACID IS SATURATED when all available carbon bonds are occupied—are "saturated"—by hydrogen. These molecules are highly stable, which means that they do not normally go rancid, even when heated for cooking purposes. They are straight in form, and for this reason they pack together easily—think of a stack of logs—so that they form a solid or semi-solid fat at room temperature.

Saturated fatty acids are found mainly in the fats of warm-blooded animals—including humans—and in plants from the tropics, such as coconut and palm fruit. Their straight structure gives stability to cell membranes and other biochemical compounds when the temperature is warm.

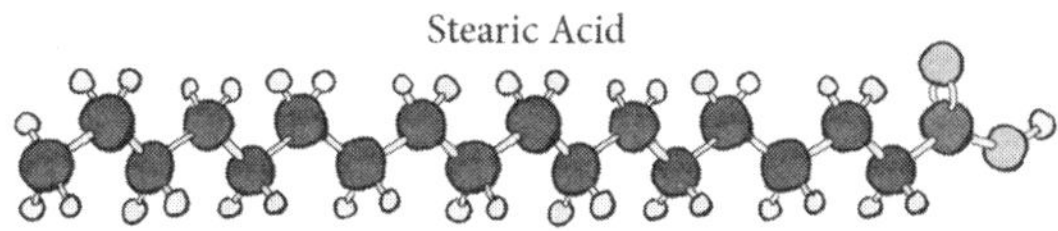

An eighteen-carbon saturated fatty acid called stearic acid. Each carbon in the chain is attached to two hydrogen molecules (basically electrons).

Monounsaturated fatty acids are missing two hydrogen atoms—instead, two carbons in the chain are joined together with a double bond. Monounsaturated fats have a kink or bend at the position of the double bond so that they do not pack together as easily as saturated fats; for this reason, they are liquid at room temperature, but congeal into a solid or semi-solid when refrigerated. Like saturated fats, they are relatively stable. They do not go rancid easily and can be used in cooking. The monounsaturated fatty acid most commonly found in our food is oleic acid, the main component of olive oil, as well as the oils from almonds, pecans, cashews, peanuts and avocados. Animal fats also contain a considerable amount of monounsaturated fatty acids.

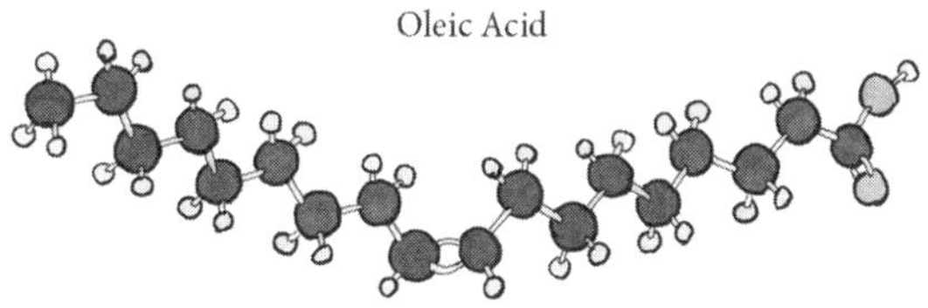

A monounsaturated fatty acid called oleic acid. Two carbons are missing one electron each, and at this position, the carbons are double-bonded to each other.

Polyunsaturated fatty acids have two or more double bonds and therefore lack four or more hydrogen atoms. The two polyunsaturated fatty acids found most frequently in our foods are linoleic acid, with two double bonds—also called omega-6; and linolenic acid, with three double bonds—also called omega-3. The polyunsaturated fatty acids have kinks or turns at the position of the double bond and therefore do not pack together easily. They are liquid, even when refrigerated.

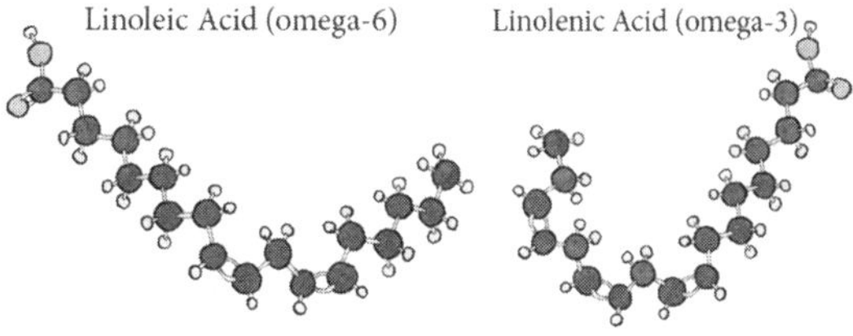

Omega-6 linoleic acid, with two double bonds (missing two electrons in two places), and omega-3 linolenic acid, with three double bonds (missing two electrons in three places).

The omega number indicates the position of the first double bond; thus, omega-3 fatty acids have the first double bond three carbons from the end of the molecule; omega-6 fatty acids have the first double bond six carbons from the end of the molecule. Monounsaturated oleic acid is an omega-9 fatty acid, with the single double bond positioned nine carbons from the end of the molecule.

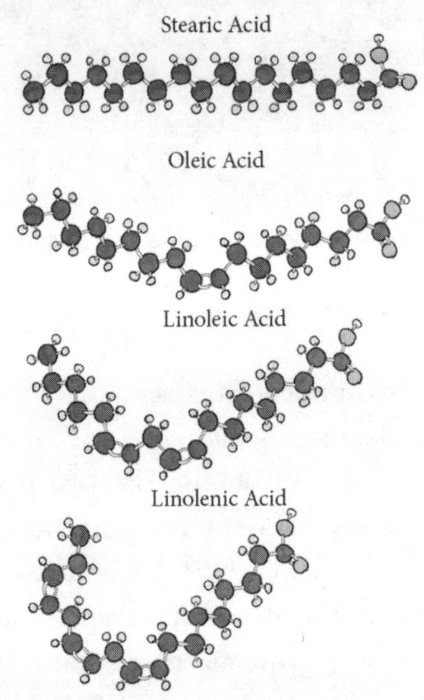

Saturated fatty acid, with no double bonds, no omega number; monounsaturated fatty acid with one double bond, omega number is 9; linoleic acid with two double bonds, omega number is 6; linolenic acid with three double bonds, omega number is 3.

In saturated fatty acids and monounsaturated fatty acids, every hydrogen is paired with another hydrogen, forming an electron cloud that is both stable and reactive. These electrons remain as pairs until conditions are right in the body for a reaction to occur.

Polyunsaturated fatty acids are less stable. Their bond structure leaves lots of hydrogen atoms sticking out at angles, which are easily broken off in conditions of heat or exposure to oxygen—such as in processing or cooking. The resulting unpaired electrons are called free radicals. In animal tissues, free radicals can damage cells and contribute to the progression of cancer, cardiovascular disease and age-related diseases. Polyunsaturated oils are considered "rancid" when they contain a lot of free radicals or have broken into pieces (called aldehydes) containing a lot of free radicals.

Your body cannot make the two basic polyunsaturated fatty acids, linoleic acid (omega-6) and linolenic acid (omega-3) so scientists call them "essential." We must obtain our essential fatty acids or EFAs from the foods we eat. Again, the nomenclature is unfortunate: polyunsaturated fatty acids are termed "essential," while saturated fatty acids and monounsaturated fatty acids are termed "nonessential." From these names alone, one might think that our bodies have no need for "nonessential" saturated or monounsaturated fats—but nothing could be further from the truth!

Our bodies need saturated and monounsaturated fatty acids in large quantities (while we only need the "essential" fatty acids in small quantities) so we have a mechanism for making our own saturated and monounsaturated fatty acids if they are not present in sufficient amounts in the diet. The body makes saturated fatty acids very easily from carbohydrates, especially from simple sugars (which is one reason people on low-fat diets tend to crave carbohydrates). The body then makes monounsaturated fatty acids from saturated fat molecules.

RESEARCHERS CLASSIFY FATTY ACIDS by their length as well as by their degree of saturation. Short-chain fatty acids have four to six carbon atoms. These fats are always saturated. Butterfat from cows contains four-carbon butyric acid (along with other fats) while butterfat from goats contains six-carbon capric acid and eight-carbon caprylic acid (along with other fats).

Medium-chain fatty acids have eight to twelve carbon atoms and are found mostly in butterfat and the tropical oils.

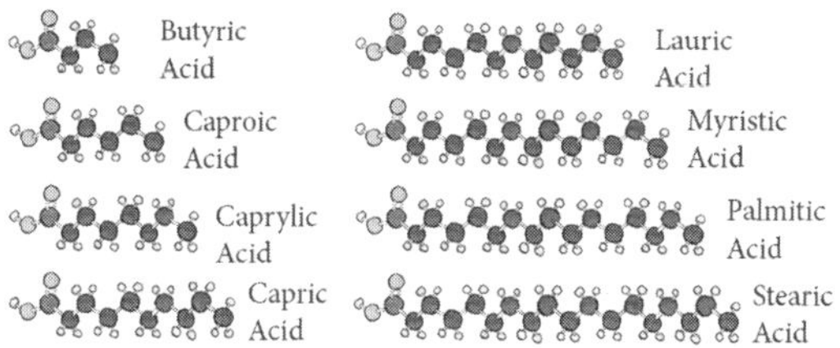

Short- and Medium-Chain Fatty Acids

Short- and medium-chain fatty acids, found in large quantities in coconut oil and in smaller amounts in butter, have recognized health benefits. They are absorbed directly into the bloodstream, provide quick energy, and do not require bile salts for digestion. For this reason, they are less likely to cause weight gain than other fatty acids, and can be helpful with weight loss. They also have antimicrobial effects in the gut—they kill pathogens, but not the beneficial bacteria—and contribute to the health of the immune system.[1]

Long-chain fatty acids have from fourteen to eighteen carbon atoms and can be either saturated, monounsaturated or polyunsaturated. Stearic acid is an eighteen-carbon saturated fatty acid found chiefly in butter and beef and lamb tallows; palmitic acid is a sixteen-carbon fatty acid found widely in animal fats and in the tropical oils, especially palm oil. Several studies have indicated that stearic acid lowers LDL-cholesterol (the so-called bad cholesterol) a little bit, while palmitic acid raises LDL-cholesterol a little bit.[2] The food industry draws on these findings to demonize palm oil—a major competitor to soybean oil, especially in Europe—but rarely mentions the seemingly beneficial effects of stearic acid in butter and meat fats.

Oleic acid, the chief component of olive oil, is an eighteen-carbon monounsaturated fatty acid. Another monounsaturated fatty acid is the sixteen-carbon palmitoleic acid, which has strong antimicrobial properties. It is found almost exclusively in animal fats. The two essential fatty acids mentioned earlier, linoleic acid (omega-6) and linolenic acid (omega-3), are also long chain, each eighteen carbons in length.

Very-long-chain fatty acids have twenty to twenty-four carbon atoms. They tend to be highly unsaturated, with four, five or six double bonds. The omega-3 and omega-6 categories represent families of fatty acids ranging from eighteen to twenty-two carbons and up to six double bonds. EFA (eicosapentaenoic acid) and DHA (docosahexaenoic acid) are omega-3 fatty acids found mostly in seafood, but also in organ meats and egg yolks. DGLA (dihomo-gamma-linolenic acid) and AA (arachidonic acid) are omega-6 fatty acids found in organ meats and animal fats. GLA (gamma-linolenic acid) is another omega-6 fatty acid found in evening primrose, borage and black currant oils. All these oils are extremely fragile and are needed by the body only in small amounts. Some people can make these fatty acids from the "parent" molecules, linoleic and linolenic acid, but others, particularly those whose ancestors consumed large amounts fish and organ meats, lack enzymes to produce them. These "obligate carnivores" must obtain them from animal foods such as organ meats, egg yolks, animal fats and seafood.

TRIGLYCERIDES ARE THREE FATTY ACIDS joined together with a glycerol molecule. This is how most fats occur, in both vegetable oils and animal fats—as three fatty acids joined as a triglyceride. During digestion the triglyceride breaks down into its three parts: two free fatty acids and one monoglyceride, which is a free fatty acid joined to a glycerol molecule. Once absorbed, the fatty acids reconnect with the three-pronged glycerol molecule, making the triglyceride whole again.

A typical triglyceride will have two fatty acids that are saturated or monounsaturated, with one unstable polyunsaturated fatty acid in place between these two. This configuration protects the polyunsaturated fatty acid from rancidity as long as it remains in the food.

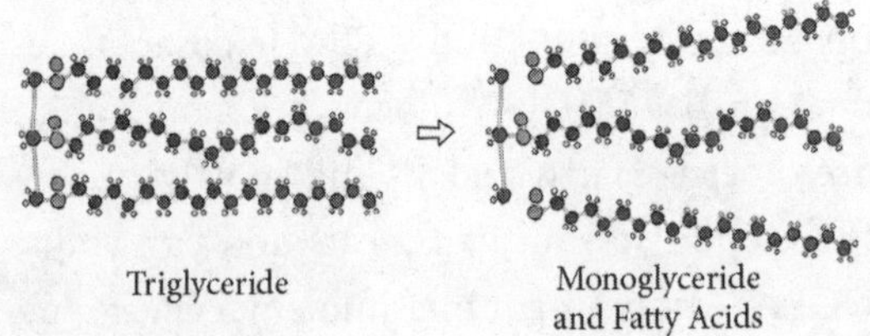

A triglyceride is three fatty acids joined to a glycerol molecule.

Triglycerides missing one or two fatty acids—diglycerides and monoglycerides—make good emulsifiers because the glycerol arms can join with a water-based compound while the fatty acid arms remains imbedded in the mixture of fatty acids, thus causing the fat to be held into the water element, rather than to separate and rise to the surface. You may have noticed mono- and diglycerides on the labels of processed foods like salad dressing, mayonnaise, spreads, custards and icing—it's a way for food manufacturers to "extend" fats by adding water. Mono- and diglycerides are actually fats, but labeling laws do not require their listing on labels as fats.

TRADITIONAL FATS AND OILS HAVE nourished mankind for millennia. Our diets have always included fats from animal sources and certain plant oils that can be easily removed from the seeds and fruit that contain them. In temperate regions, the population used olive oil, which is easily extracted using a slow-moving stone press from the oily olive fruit. In tropical regions, people used coconut oil or palm fruit oil, oils that are also easy to extract. Animal fats, olive oil and tropical oils are composed predominantly of saturated and monounsaturated fatty acids, so they are safe and stable. They do not break down during the extraction process and can be heated without any serious degradation.

Traditional cultures also used certain seed oils, including those extracted from sesame seed, flaxseed and rapeseed. These are liquid oils, containing high levels of polyunsaturated fatty acids. These seeds, however, are naturally oily and liquid oil can be extracted easily using a stone press. Typically, these oils were consumed immediately after extraction, so they were reasonably fresh and also safe when used in the context of a diet containing protective saturated fatty acids from butter, tropical oils and meat fat. Sesame oil contains unique antioxidants that are activated upon heating; flax oil is high in omega-3 fatty acids, so prone to rancidity and requires protection from high temperatures. Scandinavians and Russians valued flax oil for health-giving properties, but it was consumed freshly extracted and in small amounts—and never used for cooking.

The most problematic of the traditional seed oils is rapeseed oil, which was extracted with stone presses in large areas of India and China. It contains about 10 percent highly fragile omega-3 fatty acids, and yet it was used for cooking. In areas of selenium deficiency, use of rapeseed oil has been associated with a high incidence of fibrotic heart lesions, called Keshan's disease.[3] Animal studies suggest that when rapeseed oil is used in impoverished human diets, without adequate saturated fats from ghee (clarified butter), coconut oil or lard, then the oil's deleterious effects are magnified.[4] But in the context of healthy traditional diets that include saturated fats and adequate selenium, rapeseed oil freshly extracted using a slow-moving stone press does not appear to pose a problem.

INDUSTRIAL FATS AND OILS ARE a natural consequence of the industrial revolution and the application of modern technologies to the production of oils. Scientific innovation has helped man extract oils from traditional sources more efficiently, and created machinery that makes it possible to remove oils from seeds that will render an oil only using high heat and high pressure—namely cottonseed, corn, safflower, sunflower, soybean and canola oils.* Cottonseed oil was the first industrial oil to enter the market—an attempt to turn the waste of cotton production into an edible product. Corn oil first became available in the 1960s, to be eclipsed by soybean oil in the 1970s. Soybean oil proved more suited to the process of partial hydrogenation, and today 80 percent of the oil used in processed food is soybean oil. New oils, like grapeseed oils and rice bran oil, are also industrially extracted, and like cottonseed oil, represent an attempt to make something edible out of a waste product.

The extraction of oil from cottonseed, corn and soybeans cannot take place in a kitchen or on a street corner—these modern oils are extracted in huge factories, with the same equipment used in oil refineries. The first step is crushing the oil-bearing seeds using stainless steel presses, and then heating them to 230 degrees F. The oil is then squeezed out at pressures from 10 to 20 tons per inch, thereby generating even more heat. During this process the oils are exposed to damaging light and oxygen.

In order to extract the last fraction of oil from the crushed seeds, processors treat the pulp with a solvent—usually hexane, which is "food-grade" gasoline. The solvent is then boiled off, although up to 100 parts per million may remain in the oil. Such solvents are themselves toxic; the oils also retain the toxic pesticides adhering to seeds and grains before processing begins.

The oil that comes out of an industrial press is typically a dark, sticky, smelly gunk. The process of cleaning it up for human consumption involves even more heat and more chemicals. Steam heating removes the solvent. Additional refining consists of another heating, plus the addition of an alkaline substance, such as sodium hydroxide or sodium carbonate. These

* Safflower, sunflower and canola seeds are fairly oily and can render their oils with a cold-press or expeller-extraction method. Nevertheless, these oils are usually obtained by industrial methods.

chemicals form suds that must be washed away, and then followed by a drying process that involves more damaging heat.

The next process is degumming, which calls for the addition of phosphoric acid or citric acid and another heating. The gums precipitate out, and a centrifuge removes the dregs. Filtering the oil through fuller's earth—activated carbon or activated clays—removes the dark color.

A final step is deodorization, accomplished by passing steam over the hot oil in a vacuum at between 440 and 485 degrees F. The process distills the volatile taste and odor components from the oil. Citric acid added to the oil after deodorization inactivates trace metals left behind.

The oil that then goes into bottles looks and smells clean, but it has gone through at least six heatings: heating when pressed, heating to remove the solvents, heating during refining, heating during the drying process, heating during degumming, and heating (to very high temperatures) during deodorization.

High-temperature processing creates dangerous free radicals, aldehydes and other breakdown products. In addition, the high temperatures and pressures neutralize or destroy any beneficial antioxidants, such as fat-soluble vitamin E, which protect the body from the ravages of free radicals. Powerful industrial antioxidants, such as BHT and BHA, both suspected of causing cancer and estrogen disruption,[5] are often added to these oils to replace the vitamin E and other natural preservatives destroyed by excessive heat.

A safe, modern technique for oil extraction does exist. The "cold press" or "expeller expressed" process drills into seeds and extracts the oil and its precious cargo of antioxidants at low temperatures, with minimal exposure to light and oxygen. Safflower oil, sunflower oil, canola oil and sesame oil can be obtained with these processes. These unrefined oils will remain fresh for many months if stored in the refrigerator in dark bottles. Extra virgin olive oil is still produced by crushing olives between stone or steel rollers. This gentle process preserves the integrity of the fatty acids and the numerous natural preservatives in olive oil. When packaged in opaque containers, olive oil will retain its freshness and precious store of antioxidants for many years.

THE ADVENT OF MODERN PROCESSING, starting with cottonseed oil in the late 1800s, provided the food industry with a cheap substitute for olive oil. But manufacturers also needed a cheap substitute for saturated fats like butter, lard and tallow. Liquid cottonseed oil is too unstable for frying and too soft for processed baked goods like crackers, cookies and piecrust. The answer was partial hydrogenation, a process patented in the early 1900s, which turns liquid vegetable oils into fats that are solid at room temperature—margarine and shortening. Partial hydrogenation gave the industrial oil industry just what it needed to grow.

To produce partially hydrogenated fats, manufacturers begin with the cheapest oils—soy, corn, cottonseed or canola, which are already rancid from the extraction process—and mix them with powdered nickel oxide. The oil with its nickel catalyst is then subjected to hydrogen gas in a high-pressure, high-temperature reactor. What goes into the reactor is a liquid oil; what comes out is a semisolid that resembles gray cottage cheese and has an appalling smell. Soap-like emulsifiers and starch squeezed into the mass smooth out the lumps. High-temperature steam cleaning removes the odor. A bleaching process gets rid of the gray color. At this point the product can carry the label "pure vegetable shortening." Dyes and artificial flavors make the concoction resemble butter.* Finally, the mixture is compressed, packaged in blocks or tubs and sold as a food.

In the process of partial hydrogenation, the pressure and high temperatures in the presence of the nickel catalyst cause the hydrogen atoms on the monounsaturated or polyunsaturated fatty acid chains to change position. Before partial hydrogenation, pairs of hydrogen atoms occur together, even at the double bond, causing the molecule to bend slightly and form an electron cloud. This is called the *cis* formation, the configuration most commonly found in nature.† With partial hydrogenation, one hydrogen atom of the pair is moved to the other side so that the molecule straightens. This is called the *trans* configuration. *Trans* means "across," and partial hydrogenation causes one or more hydrogen atoms to move across the molecule, so the *cis* kink straightens out. These straight molecules pack together easily, forming a solid fat. They behave *chemically* like a solid fat; but *biochemically* they are very different from saturated fatty acids.

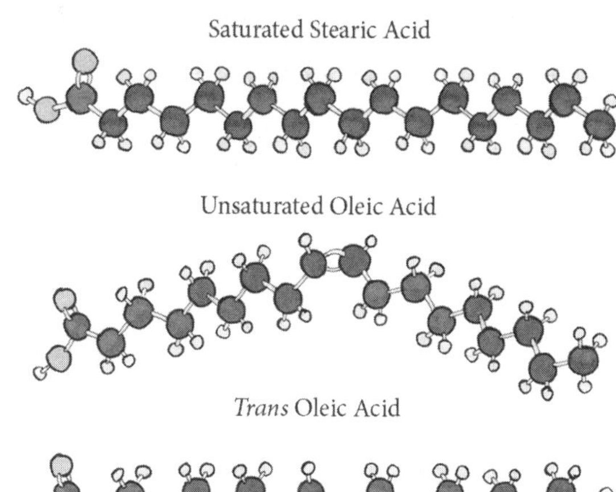

Saturated fatty acids are naturally straight; monounsaturated and polyunsaturated fatty acids have a bend at each double bond. During the process of partial hydrogenation, one of the hydrogen molecules at a double bond is moved across the molecule–"trans" means across–which causes the molecule to straighten out and behave chemically like a saturated fatty acid.

In full hydrogenation, the oil is left in the reactor longer so that all the carbon bonds are eventually filled with hydrogen, forming saturated fatty acids. The resulting artificially saturated fat is very hard and must be mixed with more unsaturated fatty acids to create a usable fat. In order to reduce the amounts of *trans* fats in processed food, manufacturers today are using more fully hydrogenated fats—that is, saturated fats artificially created out of polyunsaturated vegetable oils—a fact they are reluctant to publicize since they have spent the last one hundred years demonizing saturated fatty acids. But they can still claim that these manmade saturated fats are "cholesterol-free."

ANIMAL FATS—WHETHER THE HIGHLY saturated fats in meat and butter or the more

* Manufacturers are not allowed to use artificial colors in margarines and spreads—they must use a natural color—a comforting thought.

† Small amounts of natural *trans* fats occur in butter, meat fat and even in fish. These are not harmful but have beneficial effects.

unsaturated fats found in lard and poultry—are the main source of cholesterol in the diet. Cholesterol is often referred to as a fat or lipid, but it is actually a sterol, an organic structure with four rings. It has wax-like properties and, like fatty acids, does not dissolve in water.

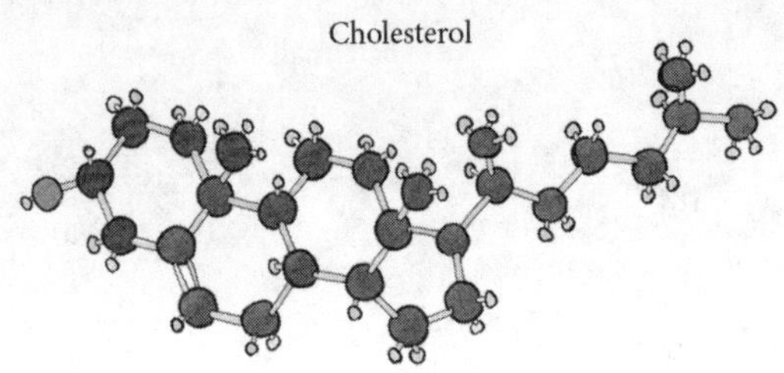

Cholesterol has a four-ring structure; it is not a fatty acid.

Cholesterol is a vital part of the cell membrane structure in all animals and humans. Cholesterol's key role is to keep the cell membrane waterproof, so that different biochemical processes are possible on the inside and the outside of the cell. It also provides powerful antioxidant protection to the cell membrane.[6] The greatest concentration of cholesterol occurs in the brain and the nervous system, and then in the muscles. Cholesterol serves as the precursor to the bile salts, necessary for digesting fats, and to vitamin D. It is the parent substance out of which all the sex hormones are made—estrogen, testosterone, progesterone—and also the many hormones produced in the adrenal cortex. These hormones regulate blood sugar levels, blood pressure and mineral uptake. They also are essential to healing, control of inflammation and stress. When we are under a lot of stress, the body calls up its reserves of cholesterol to make corticoid hormones so we can deal appropriately with the stress.* Receptors for serotonin, the body's feel-good chemical, require cholesterol to work properly,[7] which explains why very low cholesterol levels are associated with depression, violent behavior and suicide.

Since cholesterol does not dissolve in water, it needs a vehicle to carry it around in the blood—these are called lipoproteins. They serve as little submarines, with a water-soluble protein coating, carrying valuable nutrients to the cells where they are needed. The submarines dock at receptors on the cell membrane and empty their precious cargo of cholesterol, fats and fat-soluble vitamins into the cells.

Using ultracentrifugal separation of lipoproteins, researchers have been able to isolate different densities of lipoproteins. They found that LDL-cholesterol (low-density lipoprotein), which makes up the majority of lipoprotein in the body, carries cholesterol and other nutrients to the cells and HDL-cholesterol (high-density lipoprotein) carries cholesterol away from the cells and back to the liver. Put another way, LDL facilitates the entry of cholesterol, fatty acids and fat-soluble vitamins into the cells and HDL facilitates their removal.

Actually, there are four major fractions or lipoproteins: triglyceride-rich chylomicrons, very low density (VLDL), cholesterol-rich low density (LDL), and protein-rich high density

* A 1997 study of university students tracked weekly cholesterol levels. Cholesterol levels rose "proportional to the degree of examination stress." When the students were under stress, their bodies wisely made more cholesterol in order to produce hormones to help the students deal with the stress of exams.[a]

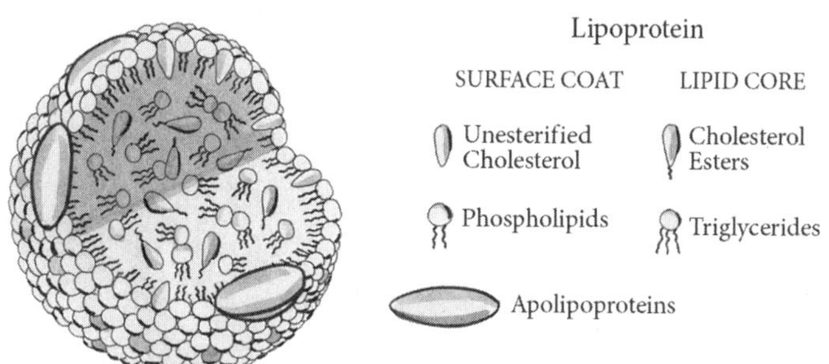

(HDL). The LDL can be further fractionated into small, dense and large "fluffy" particles. The small particles appear to infiltrate the artery preferentially. Whatever the density or fluffiness of the lipoproteins, the cholesterol they carry is all exactly the same.

While AHA literature does not mention oxidized cholesterol, many scientists believe it to be the real villain in coronary disease, as it seems to initiate the process leading to the buildup of plaque in the arteries.[8] A main cause of cholesterol oxidation in the bloodstream is highly reactive free radicals from industrial seed oils. The plot thickens.

We'll learn more about the problems of industrial fats and oils in Chapter 7.

EVERY FAT AND OIL IS a combination of saturated, monounsaturated and polyunsaturated fatty acids. In general, animal fats such as butter, lard, and tallow contain about 40–60 percent saturated fat and are solid at room temperature. Vegetable oils from temperate climates contain a preponderance of "essential" polyunsaturated fatty acids and are liquid at room temperature. But vegetable oils from the tropics are highly saturated. Coconut oil, for example, is 92 percent saturated. These fats are liquid in the tropics but hard as butter in northern climes. Plant oils are more saturated in hot climates because the increased saturation helps maintain stiffness in plant leaves. Olive oil with its preponderance of oleic acid is the product of a temperate climate. It is liquid at warm temperatures but hardens when refrigerated.

When ruminant animals like cows, sheep and goats digest their food, the process adds hydrogen to the unsaturated fatty acids naturally occurring in plants, resulting in saturated fats. These fats are predominantly saturated, with at least 50 percent of the fatty acids saturated (usually a combination of eighteen-carbon stearic acid and sixteen-carbon palmitic acid). Fat from certain parts of the animal, such as the highly prized fat around the kidneys, can be up to 75 percent saturated. The balance of fatty acids in ruminant fat is mostly monounsaturated fatty acids with a small percentage of the fat—less than 2 percent—a combination of omega-3 and omega-6 polyunsaturated fatty acids.

Fats from monogastric animals and birds—these are animals with one stomach—tend to be softer than the fat of ruminant animals because they are less saturated. Lard or pig fat is about 40 percent saturated, while the fat of birds is 30–35 percent saturated. Saturated fat content is lower, but levels of polyunsaturated fatty acids are higher, ranging from 13 to 20 percent. The balance is monounsaturated fatty acids.

Comparison of Dietary Fats

DIETARY FAT	SATURATED FAT	POLYUNSATURATED FAT: linoleic acid (an omega-6 fatty acid)	POLYUNSATURATED FAT: alpha-linolenic acid (an omega-3 fatty acid)	MONOUNSATURATED FAT: oleic acid (an omega-9 fatty acid)
Canola oil	7	21	11	61
Safflower oil	8	14	1	77
Flaxseed oil	9	16	57	18
Sunflower oil	12	71	1	16
Corn oil	13	57	1	29
Olive oil	15	9	1	75
Soybean oil	15	54	8	23
Peanut oil	19	33	*	48
Cottonseed oil	27	54	*	19
Lard	43	9	1	47
Palm oil	51	10	*	39
Butter	68	3	1	28
Coconut oil	91	2		7

*Trace   Fatty acid content normalized to 100%

Source: POS Pilot Plant Corpration

The fatty acid profile of monogastric animals will vary with the animal's diet: pigs raised in the tropics contain a lot of lauric acid in their fat, a medium-chain fatty acid they get from eating coconut meal. Pigs and poultry in the United States are fed mostly grains containing high levels of omega-6 fatty acids, so their eggs, meat and fat will contain relatively high levels of omega-6. If the animals get fish or flax meal in their feed, or if they are raised outside so that green grasses and insects form a part of the diet, the level of omega-3 fatty acids will be higher. This is also true of fish—farm-raised fish has more omega-6 and less omega-3 than wild fish.

However, it is incorrect to claim that grass feeding contributes to lower levels of saturated fat and higher levels of omega-3 fatty acids in beef. As ruminants, cows can turn unsaturated fatty acids into saturated fats very efficiently. The healthier the animal, the more efficiently it does this. Thus the fat of grass-fed animals can be slightly *more saturated* than that of grain-fed animals. Omega-3 fatty acids are slightly higher in grass-fed beef, but the amount is low to begin with and the total polyunsaturated fatty acid content (omega-3 plus omega-6) does not exceed about 2 percent. Grain-fed beef has more fat than grass-fed, with most of the increase as monounsaturated fatty acids, the same kind of fat found in olive oil.

Olive oil contains 75 percent monounsaturated oleic acid with small amounts of saturated and unsaturated fatty acids. A liquid oil that is also very stable, olive oil is the perfect oil for salad dressings, and it can also be used safely for cooking.

Fatty Acids in Grass-Fed And Grain-Fed Beef

NUTRIENTS/100 G	GRASS-FED	GRAIN-FED
WATER	68	64
TOTAL FAT	13	17
SATURATED FAT	7	7
MONOUNSATURATED FAT	5	9
OMEGA-6 FATTY ACIDS	.36	.56
OMEGA-3 FATTY ACIDS	.12	.09
OMEGA-3/OMEGA-6	1 to 3	1 to 6

Source: University of Nebraska-Lincoln/Institute of Agriculture and Natural Resources

Other "high-oleic" oils include peanut oil and sesame oil, but these do not contain more than 50 percent oleic acid, making them less suitable for frequent use.

Safflower, corn, sunflower, soybean and cottonseed oils all contain over 50 percent omega-6 fatty acids and, except for soybean oil, only minimal amounts of omega-3. Safflower oil contains almost 80 percent omega-6. Newer oils like grapeseed oil and rice bran oil have similar profiles. Whatever claims are made about these oils, they all contain dangerous levels of polyunsaturated fatty acids and therefore unsuitable for cooking.

Canola oil is very low in saturated fatty acids (about 5 percent), with 57 percent oleic acid, 23 percent omega-6 and 10–15 percent omega-3. The newest oil on the market, canola oil was developed from the rapeseed, a member of the mustard family. Researchers chose the rapeseed because it is high in oleic acid and therefore could provide a cheap alternative to olive oil—with high levels of omega-3 fatty acids considered a bonus.

Scientists once considered rapeseed oil as unsuited for human consumption—even though traditional cultures had used it for millennia—because it contains a very-long-chain fatty acid called erucic acid, which under some circumstances is associated with fibrotic heart lesions. Canola oil was created from genetic manipulation of rapeseed to contain little if any erucic acid, and nutritionists heralded the new product as the perfect heart-healthy oil—high in monounsaturated fatty acids, rich in omega-3, and very low in saturated fat. But canola oil does not live up to these claims. One study indicates that "heart-healthy" canola oil actually creates a deficiency of vitamin E, a vitamin required for a healthy cardiovascular system.[9] Other studies show that the new low-erucic-acid canola oil still can cause heart lesions, particularly when the diet is low in saturated fat.[10] Canola oil has a high sulphur content and goes rancid easily. Baked goods made with canola oil develop mold very quickly. Most seriously, during the deodorizing process, the fragile omega-3 fatty acids of processed canola oil are rendered rancid or even transformed into *trans* fatty acids, similar to those in margarine, and possibly more dangerous.[11]

Oils from cold-climate plants and cold-blooded fish living in cold waters are very low in saturated fat and high in omega-3 fatty acids, which act as a kind of antifreeze in the blood and cell membranes. Flax oil contains over 50 percent omega-3. Scandinavian folklore heralds flaxseed oil as a health food. New extraction and bottling methods have minimized rancidity problems. Flaxseed oil should always be kept refrigerated, never heated, and consumed in very small amounts in salad dressings and spreads.

Tropical oils are more saturated than other plant oils because saturated fats help maintain appropriate stiffness in plant leaves in warm climates. Palm oil is about 50 percent saturated, with 41 percent oleic acid and about 9 percent omega-6 linoleic acid. Food manufacturers in Europe, where the soybean industry has far less influence than in the United States, have avoided *trans* fats by using mostly refined palm oil in baked goods and snack foods.

Coconut oil is 92 percent saturated with over two-thirds of the saturated fat in the form of medium-chain fatty acids. Of particular interest is lauric acid, found in large quantities in coconut oil and smaller quantities in human breast milk. This fatty acid has strong antifungal and antimicrobial properties.[12] Coconut oil protects tropical populations from bacteria and fungus so prevalent in their food supply; as third-world nations in tropical areas have switched to polyunsaturated vegetable oils, the incidence of intestinal disorders and immune deficiency diseases has increased dramatically. Because coconut oil contains lauric acid, it is sometimes used in baby formulas.

Palm kernel oil, an expensive oil pressed out of the palm fruit seed, is used primarily in candy coatings; like coconut oil, it contains high levels of lauric acid.

AS THE DANGERS OF *TRANS* fats became known, followed by laws calling for *trans* fat labeling, food processors needed *trans*-free alternatives for frying and baked goods. The obvious choices were stable fats high in saturated fatty acids, such as tallow, lard and palm oil, but the influence of the soybean industry in the United States, and the perception that these stable fats are unhealthy, makes these fats a more difficult choice for the food industry.

The solution became a highly industrial process called interesterification—a process that rearranges the fatty acids in triglycerides and results in a fat with different melting and baking qualities.

Interesterification was first applied to natural fats like palm oil and lard in the 1940s. For example, in natural lard, about 2 percent of the triglycerides have three saturated fatty acids and about 24 percent have three unsaturated fatty acids. The remaining triglycerides have a combination of unsaturated and saturated fatty acids. After interesterification, the number of triglycerides with three saturates or three unsaturates are increased while the number of triglycerides with a combination of saturated and unsaturated fatty acids are decreased. The result is a higher melting temperature and "improved" baking qualities, such as more volume in cakes.

To make low-*trans* or *trans*-free margarines and shortenings, manufacturers interesterify a blend of liquid oil with fully hydrogenated oil. The resulting fatty acids are mostly eighteen-carbon stearic acid, the same as the demonized fatty acids found in beef and butter! Fully hydrogenated oil is very hard, so only a small amount is needed—about 10 percent—to blend and interesterify with the liquid oil to produce a spreadable fat.

Manufacturers use one of two basic methods for producing interesterfied oil blends. The most common calls for a chemical catalyst, such as sodium methoxide or ethoxide (dangerous and highly toxic industrial solvents), or hazardous metallic sodium or a sodium-potassium alloy. This method requires heat of 176–248 degrees F to produce interesterified fatty acids. The product must then be neutralized (to remove the caustic catalyst), bleached (to get rid of the resultant dark brown color) and deodorized (a process that can actually introduce *trans* fats into the mix). The other method uses enzymes to produce the interesterified fats. It is more expensive but results in less loss of oil through the formation of soaps, esters and mono- and diglycerides.

Whichever method is used, the final product will contain chemical residues, hexanes and many dangerous breakdown products full of free radicals.[13]

In reaction to the *trans* fat backlash, the food processing industry has moved from the frying pan into the fire. The industry considered *trans* fats the perfect solution to the problems inherent in liquid vegetable oils—the process of partial hydrogenation made these highly reactive oils into stable hardened fats. Early studies showed that the liquid oils were highly carcinogenic; *trans* fats solved the problem, or so they thought.

The evidence that *trans* fats were also carcinogenic, and also caused many other health problems, emerged slowly. But once the problems with *trans* fats became clear, the industry scrambled for alternatives. Unfortunately, rather than return to stable, saturated—and usually more expensive—animal fats, it chose either interesterified fats or simply returned to the liquid oils, using both in softer "heart-healthy" spreads. The label "*trans*-fat-free" on a product creates the impression that it is safe and healthy. Unfortunately, the effects of these "liquid plant oils" are considerably worse.

CHAPTER 3

Not Guilty as Charged

Vegetable oils, and indeed all plant foods, contain little saturated fat* and never any cholesterol, while animal fats contain both. This is a fact. Also a fact: the demonization of saturated fat and cholesterol is an obvious marketing strategy.

The attack on animal fats began with the accusation that they caused heart disease, especially myocardial infarction or heart attack. But accusers soon added other ailments to the list: stroke, high blood pressure, cancer, diabetes, obesity, autoimmune disease, kidney disease and impotence. The 1973 McGovern committee report went so far as to claim that America's ten greatest disease killers would give way with a dietary change from butter to margarine, and from lard to vegetable oils for cooking.

The accusations against cholesterol and saturated fat rely upon the following logic: In 1900, heart disease and cancer were rare; by 1970, these and other chronic diseases had reached epidemic proportions. In 1900, Americans ate very little cholesterol and saturated fat; they followed a virtuous, abstemious, low-fat diet. By 1970, Americans had become rich, spoiled, and indulgent, gorging themselves on fatty meats, bacon, sausage, butter, eggs and cream—foods new to the American diet.

But what *were* Americans eating in 1900? The 1895 *Baptist Ladies' Cook Book: Choice and Tested Recipes Contributed by the Ladies of Monmouth, Ill* gives us a good idea.[1] This collection of recipes from the turn of the century contradicts what the establishment is telling us—that the reason we have so much cancer and heart disease today compared to a century ago is because we are eating much greater levels of saturated fats from animal foods. Yet there's hardly a recipe in this little book that does not contain butter, eggs, cream or lard—beginning with the soup chapter and ending with the large collection of the desserts.

Did Americans eat lean meat in 1900? The inhabitants of Monmouth, Illinois enjoyed steaks and rib roasts—one recipe suggests cooking the roast in beef drippings. Lean roasts were "larded" to make them tender—that is

* The exception, as explained in Chapter 2, is plant foods from tropical regions, like coconut and palm fruit.

injected with bits of pig fat. Most meat and chicken recipes call for gravy made with drippings and occasionally with added cream. The good Baptist ladies cooked the whole chicken, not skinless chicken breasts.

In 1895, nobody had heard of *al dente* steamed vegetables. All the vegetable recipes in the book are cooked a long time and many call for a cream sauce. They include asparagus dressed in cream, four versions of cabbage with cream sauce, corn and eggplant fritters fried in lard, potato balls fried in "good drippings" and parsnips fried in bacon fat. Indeed, it seems that vegetables in those days were just an excuse for a sauce.

Seafood recipes include fish *à la crème*, scalloped fish, creamed salmon and creamed fish. The sauce for broiled fish calls for one large spoonful of butter and one-and-one-half cups of cream. A whole chapter devoted to oysters includes recipes for deviled oysters made with egg yolks, creamed oyster patties made with eggs and butter, oysters wrapped in bacon, scalloped oysters, oyster pie made with *one quart* of cream, oyster fritters fried in drippings, oysters fried in hot lard and scalloped oysters made with butter and whole milk.*

A chapter on organ meats includes fried veal liver and sweet breads—both creamed and fried. A scrapple recipe calls for hog's head, heart, tongue and part of the liver. This rich mixture was stored in a crock and covered with melted lard. Midwestern families consumed scrapple for breakfast, sliced and fried in lard.

There are separate full chapters for eggs and cheese.

What about salads? Only one salad recipe in the book calls for lettuce, "when available." Lettuce is a modern luxury—in the past we ate lettuce only during the growing season.† The other salad recipes feature apples, cabbage, ham, tongue, chicken, oysters, fruit, potatoes, veal, lobster, sweet breads, shrimp and nasturtium flowers.

The recipes for salad dressing are of great interest to our argument. The dressing for coleslaw features sweet cream. Three recipes for salad dressing contain egg yolk, mustard and vinegar. One recipe calls for olive oil *or* melted butter. If they didn't have olive oil in Illinois in 1895, which they probably didn't, they used melted butter instead. Another recipe includes one cup of whipped cream. Just one salad dressing recipe in the book calls for "oil." Americans at the turn of the century nourished themselves with butter, cream, egg yolks and lard, not with vegetable oil. Some Italian communities may have used olive oil—and cottonseed oil was just beginning to appear in the food supply—but Americans generally used animal fats, even on salads.

The Baptists were fond of rich desserts. Half of the book is devoted to cakes, pies, ice creams, puddings and donuts. The donuts were fried in lard, of course, and the cakes were made with butter. Two advertisements for dentists at the back of the book testify to the known negative effects of sugar and white flour on the teeth, but

* Most likely these recipes were for canned oysters from the Chesapeake Bay. Estimated oyster consumption on the East Coast in 1900 was three hundred to six hundred oysters per person per year, compared to less than one oyster per person per year in the United States today.[a]

† Lettuce was a rare food in 1900; today we consume it frequently. Heart disease and cancer were rare in 1900; today they occur at epidemic rates. The obvious conclusion is that cancer and heart disease are caused by lettuce—at least according to the logic of the diet-heart promoters.

cancer and heart disease were rare before the turn of the century. While people were sturdy and strong, true obesity was uncommon.

The argument that Americans today eat more animal fats than they did a century ago does not hold up to the facts. Quite the opposite. Today's typical American diet of lean meat, skinless chicken breasts, reduced-fat milk, margarine and vegetable oil contain little animal fat. Based on *The Baptist Ladies' Cook Book* and many other cookbooks of the period, the American diet in 1900 was far richer and more "indulgent" than it is today.

EVEN IN THE 1960s, SOME communities cooked everything in lard. In 1961, scientists studied the residents of Roseto, Pennsylvania, and the findings baffled researchers. The citizens of Roseto had exceptionally low rates of heart disease. In Roseto, men over sixty-five enjoyed a death rate of 1 percent while the national average was 2 percent. Widowers outnumbered widows, too. In his bestselling book *Outliers: The Story of Success*, author Malcolm Gladwell notes that in Roseto men and women under fifty-five years old had almost no heart disease whatsoever, and those over sixty-five suffered roughly only 50 percent as much heart disease as did average Americans. The men worked in the slate quarries where they did contract illnesses from gases and dust, but Roseto also had no crime, and very few applications for public assistance.[2]

The experts looked at genetics, geography and other factors, yet nothing explained why the inhabitants of Roseto were "outliers," that is, statistical anomalies, when it came to the rate of heart disease within the community. They did not tend to slimness, and in fact were often obese. They didn't exercise much either, and the men enjoyed their cigars.

Then the investigators looked at their diet. People in Roseto did not use olive oil; instead they cooked in lard. They preferred wine to soft drinks and milk. They piled pepperoni, sausage, salami and sometimes eggs on their pizzas. They ate hard and soft cheese. Over 40 percent of their caloric intake was from saturated fat, a large portion of it from lard. Of course, today's dietitians can't even say the word "lard" without clutching their chests in pain. So they concluded with perfect political correctness that diet was not a factor either.

Instead, scientists concluded that the close-knit community experienced a reduced rate of heart disease because of lower stress levels. They called it the "Roseto Effect." According to Dr. Stewart Wolf, one of the original study authors, "The community [of Roseto] was very cohesive. There was no keeping up with the Joneses. Houses were very close together, and everyone lived more or less alike. Elderly were revered and incorporated into community life. Housewives were respected, and fathers ran the families."[3] Many studies followed, including a fifty-year study comparing nearby towns Bangor and Nazareth. As the original authors had predicted, when the Bangor cohort shed their Italian social structure and became more Americanized in the years following the initial study, heart disease rose.[4]

The town of Roseto should hold no mysteries for the scientific community. As we discussed in Chapter 1, anyone with some scientific background in the subject of fats and oils would know that in the United States, from 1920 to 1960, heart disease skyrocketed while animal fat consumption (especially lard consumption) dropped equally drastically. They would also be familiar with the many other studies that contradict the notion that animal fats cause heart disease. Instead the politically correct pundits reached into their barrel of lame explanations and pulled out the familiar "strong family and social ties." While obesity in the Roseto folks was probably due to their lack of exercise and the sweet desserts they liked, their hearts were strong because they consumed plenty of the ideal fuel for the heart—saturated fat.

Shortly after the Roseto study, the *British Medical Journal* published a study where patients who had already suffered one heart attack were assigned to one of three groups and given polyunsaturated corn oil, monounsaturated olive oil or saturated animal fats respectively. The endpoints were further heart attack or death. Those in the corn oil group saw their blood cholesterol levels come down by an average of 30 percent, while there was no change in the other two groups. However, at the end of the two-year trial only 52 percent of the corn oil group were still alive and had avoided a second heart attack. Those on the monounsaturated olive oil fared a little better: 57 percent survived and had no further heart attacks. But those eating saturated animal fats fared the best with 75 percent surviving and without further attack.[5] Perhaps this third group had strong family ties as well?

CONTRADICTORY EVIDENCE CONTINUES TO ACCUMULATE, but the diet-heart and lipid-theory dogma persists—just changed slightly after the bad news about *trans* fats became public. The American Heart Association (AHA) and almost every other conventional medical group and government agency just tacked *trans* fats on to saturated fats, creating the bad fats brothers—Sat and Trans—both of whom raise the villainous LDL-cholesterol and therefore cause heart disease.

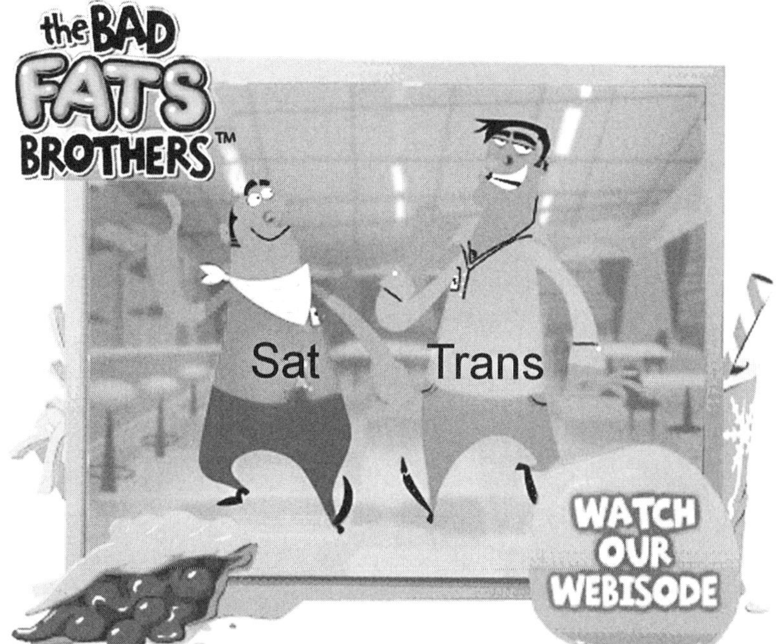

They're a charming pair, Sat and Trans. But that doesn't mean they make good friends. Read on to learn how they clog arteries and break hearts -- and how to limit your time with them by avoiding the foods they're in.

Fats: The Good, the Bad & the Ugly

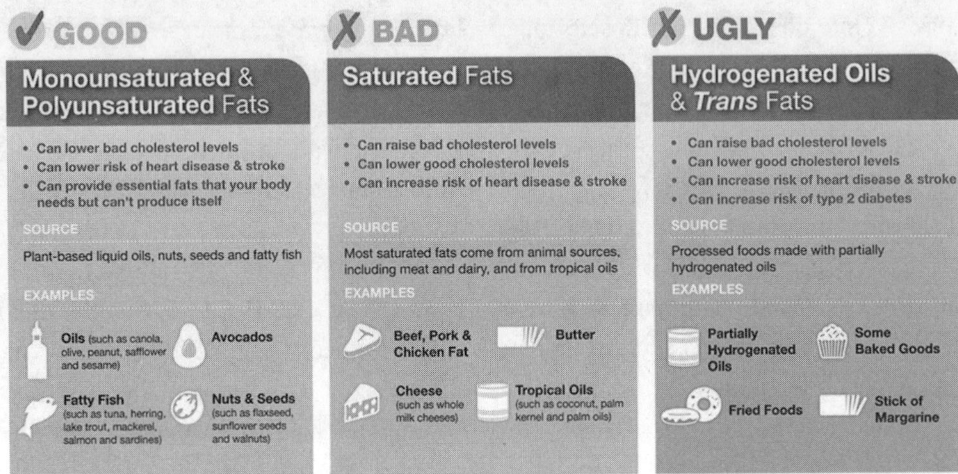

Source: The American Heart Association

In 2014, the AHA proclaimed the evidence "irrefutable that saturated fat should be decreased to 5 to 6% of calories by replacement with polyunsaturated fat to lower LDL-cholesterol and reduce CVD risk."[6] Polyunsaturated oils became the "good" replacement for both *trans* and saturated fats—anything to prevent the population from embracing delicious foods like chicken wings, butter and cheese.*

The Harvard Health website parrots the AHA, advising readers to "Choose foods with healthy unsaturated fat (fish, nuts, and most plant oils), limit foods high in saturated fat (butter, whole milk, cheese, coconut and palm oil, and red meats), and try to avoid foods with *trans* fat."[7]

Seven years earlier, in 2006, the results of the Women's Health Initiative (WHI) Dietary Modification Trial appeared in the *Journal of the American Medical Association*. The study involved more than forty-eight thousand postmenopausal women, who were randomly assigned to either a regular unrestricted diet or to a "healthy" diet that was low in fat (20 percent fat) and high in fiber, with at least five servings of fruits and vegetables and six servings of grains per day—in other words, they followed the dietary guidelines to a T.[8] The "healthy" eaters attended group sessions led by dietitians who administered "intense behavioral modification" to keep them on their diets. And the "healthy" diet women did surprisingly well, maintaining their fat intake at 24 percent of total calories and the dreaded saturated fat at 8 percent. By contrast, the control group consumed 38 percent of total calories as fat with about 12 percent as saturated fat—still low in fat compared to the traditional American diet, but way more than the amount the AHA considers safe. The "healthy" diet group also consumed more fruits and vegetables, grains and fiber. Researchers followed the women closely for more than eight years while recording cases of clinically confirmed breast cancer, colon cancer, heart disease, heart attacks and strokes, confidently predicting, for example, a 14 percent decrease in breast cancer incidence. When the results came, the benefit

* Chicken fat is mostly polyunsaturated and monounsaturated, but the AHA ignores this inconvenient fact.

from years of restrictive eating was…nothing! The two groups showed no difference in the incidence of cancer, stroke and heart disease, and no difference in weight gain either.[9]

More recently, a 2010 mega-analysis published in the *American Journal of Clinical Nutrition* combined the relative risk rates from twenty-one studies representing almost three hundred fifty thousand people whose diets and health outcomes were followed for five to twenty-three years. The conclusion: "There is no significant evidence for concluding that dietary saturated fat is associated with an increased risk of CHD (coronary heart disease) or CVD (cardiovascular disease)."[10] Not one word about this study appeared in the mainstream press. An accompanying editorial voiced outrage at the findings and repeated the same advice—avoid red meat, whole milk, egg yolks and cheese, and eat more egg whites, grains, fat-free dairy foods and seed oils. Only James H. Hodges of the American Meat Institute Foundation spoke out: "This study is critically important because of its size and statistical power. No doubt, it will be viewed with skepticism by some researchers who believe strongly in a link between heart disease and saturated fat. But when it comes to science, we must view new findings with an open mind and critical thought. Without an open mind, we risk enacting misguided public policies. While this study may not reflect prevailing nutrition advice, it is a very substantial body of work…The magnitude of this study and its findings merit both respect and thoughtful consideration."[11]

On the heels of the meta-analysis exonerating saturated fat is a prospective 2010 study from Australia which looked at adults over a period of fifteen years. People who ate the most full-fat dairy products had a 69 percent lower risk of cardiovascular death than those who ate the least; or to put it another way, people who mostly avoided dairy foods or consumed low-fat dairy had more than three times the risk of dying of coronary heart disease or stroke compared to people who ate the most full-fat dairy.[12] A 2004 study from Sweden got similar results. The researchers measured blood levels of two biomarkers for milk fat in over four hundred heart attack patients and over five hundred healthy controls. The markers, pentadecanoic acid and heptadecanoic acid,* provide a good indication of how much dairy fat a person has been eating. The researchers found that people with the highest levels of these milk fat biomarkers—that means they were consuming butter and full-fat dairy foods—were at lower risk of heart attack; for women the risk was reduced by 26 percent and for men the risk was 9 percent lower.[13] The study has particular relevance because the researchers did not rely on dietary questionnaires, which are notoriously inaccurate, but on blood markers of fatty acid consumption.

Also in 2004, researchers found that in postmenopausal women with relatively low total fat intake, a greater saturated fat intake was associated with less progression of coronary atherosclerosis, whereas carbohydrate intake was associated with a greater progression.[14]

The 2013 Sydney Diet Heart Study not only further exonerated saturated fat, but also found problems with polyunsaturated oils—the kind we are supposed to use in place

* Pentadecanoic acid is a rare fifteen-carbon saturated fat and heptadecanoic is a rare seventeen-carbon saturated fat; both occur almost exclusively in butterfat.

of saturates. It involved four hundred fifty-eight men ages thirty to fifty-nine. One group was advised to replace dietary saturated fats with omega-6 oils, while the other received no specific dietary advice. The result: all-cause mortality and mortality from coronary heart disease were *higher* in the intervention group than in controls. These findings are the more remarkable because the researchers lumped "common margarines and shortenings" with saturated fat, so the intervention group avoided not only saturated fat but *trans* fats as well. The researchers concluded, "These findings could have important implications for worldwide dietary advice to substitute omega-6 linoleic acid, or polyunsaturated fats in general, for saturated fats."[15] Not a peep about this study appeared in the major media.

Another exhaustive analysis, published in 2014, looked at nearly eighty studies and found no evidence that eating saturated fat increases the incidence of heart attacks and other cardiac events. The study did not find that people who ate higher levels of saturated fat had more heart disease than those who ate less, nor did the study find less heart disease in those dutifully eating higher amounts of polyunsaturated and monounsaturated fat.[16] "My take on this would be that it's not saturated fat that we should worry about" in our diets, said Dr. Rajiv Chowdhury, the study's lead author and a cardiovascular epidemiologist in the department of public health and primary care at Cambridge University.

Here in the United States, health officials will make sure we keep worrying. Dr. Frank Hu, professor of nutrition and epidemiology at the Harvard School of Public Health, said that the findings "should not be taken as a green light to eat more steak, butter and other foods rich in saturated fat." Prominent food Puritan Alice H. Lichtenstein, a nutritional biochemist at Tufts University, chided, "It would be unfortunate if these results were interpreted to suggest that people can go back to eating butter and cheese with abandon."[17]

A large review of existing research published in 2015 found that saturated fats were not associated with all-cause mortality, heart disease, ischemic stroke or type 2 diabetes while *trans* fats were associated with higher all-cause mortality, total CHD and CHD mortality. The authors noted wryly, "Dietary guidelines must carefully consider the health effects of recommendations for alternative macronutrients to replace *trans* fats and saturated fats." The researchers included data from forty-one studies covering more than three hundred thousand people, and twenty studies of *trans* fat intake and health outcomes that covered more than two hundred thousand individuals.

But researchers in this field still cannot bring themselves to give the green light to butter and meat fats. "This study shows that focusing on reducing saturated fats as the primary goal in eating well is not quite right," said Patty W. Siri-Tarino, of Children's Hospital Oakland Research Institute. "Eating well means replacing those saturated fats with polyunsaturated fats rather than carbohydrates, particularly refined and processed carbohydrates, which is what usually happens," she added.[18] In other words, there is nothing wrong with saturated fats but you still shouldn't eat them!

While Americans may remain fat-phobic, the anti–saturated fat mantra is crumbling in other parts of the world. In the UK, the *British Medical Journal* published an article by cardiologist Aseem Malhotra, who blasted the notion that saturated fats cause heart disease, noting that when you take satisfying fats out of the diet, the food tastes worse and you compensate by replacing saturated fat with sugar.[19] Following Malhotra's article, Joanna Blythman, writing for *The Guardian*, staunchly defended butter. "The anti-sat-fat message has been used effectively by food manufacturers to woo us away from whole, natural foods such as butter, which is only minimally processed, on to their products, which are entirely the opposite, such as margarine," she said,[20] noting the 2010 review, which found no convincing evidence that saturated fat causes heart disease.[21]

In Australia, ABC's Catalyst TV program, *Heart of the Matter*, sent the Internet abuzz with its critique of the low-fat agenda[22]: Part II, *Cholesterol Drug War*,[23] challenged the notion that we should be taking cholesterol-lowering drugs.*

And finally, Sweden has become the first Western nation to reject the low-fat diet dogma in favor of low-carb, high-fat nutrition. The switch in dietary advice followed the publication of a two-year study by the independent Swedish Council on Health Technology Assessment, which reviewed sixteen thousand studies. The conclusion: butter, olive oil, heavy cream and bacon are not harmful foods.[24]

STILL, THE FORCES ALLIED WITH the vegetable oil industry have plenty of research they can point to in support of their agenda.

During the late 1990s, when news about the dangers of *trans* fats emerged, conventional dietary gurus pointed to a study published in 1997 in the *American Journal of Cardiology*[25] to justify avoidance of red meat and butterfat, the two main sources of saturated fat in the Western diet.

Arthur Agatston, author of the best-selling *South Beach Diet*, refers to this research when he states: "The major problem I have with the Atkins Diet is the liberal intake of saturated fats. There is evidence now that immediately following a meal of saturated fats, there is dysfunction in the arteries, including those that supply the heart muscle with blood. As a result, the lining of the arteries (the endothelium) is predisposed to constriction and clotting. Imagine: Under the right (or rather, wrong) circumstances, eating a meal that's high in saturated fat can trigger a heart attack! In addition, after a high-fat meal certain elements in the blood called remnant particles, persist for longer than is healthy. These particles contribute to the buildup of plaque in the vessel wall."[26]

Agatston recommends consuming polyunsaturated and monounsaturated vegetable oils, including tub spreads, rather than animal fats like butter.

In the study Agatston describes, carried out by Robert A. Vogel and his team, ten volunteers were tested for "endothelial function" using ultrasound to measure the diameter change in the brachial artery after a high-fat and a low-fat meal, each of nine hundred calories. The high-fat meal contained 50 grams of fat and the low-fat meal contained, according to the authors, no fat at all.†

"Flow-mediated vascularity" did decrease more in the high-fat group compared to the low-fat group. Interestingly, LDL-cholesterol declined slightly for both groups, but in the low-fat group, the so-called good HDL-cholesterol also declined, whereas it remained stable in the high-fat group. Blood pressure declined in the

* These two programs disappeared from the Internet shortly thereafter, but not before several individuals put them up on YouTube.

† Actually, no food is completely devoid of fat, not even skim milk.

high-fat group, but rose in the low-fat group. Most significantly, blood glucose rose in the low-fat group, but declined slightly and then returned to baseline in the high-fat group.

For years the conventional view held that high-fat foods raise so-called bad LDL-cholesterol and blood pressure and therefore contribute to heart disease. But since that didn't happen in this study, the authors declared that an inherently subjective measurement of "endothelial function" would serve as a better marker for heart disease.

But was it saturated fat that caused the decline in endothelial function? The high-fat meal consisted of an Egg McMuffin, a Sausage McMuffin, two hash brown patties and a noncaffeinated beverage. The low-fat meal consisted of Frosted Flakes, skim milk and orange juice. According to the authors, the high-fat meal contained 50 grams of fat, of which 14 were saturated fat—so only 28 percent of the fat in the high-fat meal was saturated. The rest was a combination of *trans* fats, monounsaturated fat and polyunsaturated fat, any one of which, or all together, could contribute to the decline in endothelial function. But Agatston (along with the study authors) blames the adverse effects on saturated fats!

The low-fat meal that won the endothelial-function contest was obviously a terrible dietary choice—extremely high in sugar and devoid of nutrients. Yet it did have one thing going for it—it is unlikely that Frosted Flakes, skim milk or orange juice contained MSG, an inflammatory additive, whereas the high-fat meal certainly contained MSG in the sausage and hash browns. If the bread contained soy, which it probably did, this would be another source of MSG. The presence of MSG in the high-fat meal provides a likely explanation for the decline in endothelial function.

The subjects in this study ate junk food, and the research itself can only be described as junk. The study was designed so poorly that no conclusions should be drawn from it. In order to test the effects of saturated fat on endothelial function, the researchers should have provided two identical meals of simple whole foods, except for the addition of a mostly saturated fat such as suet or coconut oil to one of the meals. Then, to compare the effects of the various fats with saturated fat, the researchers should have repeated the experiment adding a mostly monounsaturated fat, such as olive oil, to one of the meals, a high-*trans* fat such as vegetable shortening, and finally a polyunsaturated fat such as corn oil.

To correlate their findings—a temporary decline in endothelial function—with long-term effects such as heart disease, the authors should have bolstered their argument with reference to numerous studies; but they cite only one, which postulates a chronic decline in endothelial function with atherosclerosis. They provide no evidence that the temporary decline in endothelial function observed in this study is associated with atherosclerosis in the long term or that such a decline can "trigger a heart attack."

As it becomes more and more obvious that cholesterol levels have little predictive value for heart disease—and that saturated fats in fact have little or no effect on cholesterol levels anyway—researchers who know where their bread is buttered—or rather, spread with margarine—are searching for other ways to demonize saturated fats. The study carried out by Vogel and his team can only be characterized as "garbage in, garbage out"—a grasping-at-straws attempt to stem the change in consumer eating habits toward real, whole foods.

Endothelial function returned to the news in 2006 with the publication of a study entitled,

"Consumption of Saturated Fat Impairs the Anti-Inflammatory Properties of High-Density Lipoproteins and Endothelial Function."[27] The findings indicated that a single meal rich in saturated fats disrupts arterial function and contributes to the inflammation of the blood vessels. An *Associated Press* story by Joe Milicia quoted Kansas City cardiologist Dr. James O'Keefe, who claimed the study showed that "when you eat [saturated fat], inflammation and damage to the vessels happens immediately afterward." Dr. Nicholls, principal author of the study, insisted that his research showed the "need to aggressively reduce the amount of saturated fat consumed in the diet." According to the article, that meant reducing our intake of beef, pork, lard, poultry fat, butter, milk, cheese, coconut oil, palm oil and cocoa butter, and replacing them with safflower oil, sesame oil, sunflower seeds, corn oil and soybean oil.[28] The study design? The researchers fed fourteen adults a meal of carrot cake and a milk shake on two separate occasions one month apart, one made with highly saturated coconut oil and one made with highly polyunsaturated safflower oil. Both oils were nonhydrogenated, organic, unrefined and virgin.

Despite the newspaper reports and Nicholls's attention-grabbing claims, the researchers found no clearly discernible effect of any type of fat on arterial function, and those consuming saturated fat had the best arterial function at all time points measured. In fact, the researchers did not even study the inflammation occurring in the blood vessels of the people eating the meals. Instead, they looked at isolated cells in which they found high-density lipoprotein (HDL) taken from people eating safflower oil to have greater anti-inflammatory power than HDL taken from people eating coconut oil. Without a shred of evidence, the newspaper reports attributed this observation to the saturated fat that the study subjects consumed. In fact, in the published study the authors actually made no such claim, noting that these effects might be due to the large difference in vitamin E content of the two diets. In any event, the carrot-cake-and-milkshake study has no relevance in the real world.

Along with cholesterol, a compound called homocysteine is thought to be a marker for proneness to heart disease. Researchers in the Netherlands studied the effects of different fatty acids, including saturated fatty acids and very-long-chain omega-3 fatty acids, on homocysteine levels in two age groups, forty-seven to forty-nine years old and seventy-one to seventy-four years old. The results were published in the *American Journal of Clinical Nutrition* with the following conclusion: "High intakes of SFAs [saturated fatty acids] are associated with high plasma concentrations of tHcy [homocysteine]."[29]

Here was another study that the food industry could use to bash saturated fats, but if you look closely at the tables, you find no tenable or consistent relationships between consumption of various fatty acids and homocysteine levels. By contrast, the difference in homocysteine levels was significantly associated with age, with levels ten times higher in the seventy-year-olds compared to the forty-year-olds, but the study abstract contains no mention of this important fact.

The current Cinderella study—used as damage control to counter the increasing attention on butter—is a 2014 meta-analysis of thirteen studies involving more than three hundred thousand participants. The findings: individuals who traded 5 percent of the calories they consumed from saturated fat for sources of omega-6 polyunsaturated oil lowered their risk of CHD by 9 percent and lowered their risk of death from CHD by 13 percent.[30] Every single study reviewed in the meta-analysis dates from the 1990s to the present, after decades of recommendations to consume polyunsaturated fatty acids to prevent heart disease—so the potential for bias (not to mention influence) is very great. Obtaining precise figures of 5 percent and 13 percent from a meta-analysis defies logic.

RED MEAT, AS A SOURCE of saturated fatty acids, gets repeated bashings in the media. In fact, in a recent report, the World Health Organization (WHO) ranked bacon, sausage and other cured and processed meats as "group 1 carcinogens," which puts them in the same category as tobacco, asbestos, alcohol and arsenic. It also placed fresh red meat in the "group 2A" category, which suggests that it is "probably carcinogenic" to humans.

Such accusations are becoming more common. An example is a 2009 study published in the *Archives of Internal Medicine*.[31] "Eating red meat increases the chances of dying prematurely," said the newspaper reports. "Americans who consumed about four ounces of red meat a day were more than 30 percent more likely to die during the 10 years they were followed, mostly from heart disease and cancer."[32] The report itself describes the increases in total mortality as "modest," and a careful reading of the text reveals some important details. Participants in the highest quintile of meat consumption, when compared to those in the lowest quintile, were three times more likely to smoke, 50 percent less likely to engage in vigorous exercise, were less well educated, had lower fiber consumption and ate fewer fruits and vegetables. The authors did not explore the possibility that frequent meat eaters were more likely to eat processed vegetable oils and processed food in general.

Commenters noted that the study was not designed to determine cause and effect, and its ability to determine or verify the participants' true meat intake was almost nonexistent. According to researcher Chris Masterjohn, PhD, the flawed study "emphasizes the most basic principle of science that they want us all to forget: that correlation does not prove causation. There are thus two important points we need to understand about this study to realize just how little it does to increase our knowledge: the study found a correlation between increased mortality and a population's propensity to report eating meat, not a correlation between mortality and true meat intake...these may be two completely different things; and correlation does not show causation. There is absolutely no scientific basis to conclude from this study that eating meat increases mortality."[33]

HIGH BLOOD PRESSURE IS SAID to be a risk factor for heart disease. During the 1960s, Fleischmann's Margarine ran advertisements in the *Journal of the American Medical Association* touting 100 percent corn oil unsalted margarine for "hypertensive patients." The copy ran: "The substitution of Fleischmann's Unsalted Corn Oil Margarine for butter or ordinary margarines in your hypertensive patients' dietary regimen, has the added advantage of increasing their intake of high polyunsaturates...important because of their association with hypertension and atherosclerosis." At that time, not a single study linked consumption of polyunsaturated fatty acids with protection against high blood pressure.

To lower blood pressure, doctors today

NEW...made from 100% corn oil
UNSALTED MARGARINE
FOR HYPERTENSIVE PATIENTS

- * contains only 10 mgs. of sodium per 100 grams
- * contains 50% liquid corn oil and 50% partially hydrogenated corn oil
- * has 30% linoleic acid—10 times that of butter

Because of the relationship of high-sodium intake to elevated blood pressure, new Fleischmann's Unsalted Corn Oil Margarine will prove to be a valuable addition to the dietary regimen of your hypertensive patients. It contains only 10 mgs. of sodium per 100 grams.

Fleischmann's Unsalted Margarine is made from 100% corn oil and contains both liquid corn oil and partially hydrogenated corn oil. Its linoleic acid content of 30% is three times higher than the 10% of regular margarines and ten times higher than the 3% of butter. This is the *only* unsalted margarine made from 100% corn oil.

The substitution of Fleischmann's Unsalted Corn Oil Margarine for butter or ordinary margarines in your hypertensive patients' dietary regimen has the added advantage of increasing their intake of high polyunsaturates . . . important because of their association with hypertension and atherosclerosis.

If your hypertensive patient needs sodium restriction, recommend Fleischmann's Unsalted. It has a light, delicate taste that he'll like. Tell him that it is available in his grocer's frozen food case.

Write now for physician booklet of 5 coupons—each coupon redeemable by your patient for 1 lb. of Fleischmann's Unsalted Margarine. Address Fleischmann's Unsalted Margarine, 625 Madison Avenue, N. Y. 22, N. Y. *Distribution presently limited in some areas.*

In line with the suggestion of the American Heart Association to manufacturers, we are listing the fatty acid composition of Fleischmann's Unsalted (Sweet) Margarine:

Unsaturated Fatty Acids:	
Polyunsaturates	30%
Monounsaturates	50%
Saturated Fatty Acids	20%
	100%

AVERAGE DAILY INTAKE
Two Ounces or Eight Pats of Fleischmann's Corn Oil Margarine Will Supply

Corn Oil—Liquid	22.7 Gm.
Corn Oil—Partially Hydrogenated	22.7 Gm.
Iodine Value	90-95
Sodium (dietetically sodium-free)	6 Mgs.
Linoleic Acid	13.6 Gm.
Vitamin A (Adult's Need)	47%
Vitamin A (Child's Need)	62%
Vitamin D (Adult's and Child's Need)	62%

Fleischmann's
Fresh-Frozen in the green foil package in your grocer's frozen food case

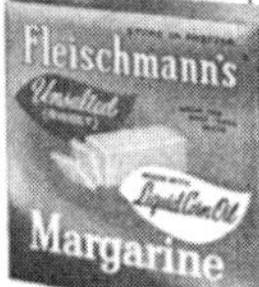

ONLY UNSALTED MARGARINE MADE FROM 100% CORN OIL

recommend the DASH (Dietary Approaches to Stop Hypertention) Diet, endorsed by the American Heart Association and the 2010 Dietary Guidelines for America. The diet calls for reducing salt, reducing processed foods containing salt, reducing meat products "high in saturated fat," and eating more whole grains, legumes, fruits and vegetables. However, studies on the diet showed that it only worked, and worked only a little bit, in people whose blood pressure was only moderately high.[34] Any one of these strategies—including the avoidance of processed foods—could take credit for the slight reduction in blood pressure.

Today, even conventional medical websites admit that intake of dietary fats has no relationship to blood pressure. For example, we read at medtv.com: "People often wonder if fats in the diet affect blood pressure. The answer is no. Fats in a person's diet do not directly affect blood pressure."[35]

Physicians operate under the assumption

that high blood pressure predisposes an individual to heart attack (as well as stroke and kidney disease). Surprisingly, no randomized clinical trial has ever proven that lowering high blood pressure reduces the risk for death from heart disease. For example, one of the goals of the Multiple Risk Factor Trial (MRFIT) was to reduce participants' blood pressure below 140/90, along with lowering cholesterol and quitting smoking, but the conscientious patients fared no differently from controls. In fact, those who took diuretics to lower their blood pressure had the highest mortality rates,[36] possibly due to potassium depletion.

The truth is, there are many causes of hypertension, including kidney disease, hormone imbalance, diabetes, atherosclerosis and a range of nutrient deficiencies—such as CoQ10, potassium and protein. *Trans* fats inhibit biochemical processes in the cell membranes and high blood pressure is a probable outcome of this biochemical chaos.

STROKE IS THE THIRD LEADING cause of death in the United States and a leading cause of disability. The American Heart Association claims that high cholesterol levels contribute to stroke and are another reason to avoid cholesterol-rich foods such as butter, egg yolks and organ meats.[37]

The fact is, researchers have not found much correlation between cholesterol levels and risk of stroke. For example, a 1995 report in which researchers pooled together the results of forty-five prospective cohort studies involving over four hundred thousand people found "a weaker relationship between cholesterol levels and the risk of stroke than with coronary artery disease."[38] The 2010 Japan Collaborative Cohort Study for Evaluation of Cancer Risk found that saturated fat intake was *inversely* associated with mortality from stroke.[39]

The association of stroke with cholesterol levels becomes clearer when we distinguish between ischemic and hemorrhagic stroke. Ischemic stroke, where a blockage closes the flow of blood, is the more common type, but the hemorrhagic stroke, where a blood vessel ruptures, is more deadly—hemorrhagic stroke patients end up with greater neurological problems and are four times more likely to die within thirty days than victims of ischemic strokes.

It turns out that as cholesterol levels go up, the risk of ischemic stroke goes up while the risk of deadly hemorrhagic stroke goes down. So cholesterol-rich foods that might raise cholesterol levels should protect against hemorrhagic stroke; the logic is that avoiding these foods will protect against the more common ischemic stroke, but the research shows otherwise. In the Honolulu Heart Study, the risk of ischemic stroke *decreased* as the intake of total and saturated fat went up.[40] And the Framingham Heart Study, which followed eight hundred men over the course of nineteen years, found that "intakes of fat, saturated fat, and monounsaturated fat were associated with *reduced* risk of ischemic stroke in men [emphasis added]."[41]

In an analysis of all the studies on stroke and cholesterol, Chris Masterjohn, PhD, argues that the likely cause of stroke is oxidized cholesterol in the blood. This means that the best protection against stroke is avoiding polyunsaturated oils, full of oxidizing free radicals, and choosing tasty and nutritious foods containing stable saturated fat—like butter, eggs and organ meats.[42]

DIABETES IS ON THE INCREASE and represents a huge burden on families and the medical system. The dietary advice from the American Diabetes Association is cloned from the American Heart Association: avoid *trans* fats found in processed foods like snacks (crackers and chips) and baked goods (muffins, cookies and cakes) made with hydrogenated oil or partially hydrogenated oil, stick margarines, shortening and some fast-food items such as French fries—but also avoid saturated fats found in lard, fatback and salt pork; high-fat meats like regular ground beef, bologna, hot dogs, sausage, bacon and spareribs; high-fat dairy products such as full-fat cheese, cream, ice cream, whole milk, 2 percent milk and sour cream; butter; cream sauces, gravy made with meat drippings; chocolate; palm oil and palm kernel oil; coconut and coconut oil; and poultry (chicken and turkey) skin. In addition, they recommend keeping your cholesterol consumption below 300 milligrams per day by avoiding high-fat dairy products (whole or 2 percent milk, cream, ice cream, full-fat cheese), egg yolks, liver and other organ meats, high-fat meat and poultry skin.*[43]

Modern advice to diabetics assures them that they do not need to worry too much about carbohydrates—their daily insulin can take care of that. But for many years, scientists and physicians recognized the fact that diabetes was a consequence of a diet rich in carbohydrates, especially simple sugars. Before the discovery of insulin, the only treatment for diabetes was a very high-fat, low-carb diet, because the body does not need insulin to process fats. In those days, the medical community recognized only one type of diabetes: type 1 or juvenile diabetes resulting from a malfunction of the pancreas. If the pancreas—worn out by a constant onslaught of sugar in the diet or simply not functioning properly due to nutrient deficiencies—cannot produce enough insulin to transfer the sugar from the bloodstream to the cells, glucose levels in the bloodstream remain abnormally high, with serious consequences.

Today, we recognize a second type of diabetes, type 2 diabetes, which is the inability of the insulin receptors on the cell membrane to efficiently uptake the glucose from the blood. The result is high levels of both sugar and insulin in the bloodstream, again with serious consequences.

Researchers and physicians are adamant that saturated fat causes insulin resistance leading to type 2 diabetes. They cite several studies, from the years 2002–2003. One was published in the *British Journal of Nutrition* entitled, "Acute effects of meal fatty acid composition on insulin sensitivity in healthy post-menopausal women."[44] In the study, four groups of subjects consumed a breakfast of Rice Krispies, banana, skim milk, "Nesquik" (a chocolate drink) and something called "Marvel," along with 40 grams of fat. The first group got mostly saturated fat from palm oil, the second group got mostly monounsaturated fat from olive oil, the third group got mostly omega-6 fatty acids from safflower oil, and the fourth group got high levels of omega-3 fatty acids from a combination of safflower oil and fish oil.

* Such a horribly restrictive diet is probably worse than all the poking, pricking and drug side effects that come with conventional diabetes treatment. Yet the American Diabetes website assures diabetes patients, "Eating well is one of life's greatest pleasures. Having diabetes shouldn't keep you from enjoying a wide variety of foods including some of your favorites. People with diabetes have the same nutritional needs as anyone else."

The researchers measured levels of insulin and glucose in the blood at intervals after breakfast and also after a so-called low-fat lunch consisting of cheese pizza (said to contain only 5.4 grams of fat), lettuce, cucumber and tomatoes. Those given the mostly saturated palm oil had higher insulin levels an hour after breakfast and lunch compared to the other three groups. However, insulin levels were the same for all groups two hours after each meal. Blood glucose levels followed a similar curve for all four groups.

The study provides a poor justification for recommending against saturated fat. All four groups consumed a very unnatural diet high in processed foods, and the fats used do not reflect the type of fatty acid profiles found in normal diets. Furthermore, the levels of insulin in the subjects were not chronically high, as one finds in a person with type 2 diabetes, and the glucose curves were normal for all groups. The study tells us nothing about what happens in real life with people eating real food.

Another 2002 study, this one published in *Diabetologia*, was titled "Substituting dietary saturated fat with polyunsaturated fat changes abdominal fat distribution and improves insulin sensitivity."[45] It looked at a small group of subjects—a total of seventeen—who received instructions to follow a diet rich in saturated fatty acids (by using more dairy products) or polyunsaturated fatty acids (by using more oils and spreads) for five weeks. The subjects on the saturated fat diet had a slightly lower measure of insulin sensitivity, but their glucose levels and body mass indices were virtually identical with those in the polyunsaturated group. Again, this study has little to do with real life. The researchers did not measure the actual amount of saturated or polyunsaturated fat (or *trans* fat) in each diet, and the number of subjects was too small to be meaningful.

Neither of these studies tells us what happens to people with or without diabetes who eat a diet high in natural saturated fats compared to those whose diets contain a lot of vegetable oils. The fact that the researchers so soundly condemn saturated fats after such trivial findings constitutes strong evidence of bias.

Another study, this one from the University of Minnesota,[46] and reported in the December 2003 issue of *Prevention* magazine, reported that "among three thousand people tested, those with the highest blood levels of saturated fats were twice as likely to develop diabetes as those with the lowest." According to Aaron Folsom, MD, one author of the study, "Saturated fats in the blood appear to affect your body's ability to effectively use insulin, the hallmark of type-2 diabetes." Naturally this report was followed by warnings not to eat saturated fats like butter, cream and the fat on meat. But Dr. Folsom makes an error common to those not trained in fatty acid metabolism. A high level of saturated fatty acids in the blood is reflective of high-carbohydrate intake and subsequent synthesis of fatty acids from excess carbohydrates. Saturated fatty acids in the blood are not an appropriate marker of dietary fat intake, but are rather a marker of carbohydrate intake. What the researchers at the University of Minnesota actually discovered (or rather, reaffirmed) was that people who eat a lot of carbohydrates are more likely to develop diabetes.

Telling people to avoid saturated fats almost invariably results in their consuming more *trans* fats or omega-6 vegetable oils, both of which have many adverse effects. *Trans* fats, for example, interfere with the insulin receptors in the cell membranes, thereby contributing to type 2 diabetes. The saturated fats, on the other hand, have no effect when appropriate comparisons are made.[47]

Regarding dairy fats, new evidence indicates that they actually have protective properties. Swedish research from 2014, presented at the annual meeting of the European Association for the Study of Diabetes (EASD), shows that people who consumed eight or more portions of high-fat dairy products per day had a 23 percent lower risk of getting type 2 diabetes than those who had fewer portions per day. The study included almost twenty-seven thousand individuals (60 percent women), ages forty-five to seventy-four.*

In spite of these interesting findings, Dr. Richard Elliott, Diabetes UK research communications manager, warned: "This study adds to research which suggests that different sources of fat in the diet affect the risk of type 2 diabetes in different ways. However, this does not mean that adding high-fat dairy products to your diet will actively help to protect against type 2 diabetes, and we would not recommend this. Consumption of dairy products can form part of a healthy diet, but it's important to be aware of the amount you consume, as they can be high in calories, which can contribute to becoming overweight, and therefore increase your risk of type 2 diabetes. More research will be needed before we change our advice that the best way to reduce your risk of type 2 diabetes is by maintaining a healthy weight through increased physical activity and a balanced diet that is low in salt, saturated fat and sugar and rich in fruit and vegetables."[48]

In summary, the results of studies into dietary fats and diabetes do not justify the advice to limit saturated fat. Type 2 diabetes is a new disease, one that has now reached epidemic proportions. Type 2 diabetes did not exist one hundred years ago when our diets were very rich in saturated fats, but appeared when *trans* fats came into the diet and became an epidemic with the consumption of more and more foods containing *trans* fats and processed food in general. And since we know that *trans* fats interfere with insulin receptors in the cells, it is clear that the blame lies with new industrial fats, not traditional saturated fats.

THE ANTI-ANIMAL FAT CAMPAIGN BEGAN with a focus on heart disease, not cancer, and relied upon a kind of logic that appealed to both physicians and laymen. Animal fat contains cholesterol, and cholesterol clogs arteries, and clogged arteries lead to heart disease. But the logic that fingers saturated fat as the culprit in other diseases, especially in cancer, is more difficult to trace. Since saturated fats are stable, protect against oxidation and play essential roles in cell membrane integrity and hormone production, scientists find it difficult to articulate just how and why saturated fats could cause cancer.

Nevertheless, the scientific literature—followed by the popular press—takes it as a given that saturated fat causes cancer, and that we can protect ourselves by eating lean meat and substituting polyunsaturated vegetable oil

* To make matters confusing, the researchers found that eating a lot of meat and meat products was linked with worse odds of getting diabetes; but meat consumption is often a marker for consumption of processed food.

for saturated fats like cream and butter. These are shocking recommendations given the fact that modern polyunsaturated oils predispose both animals and humans to cancer in study after study.

The American Cancer Society (ACS) advises us to choose fish, poultry or beans instead of red meat (beef, pork and lamb). If you eat red meat, advises the ACS, choose lean cuts and eat smaller portions. These strictures are mixed with advice that is sensible. We should avoid fried foods (since they are invariably fried in vegetable oils) and charbroiled meats (since charbroiling creates carcinogens). The ACS guidelines advise limiting the use of creamy sauces, dressings and dips with fruits and vegetables. This is good advice also, since "creamy sauces, dressings and dips" are usually concocted with vegetable oils and not real cream. But since the guidelines do not explain this fact, the reader comes away with the erroneous impression that cream is bad.

"High-fat diets are associated with increased cancer risk, so good health relies on fat-conscious eating decisions," admonishes the ACS.*[49] But what kind of fats? The kind we can see, like the butter on our bread, the fat on our meat or the yolks in our eggs, or the fats that we don't see, like the vegetable oils in fried and processed foods, in "healthy" spreads, or emulsified to make cream-like substances?

Women worried about breast cancer have become a major target of the saturated fat guilt trip. When guilt doesn't work, the food industry turns to the other potent weapon in their arsenal: fear. Take this headline, for example: "Women Who Eat High-Fat Foods Could Be Doubling Their Risk of Breast Cancer, Scientists Say." This and similar pronouncements heralded a study published in 2003 in the *International Journal of Cancer*: "Eating high-fat red meats and dairy products such as cream may increase the risk of breast cancer in premenopausal women." Nutrition researcher Eunyoung Cho said of the study: "I would not recommend that [Atkins] diet for premenopausal women unless they replace red meat with poultry and fish... Breast cancer risk increases 58 percent by eating animal fat."[50]

But a close look at the study does not raise any real alarms. The researchers found that if your diet contains 14 percent of calories as animal fat, your chances of getting breast cancer are 0.68 percent; if your diet contains 18–21 percent of calories as animal fat, your chances of getting breast cancer are 0.88 percent; and if your diet contains more than 21 percent animal fat, your chances of getting breast cancer actually go down to 0.73 percent.

Spokespersons for the study used every trick in the book to make these trivial results seem scary. In addition to the incredible hype over minor differences, they divided the subjects into unequal quintiles (the highest quintile of 21–46 percent had the greatest range); determined fat percentages by self-assessed dietary recall that was surveyed only twice during the study; and neglected to indicate the important fact that there were twice as many smokers in the group with highest animal fat consumption compared to lowest.[51]

The study authors also fail to mention a survey showing that women on low-fat diets have just as much breast cancer as those on

* These were the guidelines in the early 2000s. Today the ACS steers clear of strictures that specifically single out butter and other saturated fats, but promotes a diet that emphasizes plant foods, lean meat and limited amounts of "calorie-dense" foods.[a]

high-fat diets.[52] Two subsequent reviews have found weak or insignificant associations of saturated fat intake and breast cancer risk, and note the prevalence of confounding factors.[53]

The Women's Health Initiative Dietary Modification Trial, specifically designed to examine the effect of a low-fat diet on the development of breast cancer, showed similar rates of breast cancer in women eating a low-fat diet and in those eating a "regular" diet.[54] One recent study from the National Institutes of Health—the AARP Diet and Health Study—found a very weak positive association between fat and postmenopausal breast cancer,[55] but when other studies are considered, the overall evidence does not support a relationship between saturated fat intake and breast cancer.

WHAT ABOUT THE ACCUSATION THAT beef causes cancer, in particular cancer of the colon? The genesis of this myth involves more than just muddied thinking, but actual skullduggery. In 1965, an influential physician, Ernst Wynder, took worldwide consumption data for industrial vegetable oils, called them animal fat (which they were not) and compared them with worldwide colon cancer mortality.[56] The table he produced showed high rates of colon cancer in European countries and low rates of colon cancer in Japan, and concluded that there was a positive effect, in other words, that saturated fat, the kind found in beef, caused colon cancer. What the data *actually showed* was that consumption of polyunsaturated vegetable oils, not saturated animal fats, was associated with a higher incidence of colon cancer. And Wynder forgot to mention that Asians have much higher rates than Americans of other types of cancers, particularly harder-to-treat cancers of the liver, pancreas, stomach, esophagus and lungs.

Then in 1973, William Haenszel and his colleagues from the National Cancer Institute reported the findings from a study that relied on notoriously unreliable dietary recall and lacked matched controls—in other words, a very poorly designed study.[57] The researchers stated that they found a relationship between beef and colon cancer that fit the earlier work of Wynder. Actually, what they really found was that among Westernized Japanese Americans, those who said they consumed lots of macaroni, green beans and peas, as well as beef, had the highest rates of colon cancer; while among traditional Japanese Americans, those who said they consumed lots of dried cuttlefish, Chinese peas, bamboo shoots, rice and fermented soy products had the highest rates of colon cancer. Thus, the researchers singled out beef as the culprit from a choice of several foods associated with cancer in Westerners and ignored politically correct foods like soy products, fish and vegetables as a potential cause of cancer in Japanese Americans. Unfortunately, this second-rate and inconclusive study has become firmly fixed in the consciousness of the scientific community as providing evidence for the assertion that beef causes colon cancer.

Two American studies conducted in the 1990s did find a higher risk of colon cancer among those who eat red meat.[58] However, no study conducted in Europe has ever shown an association between meat consumption and cancer.[59] These findings suggest that European sausage and luncheon meat, included in the rubric of "meat consumption," are prepared by traditional methods that require few additives, while similar products in the United States contain many carcinogenic preservatives and flavorings. Unfortunately, the American Cancer Society's 1996 recommendation that Americans cut down on their consumption of meat—particularly fatty meat—in order to avoid cancer makes no distinction between fresh meats and those embalmed with modern chemicals.

While two U.S. studies have implicated meat consumption as a cause of colon cancer, several others contradict these findings. In 1975, researchers compared Seventh-Day Adventist physicians, who do not eat meat, with non-Seventh-Day Adventist physicians, and found that the vegetarian doctors had higher rates of gastrointestinal and colorectal cancer deaths.[60] National Cancer Institute data show that Argentina, with very high levels of beef consumption, has significantly lower rates of colon cancer than other Western countries where beef consumption is considerably lower.[61] A 1997 study published in the *International Journal of Cancer* found that increased risk of colon and rectal cancer was positively associated with consumption of bread, cereal dishes, potatoes, cakes, desserts and refined sugars, but not with eggs or meat.[62] And a 1978 study published in the *Journal of the National Cancer Institute* found no greater risk of colon cancer, regardless of the amounts of beef or other meats ingested.[63] The study also found that those who ate plenty of cruciferous vegetables, such as cabbage, Brussels sprouts and broccoli, had lower rates of colon cancer.

Actually, we do know one of the mechanisms that initiates colon cancer, and it does not involve meat, *per se*. Colon cancer occurs when high levels of industrial fats and oils, along with certain carcinogens, are acted on by certain enzymes in the cells lining the colon, leading to tumor formation.[64] This explains the fact that in industrialized countries, where there are many carcinogens in the diet and where consumption of vegetable oils and carcinogens, in addition to meat, is high, some studies have correlated meat eating with colon cancer; but in traditional societies, where vegetable oils are absent and the food is free of additives, meat eating is not associated with cancer.

Riding piggyback on the alleged link between beef and colon cancer are supposed associations with other cancers. Here the evidence shows a similarly inconsistent pattern. Cancer is a disease of rich countries where numerous factors can be fingered—altered fats, fabricated foods, low levels of protective nutrients, high levels of carcinogens—and rich countries consume lots of beef. But association is not the same as cause. Countries with more telephones have more cancer, but that does not mean that telephones cause cancer. As for prostate cancer, a 2010 meta-analysis found little correlation with red meat and even processed meat.[65] It also showed little protection from fruits and vegetables.[66]

The fats most associated with cancer are *trans* fats. In a 1999 analysis of the Nurses' Health Study, Harvard researchers found that a high intake of *trans* fats was associated with risk for non-Hodgkin's lymphoma.[67] A 2013 study found that a pooled analysis of twelve cohort studies observed no association between total fat intake and ovarian cancer risk; but further analysis revealed that omega-3 fatty acids were protective against ovarian cancer and that *trans* fats were a risk factor.[68]

In summary, beef became the fall guy for vegetable oils and other ingredients in processed foods, which flooded the marketplace, especially after the Second World War, and ushered in the epidemic of cancer—now estimated to occur in one person out of three.

DO SATURATED FATS MAKE US FAT? Do animal fats lead to lard ass and butter belly? The most cursory look at modern trends should be enough to convince us that the answer is no. The USDA dietary guidelines, implemented in the 1980s, demonized animal fats and gave Americans the green light to eat all the carbohydrates from the base of the food pyramid they wanted. Obesity rates have since doubled, from 15 percent to 30 percent of the population. Many of these high-carb foods are also high in vegetable oils, hidden fats deemed better for weight loss than animal fats. But why would animal fats cause weight gain more than vegetable oils? They are equally caloric. In fact, per weight and volume, animal fats contain slightly lower levels of calories than vegetable oils.

By analyzing menus from turn-of-the-century cookbooks, we can estimate that most diets at that time contained about 35–40 percent of calories as fat. Fats contain about twice as many calories per gram as protein or carbohydrate foods. In a diet of 2,500 calories, 35 percent of calories as fat translates to 97 grams of fat (slightly less than 1/2 cup) per day, as added fat or distributed in food. Pictures of the general populace at the time do not show large numbers of obese individuals, and in fact, they showed mostly healthy-looking people unless the scene was one of poverty.

A diet low in carbs and high in protein and fat for weight loss is not a new idea. First popularized by William Banting in 1863 in a booklet called *Letter on Corpulence, Addressed to the Public*, Banting's diet included meat, vegetables and fruit, and left out bread, potatoes and sweets. Many low-carb versions have followed, including Robert Cameron's *Drinking Man's Diet* (1964) and the immensely popular low-carb diet of Dr. Robert Atkins. But conventional weight loss advice still calls for replacing fats with carbs because—so the logic goes—fats by volume contain more than double the calories of carbohydrate foods (one tablespoon of butter contains about 100 calories, while one tablespoon of sugar contains 50).

And the high-carb school is sticking to its story. Vigorous debate broke out with the publication of science writer Gary Taubes's 2002 exposé in the *New York Times Magazine*, "What If It's All Been a Big Fat Lie?" In it, Taubes explains why the USDA-endorsed high-carb diet is more likely to make us fat (and diabetic) than a diet containing higher levels of fat, including saturated fat. Many dieters wrote to the newspapers confirming their experience that only the Atkins-type diet helped them lose weight and keep it off.

In response, low-fat guru Dean Ornish got plenty of column space to sputter about the dire consequences of a high-fat diet and prime-time exposure on Oprah Winfrey's show to warn dieters about the Atkins regime. Oprah was polite but noncommittal. According to the tabloid *Globe*, by 2002, Oprah's days of yo-yo dieting were over. She had come down to a reasonable weight of 174 pounds and was "filled with joy." Her successful dieting approach? Eliminate the "white stuff"—potatoes, white rice, pasta, refined sugar, bread and salt. Eliminating salt is probably not necessary, but the TV star seems to have found the winning combination—reasonable expectations and an elimination of all those high-carb foods that we've been told will keep us healthy and slim.

A study by Dr. Eric Westman of Duke University, presented at the annual scientific meeting of the American Heart Association, looked at one hundred twenty overweight volunteers, who were randomly assigned to the Atkins diet or the AHA's Step 1 Diet, a widely used low-fat approach. On the Atkins diet, people limited their carbs to less than 20 grams per day, and consumed 60 percent of their calories from fat. After six months, the people on the Atkins diet had lost an average of 31 pounds, compared with 20 pounds on the AHA diet, and more people stuck with the Atkins regimen. Total cholesterol fell slightly in both groups, but only those in the Atkins group saw an increase in HDL.[69] The results were relegated to a side column in the *Washington Post*.[70] Sally Squires, author of "Lean Plate Club," a weekly column, reported the good news in a few sentences, followed by paragraphs of backpedaling—the Atkins diet could cause heart disease, constipation and nutritional deficiencies. "We were surprised that women could adhere to it [the Atkins diet] as well as they did," said dietician Bonnie Brehm. "I'm not sure that there is a take-home message from this study, except that there is more research needed...We by no means are recommending the Atkins diet from this one study." But there was more than one study confirming these results.

A 2003 study conducted by Harvard School of Public Health (presented to the Association for the Study of Obesity, but not published) followed twenty-one overweight volunteers, divided into three groups. All food was prepared for the volunteers so the researchers knew exactly what they were eating. Those eating a high-fat diet (65 percent of calories as fat) lost more weight than those eating high-carb diets (23 versus 17 pounds lost), even though their calorie intake was the same. In fact, those eating a high-fat diet containing 300 more calories per day still lost more weight than the lower-calorie, high-carb group (20 versus 17 pounds lost). This interesting research received no media attention whatsoever, and all descriptions of it and its findings have disappeared from the Internet.[71]

Diets high in fat are more satisfying and can lead to voluntary calorie restriction, as shown by a 2007 study conducted by Temple University School of Medicine. The study took place in a clinical research center where every calorie eaten and spent was measured. After a week of typical eating, ten obese patients with type 2 diabetes followed a diet that limited their carbohydrate intake to 20 grams per day, but allowed unlimited protein and fat. With carbs out of the diet, the patients spontaneously reduced their daily energy consumption by 1,000 calories per day. "When carbohydrates were restricted," said lead researcher Guenther Boden, MD, "the subjects spontaneously reduced their caloric intake to a level appropriate for their height, did not compensate by eating more protein or fat, and lost weight. We concluded that excessive overeating had been fueled by carbohydrates." In addition to calorie reduction and weight loss, the subjects experienced markedly improved glucose levels and insulin sensitivity, as well as lower triglycerides and cholesterol.[72] The interesting thing about this study was the fact that the subjects did not consciously try to restrict calories or lose weight, showing that restricting carbs and increasing fat in the diet works better than will power.

Also in 2007, other researchers found that a high-fat diet is just as effective as a high-carb diet for long-term weight loss, with better HDL-cholesterol (the so-called "good" cholesterol) levels among high-fat dieters.[73] And in the same year, researchers at Louisiana State University found that participants who ate eggs for breakfast had greater weight loss results and better energy levels than those who ate two bagels, even though the number of calories in both diets was about the same.[74]

Another study that year compared popular diets and found that overweight women trying the Atkins low-carbohydrate diet plan lost more weight (ten pounds versus about six) than women following the LEARN low-fat diet, which was patterned after the government dietary guidelines, and the Ornish diet, a very low-fat, mostly vegetarian plan, and much more (ten pounds versus three) than women following the Zone diet, a high-protein, restricted-carbohydrate plan. The weight loss occurred in spite of the fact that the Atkins dieters did not follow the guidelines very well, consuming far more carbs than allowed on the plan.[75] According to Christopher D. Gardner, assistant professor at the Stanford University School of Medicine and the study's lead author, "There's something to the low-carb thing that's intriguing. Cutting back drastically on simple carbohydrates is clearly a step in the right direction to helping people lose weight." Other markers, such as blood pressure and cholesterol levels, were similar or better among Atkins dieters, in spite of the fact that these diets contained about 30 percent of calories as saturated fat—triple the recommended amount.

The results did not please proponents of low-fat diets. "Once the weight-loss stops, the effect of saturated fat would be negative," said James O. Hill, director of the Center for Human Nutrition at the University of Colorado at Denver. "There is no magic combination of fat versus carbs versus protein," said Alice Lichtenstein of Tufts University. "It doesn't matter in the long run. The bottom line is calories, calories, calories."[76] And finally, from Dean Ornish himself: "It's a lot easier to follow a diet that tells you to eat bacon and brie than to eat predominantly fruits and vegetables... I'm concerned that this study may cause people to forgo eating a healthy diet for one that's actually harmful for them."[77]

That same year, researchers in Sweden published an interesting study involving almost twenty thousand perimenopausal Swedish women over nine years. Some weight gain is a normal occurrence at menopause, in part because midriff fat produces a type of estrogen to compensate for the estrogen produced by the ovaries, which at menopause are winding down. The researchers found that participants eating cheese and full-fat dairy had a lower rate of weight gain as they grew older.[78] Like the Harvard study a few years earlier, these findings received no coverage in the press.

In a 2008 trial carried out in Israel, described by Gary Taubes as "arguably the best such trial ever done and the most rigorous," researchers found that a low-carbohydrate diet high in saturated fat resulted in the greatest weight loss and the most desirable lipid profiles. The trial compared three diets: a calorie-restricted American Heart Association (AHA) diet with about 30 percent of calories from fat, with less than 10 percent of calories as saturated fat; a calorie-restricted

Mediterranean diet, high in dietary fiber and monounsaturated fat; and a low-carbohydrate diet, described as "high in saturated fat," containing about 40 percent of calories as fat, with 12.5 percent as saturated fat. Calories were not restricted on the low-carbohydrate diet, yet after two years, this group had lost the most weight—ten pounds versus six in the low-fat diet. LDL-cholesterol reduction was best with the Mediterranean diet, while those on the supposedly heart-healthy AHA-recommended diet saw no reduction in LDL-cholesterol. Those on the low-carbohydrate diet had a moderate reduction of LDL-cholesterol, but the best results for the ratio of total cholesterol to HDL-cholesterol, with increased HDL-cholesterol, the so-called "good" cholesterol, whereas the other two groups did not. Furthermore, the low-carb dieters saw the biggest reduction in C-reactive protein, a marker for inflammation, and the nondiabetic low-carb dieters had the lowest fasting insulin levels. (Diabetics on the Mediterranean diet had the best markers for fasting glucose and insulin levels.)[79]

The two primary press sources, HealthDay and Reuters, both reported this study incorrectly. The Reuters headline: "Similar weight loss on 3 different, popular diets."[80] According to HealthDay: "Diet Plans Produce Similar Results: Study finds Mediterranean and low-carb diets work just as well as low-fat ones."[81] Tara Parker Pope of the *New York Times* minimized the results by reporting, "The results highlight the difficulty of weight loss and the fact that most diets do not work well."[82]

Still, low-fat diets do work for some people. The explanation is that when a person changes his diet from the typical American diet of processed foods to the recommended low-fat diet containing lots of whole grains and vegetables, the body is no longer taking in all the excess omega-6 and *trans* fats found in industrial foods. And he is replacing foods loaded with sugar and additives with more natural foods containing more vitamins and minerals. But most importantly, the body turns the excess carbohydrates into saturated fat. This saturated fat can replace omega-6 and *trans* fatty acids in the tissues, which is advantageous and helps the patient feel better. A high-carbohydrate diet is really a high-saturated-fat diet, and as we shall see in Chapter 4, various processes on the cellular level work better when ample saturated fatty acids are available.*

Under experimental conditions of overfeeding simple sugars (sucrose and glucose) in a diet that provided 40 percent of energy as fat, the researchers found that the carbohydrate was oxidized and turned into fat in such a manner to prevent weight loss.[83] In other words, a diet high in both fats and carbohydrates may cause weight gain, especially when these are processed vegetable oils and refined carbohydrates.

AUTOIMMUNE DISEASE IS ANOTHER CRIME laid at the feet of saturated animal fats—conditions such as MS, asthma, inflammatory bowel disease and rheumatoid arthritis. The logic goes like this: saturated animal

* Monkeys fed diets moderately high in *trans* fats gained weight in the abdomen, even though the diet was not high in calories. Perhaps "beer belly" is not the right term—maybe we should call this type of weight gain the "*trans* fat belly." (They also developed insulin resistance.)[a]

fats contain a fatty acid called arachidonic acid (AA), and arachidonic acid causes inflammation. Thus, saturated fats cause inflammation. Indeed, animal fats are our only source of this critical fatty acid—it is involved in the life-saving process that leads to inflammation, and without inflammation, we cannot heal. But AA also helps resolve inflammation. As we shall see in Chapter 5, AA is also critical to gut health and plays many important roles in the body.

The chief culprit in causing inflammation is *trans* fatty acids. In a 2002 study, human subjects who consumed stick margarine saw an increase in the production of inflammatory prostaglandins associated with atherosclerosis, while neither liquid soy oil nor butter had the same inflammatory effect.*[84]

Regarding asthma, several studies have shown that full-fat dairy products such as whole milk and butter protect against asthma, especially in children.[85] (More on this in Chapter 8.)

Most popular books on multiple sclerosis (MS), a chronic and debilitating wasting of the nervous system, warn against the consumption of saturated fatty acids. Saturated fats are said to interfere with anti-inflammatory prostaglandins, a statement that is not supported by research. In fact, analysis of almost two hundred thousand women involved in the Nurses' Health Studies found that saturated fat, animal fat and cholesterol were protective against MS.[86] A high intake of omega-6 and *trans* fatty acids—in other words, industrial fats and oils—was associated with increased risk of MS. Even consumption of monounsaturated fat, the kind found in olive oil, carried a slight increase in risk.

As for rheumatoid arthritis, just about all the "experts" say that saturated fat contributes to painful joints because it causes inflammation. This advice constitutes mere speculation; in fact, very few studies have looked at the effects of saturated versus polyunsaturated fatty acids on the symptoms of rheumatoid arthritis, and those that have cannot be used to claim that saturated fats are bad for arthritis sufferers. In one study, a group of patients consumed a diet high in polyunsaturated fatty acids supplemented with omega-3 fatty acids called EPA and DHA (more about these in Chapter 5), while the other group consumed a diet high in saturated fatty acids. The researchers found no statistical difference between the two groups in markers for inflammation and arthritis.[87]

In another study, a diet high in polyunsaturated fatty acids and low in saturated fats reduced morning stiffness and tender joints in the short term, but the control group on a diet higher in saturated fat fared better on follow-up, one to two months later.[88]

IN 2009, JUST IN TIME for Valentine's Day, an ad alerting men and their partners to the supposed link between fatty, meat-heavy diets and erectile dysfunction aired on CNN, ESPN and Lifetime, thanks to the Physicians Committee for Responsible Medicine (PCRM). The ad, titled "Room 103," depicts a romantic hotel room and a steamy sexual encounter that comes to a crashing halt because of failure to perform. The camera then pans to the remains

* The good news about butter went unmentioned in the study abstract. One of the study authors, Alice Lichtenstein, has made a career of warning people away from foods containing "evil" saturated fats.

of the couple's dinner: a meat-heavy, high-fat dinner on the room service tray. The ad ends with the tag line, "Eating meat contributes to artery blockages—and that can make you impotent." The press release specifically targets the Atkins diet, high in meat and saturated fats, as a cause of erectile dysfunction, claiming that high cholesterol levels contribute to impotence.*[89]

Impotence appears to be a huge problem these days, given the sales of performance-enhancing drugs like Viagra, but saturated fats should not get the blame for the vast inadequacies of the standard American diet. San Diego nutritionist Kim Schuette is seeing erectile dysfunction in men as young as twenty. She treats it—very successfully—by advising them to eat a half pound of butter and six egg yolks per day. They usually return to her office a month later with grins on their faces. Egg yolks are considered a fertility food in many parts of the world.

Impotence is a commonly reported side effect of cholesterol-lowering regimes because the body makes testosterone out of cholesterol. Vitamin A is key to this conversion—and cholesterol-lowering drugs block the uptake of vitamin A. Cardiovascular disease alone is associated with erectile dysfunction, but treatment with statins seems to worsen this condition.†[90]

Saturated fats are often blamed for lowered sperm count as well. "Eating a fatty diet could reduce a man's sperm count by 40 percent," declared the *Daily Mail*, "enough to put every man off his bacon and egg."[91] This dire warning referred to a 1999 study published in the *American Journal of Clinical Nutrition*[92] which claimed that saturated fat was associated with reduced semen quality among seven hundred Danish men. Zoë Harcombe, PhD, of the UK produced a brilliant analysis of the document,[93] which noted that the researchers jumped to sweeping conclusions based on differences in fat consumption that were actually very small; they could have equally concluded from the data that monounsaturated fat and polyunsaturated fat lowered sperm count. The study did reveal that the period of abstinence for those consuming more saturated fat was less, which could explain the lower sperm count. A much more interesting—and more accurate—headline would declare: "Men who eat more saturated fat have sex more frequently!"

"SATURATED FAT CAN MAKE YOU STUPID." That was the headline in a 2006 Swedish newspaper report linking saturated fat with a decline in cognitive performance.

The newspapers were referring to a study published in the *European Journal of Neurology*. Male and female rats were divided into two groups, one fed a diet of 42 percent fat from a mixture of coconut oil and corn oil; the other was fed a diet of 10 percent fat. The high-fat diet had a negative effect on "hippocampal neurogenesis," that is, the generation of nerve cells in an area of the brain called the hippocampus, but only in the male rats. The

---

* Times have changed. During the nineteenth century, Americans considered robust "natural urges" a sign of disease. At the Battle Creek sanatorium, John Harvey Kellogg promoted cereals to the American public as a way to reduce excessive sexual activity, thought to result from the overheating properties of a high meat intake!

† True to form, the pharmaceutical industry has countered the negative publicity about decreased libido on cholesterol-lowering drugs by proposing statins to treat erectile dysfunction!

authors concluded, "Our study provides the first compelling evidence that a high intake of dietary fat per se has a negative influence on hippocampal neurogenesis."[94]

But the authors did not single out saturated fats in their conclusion—these accusations appeared only in the media. In fact, the authors did not provide any information in the study about the percentage of fatty acids in the dietary mix. The mix could have been mostly polyunsaturated corn oil—and several studies have shown that polyunsaturated oil inhibits neurological development and function. Nor did the researchers indicate what kind of coconut oil they were using. Most of the coconut oil used in scientific experiments is fully hydrogenated, a process that gets rid of all the essential fatty acids. Thus, a diet of corn oil and coconut oil may have induced a deficiency in omega-3 fatty acids, another likely explanation for cognitive decline. But the interesting thing about these findings is that they occurred only in male rats, not in the females, an indication that the lack of neurogenesis was related to hormonal factors. Most rat chow is based on soy, rich in estrogenic compounds shown to have deleterious effects on male rats.

There is no way to tell from this study which factors inhibited hippocampal neurogenesis, but the least likely one to be the culprit—the normal brain contains very high levels of saturated fat—was singled out as the whipping boy for the others.

The following year in Britain, a similar article appeared in *The Daily Mail*. The article, titled, "Diet High in Cholesterol Can Trigger Onset of Alzheimer's," warned readers about studies showing that "eating lots of foods containing saturated fats, such as butter and red meat, can boost levels of proteins in the brain linked to dementia," and that "large amounts of harmful cholesterol are found in foods high in saturated fats such as red meat, butter, cheese and offal such as liver and kidneys."[95] These dire warnings are not based on studies of humans eating red meat and butter—an online search for red meat or butter plus Alzheimer's yields nothing—but are based on research in which rats are given large amounts of purified cholesterol. The article cites "growing evidence that taking cholesterol-lowering statins makes people less likely to develop Alzheimer's later in life." No reference is provided for this remarkable statement, remarkable given the many published reports of statin-induced cognitive decline.

More sobering news comes from the Honolulu-Asia Aging Study. Researchers followed more than one thousand Japanese-American men over a forty-year period, starting in 1965. They found that cholesterol levels in men with dementia and, in particular those with Alzheimer's, had declined at least fifteen years before the diagnosis and remained lower than cholesterol levels in men without dementia throughout that period. Their conclusion: "A decline in serum total cholesterol levels may be associated with early stages in the development of dementia."[96]

Another headline, this one from 2009: "High Fat Diet May Make You Stupid and Lazy." According to the article, "A new study on rats finds that ten days of eating a high-fat diet caused short-term memory loss and made exercise difficult."[97] There's just one problem with the press release: the rats in the experiment were not fed fat, they were fed oil. The fatty acid composition of the "high-fat" diet that caused memory loss and muscle weakness was 27 percent saturated, 48 percent monounsaturated, and 25 percent polyunsaturated—an oil that would be liquid at room temperature.[98] The predominant fatty acid in the mix was monounsaturated, the kind of fatty acid in olive oil, peanut oil, canola oil and high-oleic safflower oil, the kind that is supposed to be so good for us. The rats in this study encountered problems typical of those on diets high in industrially processed vegetable oils. So while the media is urging you to avoid meat, sausage and cheese, the foods you really need to avoid are cooking oils, commercial salad dressings, fried foods, chips, snack foods and bakery products like donuts and cookies. If anything will make you stupid and lazy, it is foods like these.

THE NATIONAL KIDNEY FOUNDATION WEBSITE predictably warns kidney patients to avoid "cholesterol-raising" saturated fats. The tragic epidemic of kidney failure, so common in diabetics, taxes our health care system, by some estimates accounting for half of all medical costs. What if saturated fats were the very food that could reverse kidney failure? A recent study on mice indicates the possibility. Researchers at the Mount Sinai School of Medicine in New York used mice with both type 1 and type 2 diabetes. Once kidney damage had developed, half the mice were put on a ketogenic diet, low in carbohydrates and very high in fat. After eight weeks, the researchers noted that kidney damage was reversed in those on the high-fat diet.

Such exciting results should be shouted to the skies, but health officials are administering a large dose of cold water. "This research was carried out in mice so it is difficult to see how these results would translate into any real benefits for people with diabetes at this stage," said Dr. Iain Frame, director of research at Diabetes UK. "It is too simple to say that kidney failure could be prevented by diet alone and it is also questionable whether the diet used in this model would be sustainable for humans, even in the short term."[99] Of course, Diabetes UK and its counterparts in the United States have been pushing a low-fat, high-carb diet for diabetics for decades; this study suggests that this disastrous advice may hasten kidney failure in these patients.

THE PATTERN IS CLEAR. At every turn, saturated fats get the blame for everything that ails us—from kidney disease to cancer to stupidity. What the public doesn't realize is the fact that the research simply does not support these conclusions; if anything, the science vindicates saturated fat as a cause in all of these diseases, even heart disease.

But what if saturated fats are not merely harmless, but absolutely essential for biochemical processes? That is the premise we will explore in Chapter 4.

CHAPTER 4

The Many Roles of Saturated Fat

The human body contains almost forty trillion cells; each of these cells is surrounded by a membrane, which serves to separate the interior of the cell from the exterior environment.

As microscopes have become stronger and analytical techniques more advanced, scientists have discovered the cell membrane's many marvels. The membrane's construction allows for the passive diffusion of oxygen and carbon dioxide, while other compounds can only get inside the cell (or can be released from the cell) through channels created by proteins that span the thickness of the membrane, some of which are specific for just one single chemical. The cell "mem-brain" is indeed the brain of the cell; it senses the nutrients available on the outside and makes decisions about what should cross the barrier to enter the cell as well as what will be released from the cell to the exterior.

The cell membrane is both stable and fluid, thanks to its ingenious construction. Composed of a lipid bilayer, that is, a double layer of fatty acids, each membrane contains about one trillion fat molecules. At least half of these fat molecules must be saturated fatty acids for the cell to work properly. The basic structural unit of the membrane is a phospholipid, that is, two fatty acids joined to a structure containing phosphorus, forming a kind of head with two legs. The "legs" face inward, while the "head" faces outward to interact with the watery environment inside and outside the cell.

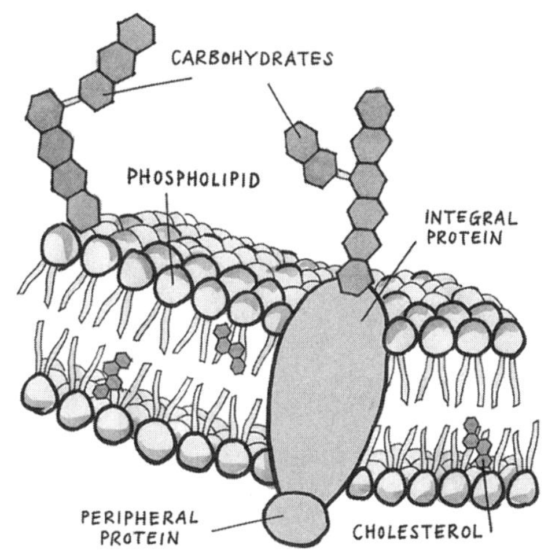

The cell membrane: Each phospholipid has two fatty acids attached to a phosphorus molecule. The fatty acids face inward while the phosphorus ends face outward to the watery environments inside and outside the cell. Specialized proteins allow the passage of compounds into and out of the cell.

The most common type of phospholipid contains one saturated fatty acid—a straight "leg"—and one unsaturated fatty acid—a bent "leg." The saturated fatty acids give the cell stability, while the unsaturated fatty acid (usually a monounsaturated fatty acid) provides flexibility. The space created by the bent leg is often filled with a cholesterol molecule, which serves as a kind of structural support and ensures that the cell is waterproof.

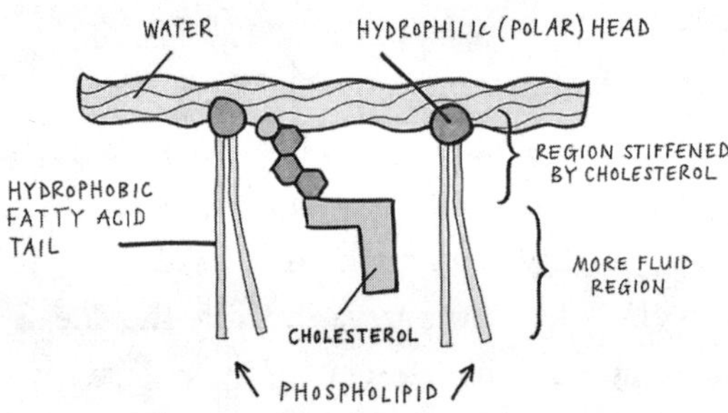

Cholesterol is packed between the fatty acids in the cell membrane to provide solidity and waterproofing.

Dotted throughout the cell membrane are structures called lipid rafts, which are rich in cholesterol and molecules called sphingolipids. In these areas, more of the fatty acids are saturated, and they tend to be longer, making the rafts thicker than other parts of the bilayer. These slightly thicker and stiffer areas on the cell membrane can better accommodate certain membrane proteins necessary for numerous processes in the cell.

Trans fatty acids have many deleterious effects on the cell membrane, including blocking receptors and inhibiting enzyme function. Interestingly, saturated fats protect the cells from these effects. In experiments with swine, the undesirable effects of *trans* fats are mitigated when the proportion of saturated fats is high.[1] This research indicates that if your diet contains liberal amounts of butter and other animal fats, you could actually eat French fries every now and then without causing much harm!

Inside the cells are mitochondria—called the powerhouses of the body, because they produce a fuel called adenosine triphosphate (ATP), the body's main energy source.* A membrane also surrounds each of the mitochondria, very similar to that surrounding the cell. These membranes also require saturated fatty acids for stability and structure.

Thus, in the most basic sense, at the level of our cells and mitochondria, and in incalculable numbers, saturated fat molecules are essential for life. Without ample saturated fats, cell membranes lack stability—you might describe them as "floppy." At the cellular level, a deficiency of necessary saturated fats leads to unpredictable, but certainly adverse, consequences.

In humans, a large fraction of the fatty acids in our cell membranes must be saturated because we are warm-blooded. We need larger amounts of saturated fats just like tropical plants, such as coconut and date palms, need larger amounts of saturated fatty acids in their leaves and fruit to provide needed stiffness in a hot climate. On the opposite end of the spectrum, cold-blooded animals from northern climates rely on unsaturated fatty acids, especially the longer and more unsaturated fatty acids, to

* The body produces ATP much more efficiently from fats than from carbohydrates. One molecule of glucose produces about 40 units of ATP in the mitochondria, while one molecule of fat produces more than 140. Furthermore, the production of ATP from glucose requires three times more enzymes and larger amounts of vitamins and minerals than the production of ATP from fat.

serve as a kind of antifreeze—like DHA and EPA, two long and highly unsaturated fatty acids found in fish from Arctic waters.

The digestive tracts of warm-blooded ruminant animals are designed to create saturated fatty acids from the unsaturated fatty acids naturally occurring in grasses and grains. Thus, the body of a warm-blooded vegetarian cow will be laced with highly saturated fat. With her high body temperature—101 degrees F—the cow needs even more saturated fatty acids than humans do to function properly. Efforts to increase the omega-3 content of beef are misguided—the cow does not need antifreeze; she needs stable saturated fats. That is why the omega-3 content in the fat of beef, lamb, and goat is very low—usually less than 1 percent, with levels largely resistant to dietary changes.

When saturated fats are not available, or when we mistakenly avoid them thinking they are not good for us, the body has a backup plan—it makes saturated fats out of carbohydrates, especially refined carbohydrates like sugar and white flour. This process is called *de novo lipogenesis* (DNL). A high-carbohydrate diet is thus a high-fat diet! In fact, avoiding saturated fat is a recipe for creating carb cravings—the body needs saturated fats so fundamentally, that it will get them one way or the other. Diets low in both saturated fat and carbohydrates—such as the South Beach Diet or low-fat versions of the paleo diet—pose a real danger and usually fail as the dieter gives in either to saturated fat or to carbohydrates in order to supply the basic building blocks for our cells.

While the body can make saturated fat by *de novo lipogenesis*, it is better to get it from the diet. To create saturated fat, DNL uses up the hydrogen ions and electrons carried by niacin (vitamin B_3), making this essential nutrient much less effective.[2] When niacin levels are depleted for DNL, it is no longer available to defend antioxidants and recycle folate and vitamin K—processes that protect us against heart disease.

SATURATED FATTY ACIDS ARE NO LESS IMPORTANT inside the cell, where they play many roles, especially in a process called protein acylation, which uses the fourteen-carbon saturated fat myristic acid and the sixteen-carbon saturated fat palmitic acid.

Myristoylation involves the attachment of myristic acid to the protein glycine. The resulting compound allows for many important reactions and signaling pathways inside the cell, the movement of proteins, and the interaction of proteins with the cell membrane.[3] Myristoylation is an integral part of apoptosis, or programmed cell death.

Apoptosis is necessary for cell homeostasis and occurs when cells are under stress. Thus, myristic acid facilitates the regular functioning of the cell; and when apoptosis does not occur, we become vulnerable to cancer. Myristic acid also supports the conversion of the basic omega-3 fatty acid, linolenic acid, into the elongated forms DHA and EPA.[4] Thus, a deficiency of myristic acid from the diet can have unfortunate consequences, including cancer, mental decline and immune system dysfunction.

Myristic acid is also involved in the amplification of important hormone signals, such as the hormone adrenaline. When the adrenal gland produces adrenaline, myristic acid acts to get the hormone to the parts of the body needed for action; the heart beats faster, the blood flow to the gut decreases while the blood flow to the muscles increases, and the production of glucose increases.[5]

The body makes myristic acid very slowly, and in times of great need, requires this fat from food. The most common source of myristic acid is butter, followed by cheese. It occurs in smaller amounts in meat fats and in tropical oils from the coconut and palm fruit.*

Sixteen-carbon palmitic acid is also important for cellular function. In the cell, palmitic acid binds with cysteine and other proteins, allowing them to attach to the cell membrane, where they can do their work. Palmitoylation helps proteins move around and interact with other proteins. Palmitoylation also plays an important role in regulating neurotransmitter release and memory formation.

Palmitic acid is the most prevalent fatty acid in animal fats (usually 30–40 percent of the total), and it is the fatty acid that the body makes first. It is frowned upon in cardiovascular circles, as research has shown that palmitic acid can raise LDL and total cholesterol slightly in feeding experiments. Myristic acid (fourteen carbons) and lauric acid (twelve carbons) do as well.[6] These findings provide the vegetable oil industry with a platform to further demonize traditional fats, as dairy fat is a major source of myristic acid, coconut oil is a major source of lauric acid, and palm oil is especially rich in palmitic acid. Eighteen-carbon stearic acid, found predominantly in meat, poultry and fish, does not raise cholesterol in feeding experiments, and is thereby acceptable in "healthy" dietary guidelines, especially as stearic acid levels are greater in lean meat than fatty meat. Cocoa butter is rich in stearic acid, a fact that makes the chocolate makers happy.

A recent discovery indicates that eighteen-carbon stearic acid also plays important roles inside the cell—along with its fourteen-carbon and sixteen-carbon brothers. Researchers developed a genetic line of flies whose cells were not able to produce stearic acid naturally. Flies with the defect did not develop beyond the pupal stage. It turns out that stearic acid is involved in signaling functions, and without it, the cells' mitochondria cannot function.[7]

Mitochondrial dysfunction is a recent disorder, occurring with increasing frequency in humans. Symptoms include just about everything that can ail us—poor growth, loss of muscle coordination, muscle weakness, visual problems, hearing problems, learning disabilities, heart disease, liver disease, kidney disease, gastrointestinal disorders, respiratory disorders, neurological problems, autonomic dysfunction and dementia. Conventional medicine blames the disorder on faulty genes, but new discoveries about the role of saturated stearic acid in the mitochondria point the finger at diets low in animal fats.

THE KIDNEY IS ONE OF the body's most important organs and systems. Properly functioning kidneys are essential for maintaining normal blood volume and composition; for filtering and excreting or saving various chemical metabolites; and for helping to maintain proper blood pressure. Hypertension (high blood pressure) can result from improperly functioning kidneys. Research carried out during the last few years indicates that both saturated fat and cholesterol play important roles in maintaining kidney function, as do the omega-3 fatty acids.

---

* The richest source of myristic acid is nutmeg. Myristic acid takes its name from the botanical name of nutmeg, *Myristica fragrans.*

The kidneys need stable fats both for their cushioning and as their energy source. The fat around the kidneys is very hard, because it has a higher concentration of saturated fatty acids than are found in any of the body's other fat deposits. These saturated fatty acids are myristic acid (the fourteen-carbon saturate), palmitic acid (the sixteen-carbon saturate), and stearic acid (the eighteen-carbon saturate). When we consume various polyunsaturated fatty acids in large amounts, they are incorporated into kidney tissues, usually at the expense of oleic acid, because the body resists changing the normal high level of saturated fatty acids in the kidney fat.[8] Myristoylation is a particularly active process in kidney function, so saturated fat supports the internal workings of the kidney as well.

"WHATEVER IS THE CAUSE OF heart disease," wrote the eminent biochemist Michael Gurr, "it is not primarily the consumption of saturated fats."[9] In fact, a careful look at the scientific literature indicates that saturated fats play a *beneficial* role in cardiovascular health. For example, a strong marker for proneness to heart disease is something called lipoprotein-a or Lp(a), which tends to be higher in those with coronary heart disease (CHD), cerebrovascular disease (CVD), atherosclerosis, thrombosis and stroke.[10] High Lp(a) predicts risk of early atherosclerosis independently of other cardiac risk factors, including LDL. One study from Tanzania found that vegetarians have higher levels of Lp(a) than fish eaters, leading to speculation that the types of fats in fish oil could be helpful to lower Lp(a).[11]

But the real surprise is the finding that saturated fats actually *lower* Lp(a).[12] Other research indicates that saturated eighteen-carbon stearic acid and sixteen-carbon palmitic acid are the preferred foods for the heart, which is why the fat around the heart muscle is highly saturated, just like the fat around the kidney.[13] The heart draws on this reserve of fat in times of stress. These findings—that saturated fat lowers Lp(a) and serves as the preferred food for the heart—are buried in their respective scientific reports, and not mentioned in the abstracts.

We've all heard the accusation "Saturated fats clog the arteries," as though our arteries were some kind of pipe and saturated fats build up in the arteries the way that grease does when poured down the drain. Actually, the artery "clogs" occur inside the intima, that is, inside the lining of the artery, as biological tissue and not as pure fat stuck to the smooth warm arteries. The fat in artery "clogs" is actually only about 26 percent saturated. The rest is unsaturated, of which more than half is polyunsaturated—a very unnatural situation in human biochemistry.[14] In most human tissues, polyunsaturated fatty acids comprise less than 10 percent of the total.

One recent study blames saturated fat for blood vessel inflammation. Published in the American Heart Association journal *Circulation Research* and entitled, "Pro-inflammatory Phenotype of Perivascular Adipocytes: Influence of High-Fat Feeding," the authors found more markers of vascular inflammation in mice placed on a "high-fat Western diet."[15] But nowhere in the article or the accompanying press release do the authors disclose the type of fat they fed to the mice.

After an e-mail query, Neil Weintraub, the principal study author, revealed the feeding formula they used—the fat used was indeed an animal fat, what the industry calls anhydrous milk fat; that is, butterfat with most of the moisture removed. The other main components of the formula were casein (20 percent by weight), sucrose (34 percent by weight) and cornstarch (15 percent by weight)—all problematic ingredients that could have contributed to the resulting inflammation. As there was no control group fed the same formula but with polyunsaturated oil instead of anhydrous milk fat, the researchers could not compare the effects of mostly saturated versus mostly polyunsaturated fatty acids.

And anhydrous milk fat may not even have the same fatty acid profile as butter. The industry has figured out how to add polyunsaturated fatty acids to milk fat through a process called enzymatic interesterification. But Weintraub believes that his results prove that "high-fat diets" can predispose individuals to heart disease even if they do not have high cholesterol levels. "Many patients who consume high fat diets do not exhibit abnormal lipid profiles, but still develop atherosclerosis nonetheless. These new findings suggest a direct link between poor dietary habits and inflammation of blood vessels." The study was again funded by the National Institutes of Health, which preaches that "poor dietary habits" mean consumption of foods like meat, butter and cheese, all high in saturated fat.

As saturated fats are stable, they do not become rancid easily, do not call upon the body's reserves of antioxidants, do not initiate cancer and do not irritate the artery walls. Contrary to everything you hear in the media, saturated fats are safe and healthy. *Trans* fats from partially hydrogenated vegetables oils and free radicals in processed liquid oils are the likeliest culprits in the current epidemic of chronic disease—a subject we will explore in more detail in Chapter 7.

Even monounsaturated fatty acids—the kind found in olive oil—can be problematic when not supported by adequate saturated fat. According to a 1998 report, mice fed a diet containing monounsaturated fats were more likely to develop atherosclerosis than mice fed a diet containing saturated fat. In fact, the mice fed monounsaturated fatty acids were more prone to heart disease than those fed polyunsaturated fatty acids.[16]

How much total saturated fat do we need? During the 1970s, researchers from Canada found that animals fed rapeseed oil and canola oil developed heart lesions. This problem was corrected when they added saturated fat to the animals' diets. On the basis of this and other research, they ultimately determined that the diet should contain at least 25 percent of fat as saturated fat. Among the food fats that they tested, the one found to have the best proportion of saturated fat was lard, the very fat we are told to avoid under all circumstances![17]

SATURATED FATS PLAY NUMEROUS OTHER roles within the body. For one, they contribute to the health of our bones. To effectively incorporate calcium into the skeletal structure, at least 50 percent of the dietary fats should be saturated.[18]

Also, several studies have shown that saturated fat can protect the liver from the effects of alcohol and other toxins, such as Tylenol.*[19] For example, a study published in the *Journal of Nutrition* found that saturated fat from beef tallow reduced alcoholic liver toxicity in rats whereas corn oil increased markers of liver

* Thus supporting the folk custom of eating butter or drinking whole milk before a big night on the town.

toxicity.[20] Moral: if you drink, eat plenty of butter and fatty meats—your liver will thank you.

Yet saturated fat often gets the blame for liver dysfunction. One example is a 2006 study entitled, "Saturated Fatty Acids Promote Endoplasmic Reticulum Stress and Liver Injury in Rats with Hepatic Steatosis," published in *Endocrinology.*[21] In this study, markers for liver function worsened in rats on a diet high in sucrose (68 percent sucrose, 12 percent corn oil and 20 percent casein) or high in lard (45 percent lard oil, 35 percent cornstarch and 20 percent casein) compared to a high-starch diet (68 percent cornstarch, 12 percent corn oil and 20 percent casein) or a high polyunsaturated diet (35 percent cornstarch, 45 percent corn oil and 20 percent casein). The lard oil diet was described as high in saturated fat, hence the title of the study, which fingers saturated fatty acids. The title contains no mention of the similar adverse effects from the high-sucrose diet; but even worse is the characterization of lard oil as high in saturated fat. The definition of lard oil is "oil consisting chiefly of olein that is expressed [extracted] from lard." Olein is a monoglyceride of monounsaturated oleic acid; that is, oleic acid joined to a glycerol molecule. Thus the diet described as high in saturated fatty acids was actually high in monounsaturated fatty acids! (And none of the diets could be called normal diets, representative of how and what we actually eat.)

Saturated fats enhance the immune system.[22] Transplant patients get specific instructions to avoid saturated fats because they increase the chances of organ rejection—polyunsaturated vegetable oils depress the immune system, resulting in lower rates of organ rejection. Those of us who have not had organ transplants should stick with saturated fats, not polyunsaturated oils, so that our immune systems will function properly and reject whatever is foreign or harmful to the body.

A key component of our immune systems is white blood cells, also called T-cells. When researchers looked at the fatty acid composition of the phospholipids in the T-cells, from both young and old donors, they found that a loss of saturated fatty acids in the lymphocytes was responsible for age-related declines in white blood cell function; they also found that they could correct cellular deficiencies in palmitic acid and myristic acid by adding these saturated fatty acids to the diet.

DHA and EPA are vital for many processes in the body. Saturated fats, especially myristic acid, support the production of these elongated omega-3 fatty acids and are needed for the proper utilization of essential fatty acids.[23] Elongated omega-3 fatty acids are better retained in the tissues when the diet is rich in saturated fats.[24] Short- and medium-chain saturated fatty acids, such as those found in butter, have important antimicrobial properties. They protect us against harmful microorganisms in the digestive tract.[25]

Saturated fats support hormone production.[26] One study showed that in men, decreasing dietary saturated fat and increasing polyunsaturated fatty acids reduced the amount of androstenedione, testosterone and free testosterone in the bloodstream. Similar results hold for women—consumption of more saturated fat results in higher production of various types of estrogen.[27]

Finally, let us consider the lungs. Proper lung function depends on a compound called lung surfactant, a soap-like substance that allows the passage of air into and out of the lungs—oxygen-rich air coming in and carbon dioxide-rich air coming out. Surfactant is composed primarily of phospholipids, that is, two fatty acids joined to a phosphate group (a structure similar to the phospholipids that make up the cell membrane). The most common phospholipid in the surfactant contains two sixteen-carbon palmitic fatty acids. This is the ideal structure for air to pass through the surfactant membrane. The passage of air is impeded when the phospholipids incorporate *trans* fatty acids rather than saturated fatty acids; the membrane tends to break if polyunsaturated fatty acids predominate in the phospholipids.[28] Thus saturated fats are essential for lung function—a fact that helps explain the results of several studies showing that children on whole milk and butter diets have less asthma than children eating reduced-fat milk and margarine.[29]

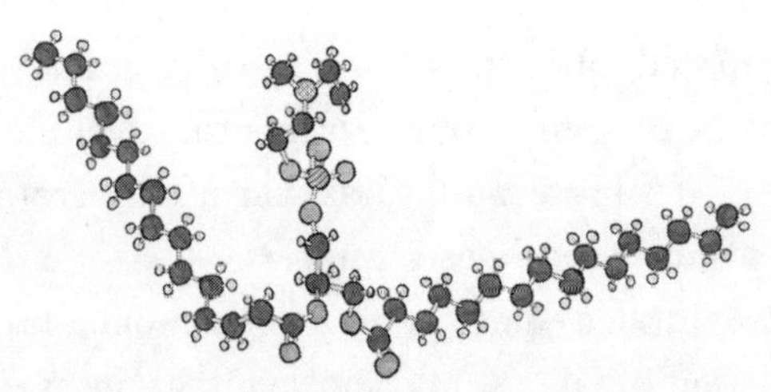

A molecule of lung surfactant is typically composed of two sixteen-carbon saturated fatty acids.

Current thinking blames lung cancer on smoking or exposure to secondhand smoke, but lots of people get lung cancer who have never smoked and who live in smoke-free houses. Many people who live a "healthy lifestyle" have been shocked to receive a diagnosis of lung cancer. Although the percentage of Americans who smoke has declined by half, we have seen only a slight drop in the rate of lung cancer. Currently, more than one hundred fifty thousand American men and women die of lung cancer every year; it is the leading cause of cancer death and the second most common type of cancer. Lung cancer patients usually receive admonitions to avoid sources of saturated fat, like red meat, but given the basic facts of lung biochemistry, avoiding industrial fats and oils and consuming natural animal fats seems a more rational dietary strategy.

CHOLESTEROL GETS TARRED WITH THE same brush as saturated fat, although the molecules are very different. Both saturated fat and cholesterol are insoluble in water, but they play very different roles in the body's chemistry.

The richest dietary source of cholesterol is animal fats, but your body can also make cholesterol—about 2,000 milligrams per day. In general, the average American absorbs about 100 milligrams of cholesterol per day from food. So in theory, even reducing animal foods to zero will result in a mere 5 percent decrease in the total amount of cholesterol available to the blood and tissues.

It is worth repeating that cholesterol is vital to the integrity of the cell membrane—but that is only one of its many important roles. Cholesterol acts as a precursor to vital corticosteroids, hormones that help us deal with stress and protect the body against heart disease and cancer; and to the sex hormones like androgen, testosterone, estrogen and progesterone. When cholesterol levels are low, the body cannot make these hormones, especially in times of stress. Infertility, impotency and difficulty dealing with stress are the logical consequences.

Cholesterol is a precursor to vitamin D, a vital fat-soluble vitamin needed for healthy bones and nervous system, proper growth, mineral metabolism, muscle tone, insulin production, reproduction and immune system function; and it is the precursor to bile salts, which are vital for digestion and assimilation of fats in the diet.

The subject of antioxidants is everywhere in the news these days, as people look to increase their fruit and vegetable intake to protect themselves against cancer. But we never hear about the role of cholesterol as an antioxidant. Research shows that cholesterol acts as a vital antioxidant in the cell membrane.*[30] As an antioxidant, cholesterol protects us against free radical damage that leads to heart disease and cancer.

Cholesterol is the body's repair substance, manufactured in large amounts when the arteries are irritated or weak. Scar tissue is rich in cholesterol. Blaming heart disease on high serum cholesterol levels is like blaming firemen who have come to put out a fire for starting the blaze.

Cholesterol nourishes the digestive tract and supports digestive function. Dietary cholesterol plays an important role in maintaining the health of the intestinal wall,[31] which is why low-cholesterol vegetarian diets can lead to leaky gut syndrome and other intestinal disorders. And cholesterol helps protect against infection and endotoxins from pathogenic bacteria—especially the vilified LDL-cholesterol, the so-called "bad" cholesterol.[32]

Cholesterol is needed for proper function of serotonin receptors in the brain.[33] Serotonin is the body's natural "feel-good" chemical. This explains why low cholesterol levels have been linked to aggressive and violent behavior, depression and suicidal tendencies. (More on this in Chapter 9.)

Mother's milk is especially rich in cholesterol and contains lipase enzymes to ensure that the baby absorbs 100 percent of this nutrient.[34] Babies and children lack the enzymes to make cholesterol and require cholesterol-rich foods throughout their growing years to ensure proper development of the brain and nervous system.

Low cholesterol levels are a definite marker for cancer,[35] a fact that scientists recognized before the anticholesterol agenda was applied to every man, woman and child in the country. We can do no better than quote verbatim from a 1974 paper on leukemia: "Leukemia in mice and humans is accompanied by a marked deficiency of unesterified cholesterol in the surface membrane of leukemic cells as compared to normal leukocytes. This deficiency induces a significant reduction in their membrane microviscosity. Since cholesterol in the cell surface membrane is exchangeable with the cholesterol in the serum lipoproteins, concomitant to the cellular deficiency of cholesterol, the average levels of cholesterol in the blood serum of leukemic patients is substantially below the average normal level." And from the conclusion: "A controlled reduction of cholesterol level in normal leukocytes may

* This is the likely explanation for the fact that cholesterol levels go up with age—we need more protection from this vital antioxidant.

thus sensitize immune response processes or phagocytic activity above threshold level beyond which malignant transformation and the development of leukemia may occur. On the other hand, a controlled enrichment of cellular cholesterol in leukemic cells may prevent the development of latent leukemia and may hopefully remit leukemia in its active form."[36] In other words, low cholesterol predisposes to leukemia, and higher cholesterol prevents this terrible disease.

More recently, scientists have discovered a novel role for cholesterol, one that explains why low cholesterol is linked to cancer and many other diseases. Cholesterol in cell membranes appears to anchor a signaling pathway linked to cell division and cancer. "Cell signals have to be tightly controlled," says Dr. Richard G.W. Anderson, chairman of cell biology at UT Southwestern Medical Center. "If the signaling machines do not work, which can happen when the cell doesn't have enough cholesterol, the cell gets the wrong information, and disease results."[37] The cholesterol-containing regions of the cell membrane are more rigid than the other areas and play a critical role in organizing signaling machinery at the cell surface. The correct arrangement of signaling modules in these domains is vital for communication inside the cell and is dependent on proper levels of cholesterol.

The fact is, higher cholesterol levels are associated with a longer life, especially in the elderly and in women of all ages—a finding confirmed in numerous studies.[38] So why is high cholesterol associated with increased risk of heart disease in young and middle-aged men? The likely explanation is the fact that at this age, men are in the midst of their careers and subject to high levels of stress. Since cholesterol provides the building blocks of stress hormones, cholesterol levels rise to provide protection—obviously not always successfully. Sometimes the effects of a stressful lifestyle are so great that they overwhelm the protective system that cholesterol provides.

THE HUMAN TONGUE HAS REMARKABLY sensitive receptors for fat. Test subjects showed a response in the blood when they tasted potatoes mashed with butter, but no response when they tasted mashed potatoes without fat, or mashed potatoes made with fat substitutes.

The biochemical response to tasting mashed potatoes with butter was elevated triglycerides, which investigators say is a bad thing. But if the human tongue has a taste for fat, that must mean humans need fat. Perhaps the fat taste buds steer people toward foods that contain essential fatty acids, say puzzled investigators. But most natural nonfatty foods contain some essential fatty acids—even potatoes. The logical conclusion is that the human body knows better than thousands of politically correct nutritionists that humans need high-fat foods, so much so that it possesses a delicate instrument for determining which foods contain lots of fat. So precise is the human taste for fat that it can distinguish real fat from imitation fat substitutes like Olestra.[39]

How long can medical orthodoxy oppose the consumption of saturated fat and cholesterol in the face of contradictory evidence? Animal foods containing saturated fat and cholesterol provide vital nutrients necessary for growth, energy and protection from degenerative disease. Like sex, animal fats are necessary for reproduction. Humans are drawn to both by powerful instincts. Suppression of natural instincts leads to weird nocturnal habits, fantasies, fetishes, bingeing, purging and splurging.

Young people these days, especially young women, grow up in a culture of fat phobia. Our natural appetite for fats gets suppressed in the fearmongering and finger wagging that permeates the media and the classroom—from nutrition lessons to fashion magazines. The result is eating disorders and a culture of thinness. Those who can resist the lure of satisfying fats keep themselves too thin, and those who can't resist give in instead to carb bingeing and let themselves get fat.

Fat cells, called adipocytes, are often blamed for conditions like diabetes, cancer and heart disease, but they may actually protect us against these illnesses. Researchers at Purdue University have discovered that pig fat cells (very similar to human fat cells) help regulate energy metabolism, anti-inflammatory pathways and certain aspects of the body's immune response that protect us against bacterial toxins. In addition, normal adipocytes produce factors that promote insulin regulation of glucose levels. These regulatory mechanisms are absent in people who are too thin, and are thwarted in the case of obesity, when the adipocytes enlarge due to lipid accumulation.[40]

This research gives new meaning to the phrase "pleasingly plump." A nice layer of fat—not too much but also not too little—goes a long way to ensuring good health.

Animal fats are nutritious, they are satisfying, and they taste good. And yet the high priests of the lipid hypothesis continue to lay their curse on the fairest of culinary pleasures—butter and béarnaise, whipped cream, soufflés and omelets, full-bodied cheeses, juicy steaks and pork sausage. Our bodies know better; they know that the very foods that we love to eat also support everything from breathing to energy production to feeling good. Those who deny themselves these pleasures tend to live with chronic sadness or smoldering rage.

CHAPTER 5

AA and DHA

Fats from warm-blooded animals contain lots of saturated fat, but their value doesn't stop there—they are also unique sources of a highly unsaturated fatty acid called AA (arachidonic acid). In addition, warm-blooded animals (along with seafood) provide another important unsaturated fatty acid called DHA (docosahexaenoic acid).

Shaped like a hairpin, AA belongs to the omega-6 family of fatty acids. It contains twenty carbons, elongated from the eighteen-carbon "parent" omega-6 molecule (linoleic acid) and desaturated from the original two double bonds to four.* Likewise DHA is a highly unsaturated "curly" molecule, which belongs to the omega-3 family and contains twenty-two carbons and six double bonds.

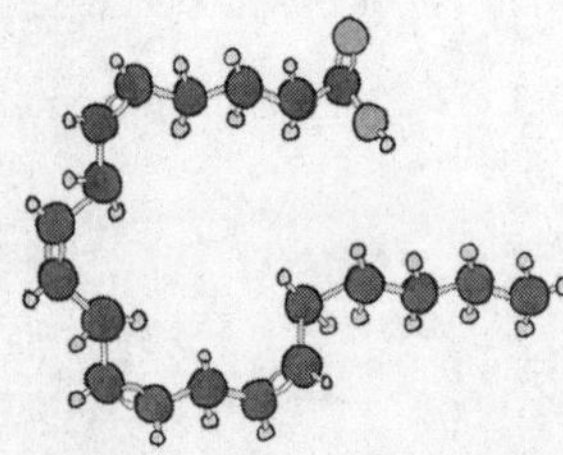

Arachidonic acid (AA) is an omega-6 fatty acid that contains twenty carbons and four double bonds.

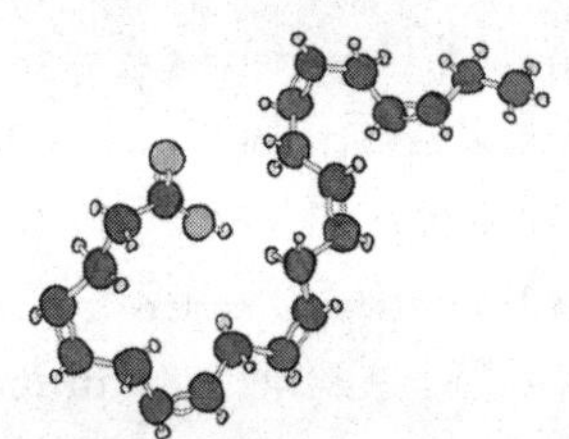

DHA (docosahexaenoic acid) is an omega-3 fatty acid that contains twenty-two carbons and six double bonds.

According to Barry Sears in his popular book *The Zone*, arachidonic acid in food is unhealthy. AA is a precursor to the Series 2 prostaglandins or eicosanoids, which are involved in swelling, inflammation, clotting and dilation. (Prostaglandin Series 1 and Series 3 groups are said to have the opposite effect, with anti-inflammatory characteristics.) According to Sears, the Series 2 family includes "bad" eicosanoids—he warns readers against eating liver and butter, sources of arachidonic acid.[1] Not only is AA inflammatory, he claims, but it "is so potent and so dangerous that when you inject it into the bloodstream of rabbits, the animals die within

* The term "arachidonic acid" comes from the modern Latin stem *arachid-*, which means "peanut." Arachidic acid is a twenty-carbon saturated fatty acid that occurs uniquely in peanut oil.

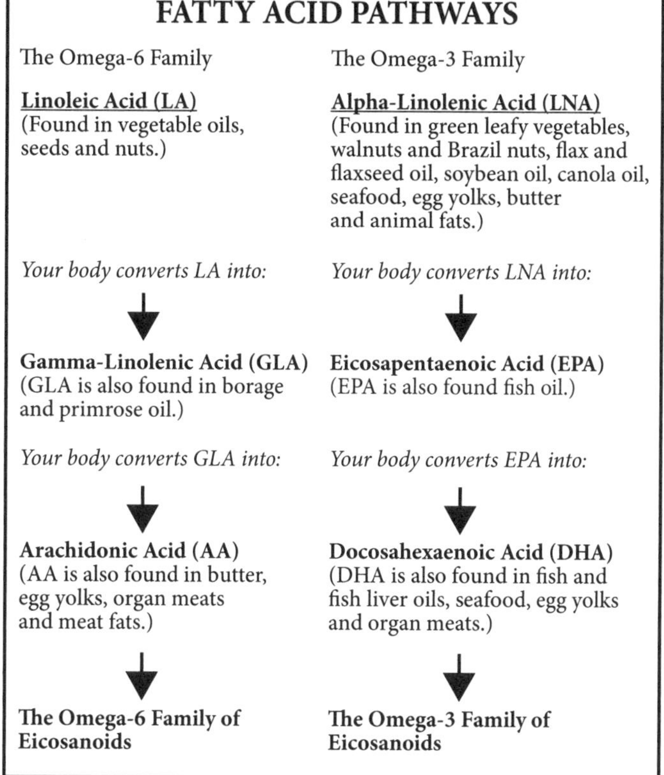

In principle, our bodies can make AA out of eighteen-carbon linoleic acid and DHA out of eighteen-carbon linolenic acid. However, many factors can interfere with this conversion, and some people even lack the enzymes to make these changes. Our best option is to obtain AA and DHA from food.

three minutes."[2] In fact, it is the presence of arachidonic acid in animal fats that researchers point to when they accuse animal fats of causing dangerous inflammation.

Fortunately, humans and animals get the AA they need by eating food or by making it, not by injecting it into the bloodstream. And to say that AA is inflammatory represents a simplistic view of the complex interactions that create inflammation in the body—a process, by the way, that is highly necessary for our survival.* Like all systems in the body, the many eicosanoids work together in an array of loops and feedback mechanisms of infinite complexity. AA is pro-inflammatory in situations requiring inflammation and anti-inflammatory in situations requiring suppression of inflammation.

* Inflammation and swelling cushion damaged and healing tissue. Without it, injuries would be excruciatingly painful, rather than merely sore and uncomfortable. Inflammation occurs in the arteries as a life-saving response to injury, usually from oxidized unsaturated fatty acids. Inflammation is also involved in the process of combating harmful microbes.

Arachidonic acid deficiency actually produces a number of inflammatory symptoms, including dandruff, hair loss, infertility and irritated, red, sore, swollen and scaly skin.[3] Over-the-counter nonsteroidal anti-inflammatory drugs (NSAIDs) work by inhibiting supposedly "inflammatory" compounds made from arachidonic acid, ironically with several inflammatory side effects. One side effect is intestinal pathologies, which closely resemble celiac disease in laboratory animals when given gluten or even egg white,[4] and they interfere with the resolution of autoimmune conditions.[5]

Our bodies can make AA from the "parent" omega-6 fatty acid, but we do so slowly and inefficiently, and in many circumstances—nutrient deficiencies, malnutrition, diabetes, low thyroid function, genetic defects—we cannot make it at all. In these common situations, arachidonic acid is "essential," meaning that we must get it from food. Egg yolk—especially duck egg yolk—and liver are our best sources of AA, followed by butter and meat fats like lard—all "forbidden" in government dietary guidelines.[6] AA occurs in most meats—probably as a component of the cell membrane—and also in seafoods. Poultry and poultry fat are excellent sources, with highest levels most probably in duck and goose fat.

Arachidonic acid is an important constituent of cell membranes, particularly abundant in the brain, muscles and liver. It is involved in cellular signaling and is necessary for the repair and growth of skeletal muscle. Thus, body builders have high requirements for AA, as do pregnant and lactating women, infants and growing children. Higher concentrations of AA in muscle tissue may also be correlated with improved insulin sensitivity.[7]

A key role of this maligned fatty acid is the formation of tight cell-to-cell junctions in the skin and intestinal tract, which can then act as physical barriers against toxins and pathogens.[8] It is AA in the cells lining the gut that allows our immune system to react to food proteins with tolerance instead of mounting an immune response,[9] and to make important molecules called lipoxins that help resolve existing inflammation.[10] It's no wonder that we are seeing so many food intolerances in our fat-phobic era, as children brought up on low-fat diets, and adults avoiding animal fats do not have the basic material they need to create a healthy, impervious gut wall. Without arachidonic acid, the gut wall can become leaky—and so can our skin. Without tight cell-to-cell junctures, the skin loses water and becomes dry and flaky. Our skin needs many compounds to be healthy, but one of the most important for glowing, buttery skin is AA.

Arachidonic acid is one of the most abundant fatty acids in the brain, and is present in similar quantities to its omega-3 cousin docosahexaenoic acid (DHA). The two molecules account for approximately 20 percent of the brain's fatty acid content.[11] Neurological health requires sufficient levels of both DHA and AA. Among other things, arachidonic acid helps to maintain cell membrane fluidity in the hippocampus, the seat of memory formation.[12] It works to protect the brain from oxidative stress[13] and also activates a protein involved in the growth and repair of neurons.[14]

Bodybuilders know about AA, often taking it as a supplement. A placebo-controlled study found that supplementation of arachidonic acid (1,500 milligrams per day for eight weeks) increased lean body mass, strength and anaerobic power in experienced resistance-trained men.[15] Another study found that 1,000 milligrams per day of arachidonic acid for fifty days enhanced anaerobic capacity and performance in exercising men.*[16]

We know that omega-3 fatty acids can protect us against heart disease, but so can omega-6 AA. A meta-analysis by Cambridge University looking for associations between heart disease risk and individual fatty acids reported a significantly reduced risk of heart disease with higher levels of omega-3 EPA (eicosapentaenoic acid) and DHA, but also with omega-6 AA.[17]

As mentioned, key signs of AA deficiency include dry, scaly, itchy skin, hair loss and dandruff, but these often clear up easily by eating good fats like butter and egg yolks. Other consequences of AA deficiency include reproductive difficulties, digestive disturbances, food intolerances, kidney disease, inability to maintain weight, poor immunity and poor growth in children. Ironically, even though AA is considered "inflammatory," deficiency can result in inflammation.[18]

What's clear is the fact that the demonized fats like butter, egg yolks, poultry fat and lard supply vital factors like AA for growth and health—conventional dietary advice has led health seekers down the wrong road!

UNLIKE THE LESSER-KNOWN ARACHIDONIC ACID, DHA is almost a household word. Popular wisdom rightly values DHA for brain function.

As with AA, our bodies can, in principle, make DHA from the eighteen-carbon omega-3 fatty acid. But in practice, this is a slow and inefficient process, and many people lack the enzymes needed to elongate and desaturate the parent molecule. These "obligate carnivores" must obtain their DHA fully formed from seafood, as well as from organ meats, egg yolks and animal fats like butter.[19] Babies get DHA from mother's milk, which ranges from a trace (0.07 percent) to greater than 1 percent, depending on the mother's diet.[20] A growing body of research indicates that DHA in the diet of infants and growing children contributes to optimal neurological development and keen vision.[21]

DHA serves as a primary structural component of the human brain, cerebral cortex, skin, sperm, testicles and retina. DHA deficiency is associated with cognitive decline[22] and depression—the brain tissue of severely depressed patients often shows reduced DHA levels.[23] Other studies have indicated that DHA benefits a range of nervous system functions, cardiovascular health and potentially other organs; supplements may be of benefit for stroke victims. DHA appears important in the formation of the acrosome, an arc-like structure on the top of sperm, which is critical in fertilization because it houses a variety of enzymes that sperm use to penetrate an egg.[24]

While skin problems, digestive disorders and food intolerances can indicate AA deficiency, DHA deficiency manifests primarily as neurological disorders including numbness and tingling, weakness, pain, psychological disturbances, poor cognitive function and difficulty learning. Other signs of deficiency include poor visual acuity, blurred vision, poor immunity, poor growth and inflammation.[25] Our tissues use DHA to synthesize compounds called "resolvins," which help bring inflammation to an end when it is no

* In the early days of bodybuilding, men in training got their arachidonic acid naturally by eating egg yolks and liver.[a]

longer needed.[26] A number of investigators have postulated that DHA deficiency may be a major cause of widespread declines in cognitive function, increases in mental disorders and epidemic levels of degenerative disease.

MANY OF US ARE ALREADY familiar with the concept of balancing omega-6 and omega-3 fatty acids in the diet. The modern diet contains about twenty times more omega-6 than omega-3, whereas the ratio should be more like two or three to one. Of even more importance is a balance of the elongated and desaturated versions of omega-6 and omega-3: AA and DHA. Too much of one will result in deficiency symptoms of the other. In addition, too much EPA, the other common elongated omega-3 fatty acid, found mostly in seafood and fish oil supplements, can result in deficiency symptoms of both AA and DHA.

Vegetarians and vegans have substantially lower levels of DHA in their bodies,[27] and often resort to fish oil supplements to correct the imbalance. Unfortunately, short-term supplemental fish oils have been shown to increase EPA, but not DHA. In addition, such supplementation leads to decreased levels of AA.[28] It isn't a long-term solution.

Our bodies use the same enzymes to convert the parent omega-3 fatty acid to DHA as they use to convert the parent omega-6 fatty acid to AA. An excess of one precursor can therefore outcompete the other for the enzymatic machinery. Large amounts of either parent omega-6 or omega-3—from the consumption of vegetable oils (high in omega-6), flax oil (high in omega-3) or even fish oil (high in EPA) will cause the cell to make fewer of these enzymes, resulting in deficiencies of either AA or DHA.[29]

This competition and cellular confusion can be avoided altogether by providing small amounts of preformed AA and DHA through the diet—and the key point is that these come from animal fats: egg yolks, organ meats, butter, animal fats, fatty fish and small amounts of cod liver oil or shark liver oil. Avoiding polyunsaturated vegetable oils and including adequate saturated fat in the diet will ensure that these highly unsaturated fatty acids are protected from oxidation and incorporated and preserved in the body. Other dietary factors that ensure the right balance of DHA and AA include avoiding refined sugar, consuming adequate calories and protein and plentiful intake of vitamin B_6, biotin, calcium, magnesium and fresh, whole foods abundant in natural antioxidants. Deficiencies of DHA and AA are commonly linked with alcoholism, diabetes, insulin resistance, certain genetic variations and strict vegetarianism.[30] Liberal amounts of egg yolks, butter and liver containing preformed arachidonic acid provide protection against the adverse effects of too much EPA (often the result of taking lots of fish oil supplements). The key is balancing nutrient-dense foods from land and sea—organ meats, egg yolks and animal fats like butter for AA, which nourishes the skin and digestive tract, and seafood, including small amounts of cod liver oil, for DHA, which nourishes the nervous system, the brain and the eyes.

Unfortunately, current dietary advice urges people to eat "good" polyunsaturated oils (soybean, corn, safflower, canola, olive and sunflower) along with supplements of fish oil. "Fats found in fish and plants may help older adults liver longer," say the headlines.[31] This combination is a recipe for deficiencies of both

AA and DHA since the omega-6 fatty acids in vegetable oils and the EPA in fish oil can interfere with the body's own production of AA and DHA.

IN THE EARLY 1980s, NASA sponsored scientific research to find a plant-based source of DHA for long-duration space flights. The researchers discovered that certain species of marine algae could produce an oil that contains both DHA and AA (sometimes called ARA).[32] These plant-derived, industrially produced versions are used in many DHA and AA supplements, and they are also added to baby formula. A number of studies have found problems with the algae-derived supplements, such as digestive disorders and neurological problems including hearing loss, with no real benefit to growing infants.[33] Nurses have described infant formula to which manufactured AA has been added as the "diarrhea formula," and the FDA has received hundreds of reports of adverse reactions in babies.[34] Women given DHA derived from egg yolks had higher levels of DHA in their milk than mothers given DHA derived from algae.[35] The plant-based AA and DHA are extracted with toxic hexane, and traces always remain in the product.[36] And it is highly likely that the industrially processed versions of these fragile fatty acids are highly oxidized—in other words, rancid.

This is just one of many examples in which plant-based or plant-derived substitutes for animal products fail to make the grade. It remains much better—and much more fun—to get the AA and DHA we need from delicious animal foods like pâté and caviar. In fact, many delicious traditional food combinations provide the synergistic combination of DHA from the omega-3 family with AA from the omega-6 family: lox and cream cheese, caviar and sour cream, liver and bacon, salmon with béarnaise sauce, and Welsh rarebit made with egg yolks and cream. Such foods not only taste delicious; they also nourish the body and mind.

CHAPTER 6

Remember the Activators!: The Fat-Soluble Vitamins A, D and K_2

"Many empty calories that Americans eat come from foods and beverages that provide calories but few nutrients—such as desserts, sodas, and candies." This statement appeared in 2016 at choosemyplate.gov, the USDA website dedicated to promoting the principles of the U.S. dietary guidelines.

On the surface it's a statement we can all agree with—but then the "solid fats" are slipped in. "A great way to help you manage your body weight is to eat fewer empty calories. Empty calories are calories from solid fats, added sugars, or both... Added sugars and fats load these choices with extra calories you don't need. Some foods and beverages provide essential nutrients, but may also contain some empty calories. For example, a cup of whole milk contains about 150 calories, with over 60 of them empty calories from fat. Fat-free milk has the same amount of calcium and other nutrients as whole milk, but with less than 90 calories and no fat or empty calories."

Here's how the guidelines define solid fats: "Solid fats are fats that are solid at room temperature, like beef fat, butter, and shortening. Solid fats mainly come from animal foods and can also be made from vegetable oils through a process called hydrogenation." Along with a picture of butter on a plate, the website lists the following as empty, solid fats: butter, milk fat, beef fat (tallow, suet), chicken fat, cream, pork fat (lard), stick margarine, shortening, hydrogenated and partially hydrogenated oils, coconut oil, palm and palm kernel oils.*

Thus "solid fats" containing *trans* fats and made from vegetable oils—which are rightly condemned—get lumped in with "solid fats" from animal sources, like butter and lard; and healthy, natural whole milk gets lumped with sugary sweets.

The guidelines continue: "Besides contributing to weight gain... Animal products containing solid fats also contain cholesterol. Saturated fats and *trans* fats tend to raise "bad" (LDL) cholesterol levels in the blood. This, in turn increases the risk for heart disease. To lower risk for heart disease, cut back on foods

* Coconut oil, palm oil and palm kernel oil contain valuable nutrients also, but a discussion of their benefits is beyond the scope of this book.

containing saturated fats and *trans* fats." Thus, according to official dogma, solid fats, no matter where they come from, contribute to obesity and heart disease.

But there is only one way officials can declare that animal fats are "empty" fats—by turning their backs on decades of scientific research into the important vitamins and other nutrients found uniquely in animal fats, including the fats in whole milk.

THE FORTUNES OF VITAMINS GO up and down. If there were a vitamin hit parade, vitamin A would be somewhere near the bottom today, maligned and misunderstood, but during the early 1900s, it stood at the top.

The discovery of vitamin A, and the history of its application in human nutrition, together represent a marriage of scientific inquiry at its best with worldwide cultural traditions. A key player in this fascinating story is the dentist, Weston A. Price, who traveled the world in the 1930s and 1940s to study healthy indigenous cultures. He discovered that the diets of healthy traditional peoples contained at least ten times more fat-soluble vitamins—vitamins found uniquely in animal foods—than the American diet of his day. His work revealed vitamin A as one of several "fat-soluble activators" present only in the fats and organ meats of land and sea animals, and necessary for the assimilation of minerals in the diet. Price noted that the foods held sacred by the peoples he studied, such as spring butter, fish eggs, seal fat and shark liver, were exceptionally rich in vitamin A. It is this same, essential vitamin A that exists in the butter fat in "empty, calorie-rich" whole milk, which ensures all the minerals in the milk are absorbed—nature doesn't make mistakes.

Government agencies claim that fruits and vegetables contain vitamin A, but in fact only animal foods supply true vitamin A. The best sources include butter, cream and cheese from cows eating green grass, liver from various animals, egg yolks from chickens raised on pasture, and a number of seafoods, such as fish eggs and especially fish liver oil—all fatty animal foods and most of them rich in "solid fats."

Vitamin A gets its proper name, retinol, from the role it plays in supporting vision in the retina. Many traditional cultures recognized the fact that certain foods could prevent blindness. In his pioneering work, *Nutrition and Physical Degeneration*, Dr. Price tells the story of a prospector who, while crossing a high plateau in the Rocky Mountains, went blind with xerophthalmia, due to a lack of vitamin A. As the man wept in despair, he was discovered by an American Indian, who caught a trout and gave him "the flesh of the head and the tissues back of the eyes, including the eyes."[1] Within a few hours the prospector's sight began to return and within two days his vision was nearly normal.

Several years previous to the travels of Weston A. Price, scientists had discovered that the richest source of vitamin A in the entire animal body is that of the retina and the tissues in back of the eyes. Many cultures used liver, another excellent source of vitamin A, to prevent and treat various types of blindness.[2] The Egyptians described a cure at least thirty-five hundred years ago: liver was first pressed to the eye and then eaten, a ritual through which the patient directed the healing powers of liver to the afflicted sense organ. Similar practices have been described in eighteenth-century Russia, rural Java in 1978 and among the inhabitants of Newfoundland in 1929. Other cultures used shark liver. Hippocrates (460–327 BC) prescribed liver soaked in honey for blindness in malnourished children. Assyrian texts dating from 700 BC and Chinese medical writings from the seventh century AD both call for the use of liver in the treatment of night blindness. A twelfth-century Hebrew treatise recommends pressing goat liver to the eyes and then eating it.

During the era of exploration and trade using sailing vessels, night blindness was a recurring problem among sailors on long voyages—by the advent of the great European navies, most people had forgotten the wisdom of traditional liver therapy. It took brave dedication to the scientific method to confirm the validity of the ancient treatments. The first to do this was Eduard Schwarz (1831–1862), a ship's doctor on an Austrian frigate that was sent around the world for scientific exploration. Before the voyage, several physicians had asked Schwarz to test the old folk remedy of using boiled ox liver to combat night blindness. On the voyage, seventy-five of the three hundred fifty-two men developed the condition. Every evening when dusk came, they lost their vision and had to be led about like the blind. Schwarz fed them ox or pork liver, which restored the night vision of every sailor afflicted.

The cure was "a true miracle," said Schwarz in his published report, which stated emphatically that night blindness was a nutritional disease. For this he came under vicious attack by the medical profession, which accused him of "frivolity" and "self-aggrandizement." Three years after his return from the expedition, the discredited physician died of TB. He was thirty-one. The use of vitamin-A-rich foods for tuberculosis lay in the future.

In 1904, the Japanese physician M. Mori described xerophthalmia in undernourished children whose diet consisted of rice, barley, cereals "and other vegetables." Xerophthalmia is a condition that progresses from night blindness to dissolution of the cornea and finally bursting of the eye. He treated the children using liver and cod liver oil, with excellent results. In fact, he found that cod liver oil was even more effective than liver in restoring visual function. Mori described it as "an excellent, almost specific medication... Indeed, in most cases, the effect is so rapid that by evening the children with night blindness are already dancing around briskly, to the joy of their mothers." Cod liver oil also helped reverse keratomalacia, a condition associated with severe nutritional deficiencies and characterized by corneal ulceration, extreme dryness of the eyes and infection.

At the end of the First World War, a physician named Bloch discovered that a diet containing whole milk, butter, eggs and cod liver oil cured night blindness and keratomalacia. In one important experiment, Bloch compared the results when he fed one group of children whole milk and the other margarine as their only fat. Half of the margarine-fed children developed corneal problems while the children receiving whole milk remained healthy.

The actual discovery of vitamin A is credited to a researcher named Elmer V. McCollum. He was curious why cows fed wheat did not thrive, became blind and gave birth to dead calves, while those fed yellow corn had no health problems. The year was 1907, and by this time, scientists were able to determine the levels of protein, carbohydrate, fat and minerals in food. The wheat and corn used in

McCollum's experiments contained equal levels of minerals and macronutrients. McCollum wondered whether the wheat contained a toxic substance, or whether there was something lacking in the wheat that was present in yellow maize.

In order to solve the puzzle, McCollum hit upon the idea of using small animals like mice or rats rather than cows for nutrition experiments—rats ate less, took up less space, reproduced rapidly and could be given controlled diets. Like many good ideas, this one met with considerable opposition. McCollum worked for the Wisconsin College of Agriculture, whose dean ordered him "to experiment with economically valuable animals—the rat was a pest to farmers!" But McCollum worked secretly in the basement of the Agriculture Hall, where he studied the effects of various diets on colonies of rats. He discovered that rats fed pure protein, pure skim milk, sugar, minerals and lard or olive oil for fat failed to grow. When he added butterfat or an extract of egg yolk to their diets, their health was restored. He discovered a fat-soluble factor in certain foods that was essential for growth and survival, which he called "fat-soluble factor A" as opposed to other accessory dietary factors, called "water-soluble B."

Research by Osborne and Mendel, published just five months after McCollum's study, found that cod liver oil produced the same results as butter in rat studies, thus confirming the early work of Mori in Japan. Continued experiments helped scientists determine that "fat-soluble factor A," or vitamin A, is colorless, but often present in foods containing beta-carotene, which is yellow. In the 1930s, researchers determined that colorless vitamin A is formed by the conversion of yellow beta-carotenes in the intestinal mucosa of animals and humans.

A number of brilliant scientists labored to elucidate the role of vitamin A in vision, beginning in 1877 with a German, W. Kuhne, who discovered that the purple retinas from dark-adapted frogs turned yellow when exposed to light. The purple color is then restored in a complex biochemical cycle involving vitamin A, and it is this process that makes vision possible. Other scientists demonstrated the role of vitamin A in cell differentiation, bone development, reproduction, hormone production and immune system function.

Due to the outstanding scientific work of these and many other researchers, the administration of cod liver oil to growing children—a tradition found among Arctic peoples such as the Scandinavians and Eskimos—became standard practice until after the Second World War. We can credit the widespread use of cod liver oil—given to reluctant children in schools, in refugee camps, at doctors' offices and even at Sunday school—to the decline in deaths and side effects from measles. Early advertisements for cod liver oil recognized its role in supporting robust growth, strong teeth and strong bones in children, as well as in protecting them against infectious disease.

Ironically, while Americans have stopped giving cod liver oil to their children, or even feeding them butter, whole milk and eggs, programs to administer vitamin A to children in Africa and Asia have had astonishing success in preventing blindness and infectious disease. This vitamin A treatment program was the brainchild of Alfred Sommer, an ophthalmologist at Johns Hopkins University, whose work on vitamin A in the 1970s and 1980s, which showed

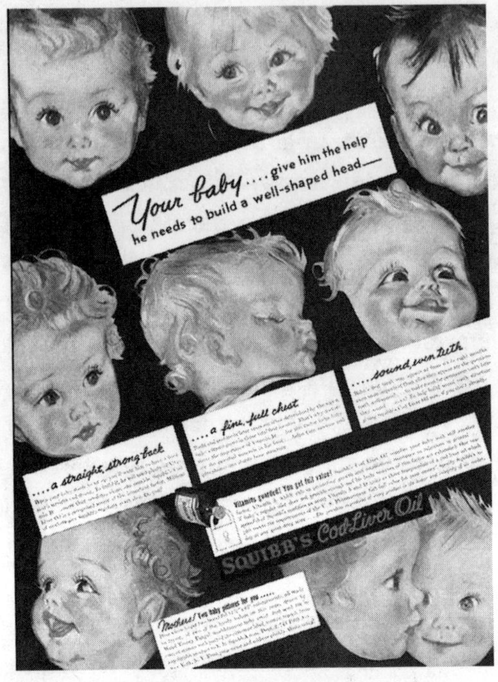

Ad for Squibb's cod liver oil: "Your baby... give him the help he needs to build a well-shaped head–a straight, strong back... a fine, full chest... sound, even teeth... daily use is important." Until after the Second World War, the medical profession recognized the importance of vitamin A in cod liver oil for optimal growth and development.

wonderful effects of vitamin A supplementation in Indonesia and Nepal, led him to lobby for an international supplementation program.

In recent decades, much vitamin A research has focused on its role in preventing cancer, and its use in combination with nontoxic therapies in the treatment of cancer. Unfortunately, few if any practicing oncologists today recognize the anticarcinogenic properties of vitamin A. Perhaps the most tragic example is Dr. Max Gerson, who treated many cases of terminal cancer with excellent results using raw liver juice, a rich source of vitamin A. In 1946, he testified before a U.S. congressional committee on the success of his treatment, but it was subsequently ignored.[3] In 1973, Dr. Kanematsu Sugiura of the Sloan Kettering Institute published the results of studies on mammary tumors in mice using high doses of vitamin A and a derivative of apricot seeds called laetrile. He observed complete regression of all the tumors in a total of five mice. The final report noted that "Dr. Sugiura has never observed complete regression of these tumors in all his cosmic experience with other chemotherapeutic agents." Nevertheless, just a few months later, spokesmen for Sloan Kettering flatly denied any value in the therapy.[4]

While the ongoing research into vitamin A and its effects is a boon to children and adults throughout the world, modern food processing conglomerates do not act on this knowledge. The food processing industry would rather use cheap vegetable oils than expensive animal fats. Some vegetable oils contain carotenes, but they do not contain true vitamin A. Yet healthy eating advocates continue to demonize natural "solid fat" sources of vitamin A, ignoring our cultural history and scientific understanding of its benefits.

UNFORTUNATELY, THE VAST MAJORITY OF popular books on nutrition insist that humans can obtain vitamin A from fruits and vegetables. Even worse, FDA regulations allow food processors to label carotenes as vitamin A. Just look at any can of tomatoes—the label clearly says it contains vitamin A, even though the only source of true vitamin A in the tomatoes comes from microscopic insect parts. The food industry, and the low-fat school of nutrition that the industry has spawned, benefit greatly from the fact that the public has only vague notions about vitamin A and where it occurs naturally.

Under optimal conditions, humans can indeed convert carotenes to vitamin A. This biochemical process occurs in the upper intestinal tract by the action of bile salts and fat-splitting enzymes. Of the entire family of carotenes, beta-carotene, found in carrots and many other fruits and vegetables, is most easily converted. Early studies indicated an equivalency of four to one of beta-carotene to retinol. In other words, four units of beta-carotene were needed to produce one unit of vitamin A. This ratio was later revised to six to one, and recent research suggests an even higher ratio.[5] This means that you have to eat an awful lot of vegetables and fruits to obtain even the daily minimal requirements of vitamin A, assuming optimal conversion.

But the transformation of carotene to vitamin A is rarely optimal. Diabetics and those with poor thyroid function, a group that could well include at least half the adult U.S. population, cannot make the conversion. Children make the conversion very poorly and infants not at all—they must obtain their precious stores of vitamin A from animal fats[6]—yet today a low-fat diet is recommended for children. Strenuous physical exercise, excessive consumption of alcohol, excessive consumption of iron (especially from "fortified" white flour and breakfast cereal), use of a number of popular drugs, excessive consumption of polyunsaturated fatty acids, zinc deficiency and even cold weather can hinder the conversion of carotenes to vitamin A,[7] as does the low-fat diet.

Carotenes are converted by the action of bile salts, and very little bile reaches the intestine when a meal is low in fat. The epicure who puts butter on his vegetables and adds cream to his vegetable soup is wiser than he knows. Butterfat stimulates the secretion of bile needed to convert carotenes into vitamin A, and at the same time supplies easily absorbed true vitamin A. Polyunsaturated oils also stimulate the secretion of bile salts but may cause rapid destruction of easily oxidized carotenes.[8]

Humans can only obtain sufficient, usable vitamin A from the fats and organ meats of land and sea animals. Depending on carotenes for vitamin A forces the body to call on large reserves of enzymes to make the conversion. In their fascinating book *Nutrition and Evolution*, Michael Crawford and David Marsh note that in animals, "If any function can be delegated to another organism it leaves the disk space free to perform some new function or to perform an old one better." For example, cats do not synthesize vitamin A from carotenes. "If they had to synthesize their own vitamin A... it would take up a significant amount of their disk space."[9] Cats get vitamin A from their prey, whose ability to synthesize vitamin A from carotenes compromises other functions, such as night vision and quickness of movement. While medical orthodoxy claims that consumption of large amounts of carotenes has no downside, it is possible that dependence on carotenes for vitamin A, even in those who are good converters, compromises other biochemical functions in subtle ways.*

Studies led by the Agricultural Research Service during the past five years have found

* What about the notion that eating carrots can improve eyesight? This was actually a piece of propaganda during the Second World War. The British did not want the Germans to know that they had developed advanced radar techniques, so they floated the rumor that British pilots were eating lots of carrots in order to be able to see German planes at night![a]

significant differences in beta-carotene uptake and conversion by physically similar volunteers. About half of the forty-five volunteers participating in one study didn't take up much beta-carotene at all, and about half of the volunteers didn't form much vitamin A from the beta-carotene they did absorb.[10] Similar results were obtained by researchers at the USDA Western Human Nutrition Research Center, who found that only about half those studied converted significant amounts of beta-carotene.[11] They also noted that the vitamin A activity of beta-carotene is surprisingly low in women.

The enzyme responsible for the conversion of beta-carotene to vitamin A is called beta-carotene 15, 15'-monoxgenase (BCOM1). Scientists from Newcastle University have found that almost 50 percent of females have a genetic variation that reduces greatly levels of BCOM and their ability to convert beta-carotene. "Vitamin A is incredibly important," notes Dr. Georg Lietz, who participated in the study. "It boosts our immune system and reduces the risk of inflammation such as that associated with chest infections. What our research shows is that many women are simply not getting enough of this vital nutrient because their bodies are not able to convert the beta-carotene... Worryingly, younger women are at particular risk," said Leitz. "The older generations tend to eat more eggs, milk and liver, which are naturally rich in vitamin A, whereas the health-conscious youngsters on low-fat diets are relying heavily on the beta-carotene form of the nutrient."[12]

Carotenes from plant foods not only fail to meet our requirements for vitamin A, but may also reduce the effectiveness of true vitamin A. A team of researchers from Ohio State University has found that beta-carotene molecules can block certain actions of the true vitamin A.[13] According to head researcher Earl Harrison, "These materials definitely have anti-vitamin-A properties, and they could basically disrupt or at least affect the whole body metabolism and action of vitamin A." The discovery could explain why previous clinical trials have found that people who supplemented with beta-carotene had a higher incidence of lung cancer than participants who took no beta-carotene.[14] Because vitamin A provides its health benefits by activating hundreds of genes, compounds contained in beta-carotene supplements could lower the activity of vitamin A. Says Harrison, "Too much beta-carotene could paradoxically result in too little vitamin A."[15]

IT IS THEREFORE VERY UNWISE to depend on plant sources for vitamin A. This vital nutrient is needed for so many key bodily functions: it supports the growth and repair of body tissues, it helps protect mucous membranes of the mouth, nose, throat and lungs; it prompts the secretion of gastric juices necessary for proper digestion of protein; it helps build strong bones and teeth and supports the formation of rich blood; it is essential for good eyesight; it aids in the production of RNA; and contributes to the health of the immune system. Your health is at risk if you're not getting enough.

Vitamin A is also involved in the conversion of cholesterol into sex hormones—estrogen, testosterone, progesterone, DHEA and many others.[16] Without it, expect infertility, erectile dysfunction and problems of endocrine disruption, such as fibroid tumors and endometriosis. In one study, vitamin A and iron given to boys of short stature was just as effective as testosterone supplements in inducing growth.[17] Various adrenal hormones that regulate the uptake of minerals, blood pressure and blood sugar levels also require vitamin A, as do the corticoid hormones that we need for healing and dealing with stress.[18] Without plentiful vitamin A in the diet, we cannot heal properly; instead we must resort to alternatives like synthetic steroids, such as prednisone—with all their side effects—to resolve inflammation and manage pain. When we are under stress, we need even more vitamin A, and when vitamin A is lacking, every little thing can be stressful. The "solid," vitamin A–containing saturated fats in butter support the efficient conversion of cholesterol into these vital hormones.

Vitamin A stores can rapidly deplete during exercise, fever, exposure to cold and periods of stress.[19] Vitamin A is especially important for expectant mothers. Deficiency during pregnancy can result in offspring with eye defects, displaced kidneys, harelip, cleft palate and abnormalities of the heart and larger blood vessels.

Foods high in vitamin A are especially important for diabetics and those suffering from thyroid conditions. In fact, the thyroid gland requires more vitamin A than any of the other glands, and cannot form thyroid hormones without it.[20] A diet rich in vitamin A will help prevent diabetes, and will protect those with diabetes from degenerative conditions associated with the disease, such as difficulty healing and deterioration of the retina and kidneys.[21]

Weston A. Price considered the fat-soluble vitamins, especially vitamin A, to be the catalysts on which all other biological processes depend.[22] Efficient mineral uptake and utilization of water-soluble vitamins require sufficient vitamin A in the diet. Vitamin A supports the assimilation of iron, for example, and helps prevent anemia.[23] Price's research demonstrated that generous amounts of vitamin A ensure healthy reproduction and offspring with attractive wide faces, straight teeth and strong sturdy bodies. He discovered that healthy nonindustrialized peoples especially valued vitamin A–rich foods for growing children and pregnant mothers. The tenfold disparity that Price discovered between primitive diets and the American diet in the 1940s is almost certainly greater today, as Americans have forsworn butter and cod liver oil for empty, processed polyunsaturates.

Vitamin A deficiencies are widespread in Third World communities that have come into contact with the West. They contribute to high infant mortality, blindness, stunting, bone deformities and susceptibility to infection.[24] These deficiencies occur even in communities that have access to plentiful carotenes in vegetables and fruits. As described by Price, a scarcity of good-quality dairy products, a rejection of organ meats as old-fashioned or unhealthful and a substitution of vegetable oil for animal fat in cooking all contribute to the physical degeneration and suffering in many developing nations that have adopted a Western diet high in processed foods.

Supplies of vitamin A are so vital to the body that humans are able to store large quantities of it in the liver and other organs. Thus it is possible for an adult to subsist on a fat-free diet for a considerable period of time before overt symptoms of deficiency appear. But during times of stress, vitamin A stores are rapidly depleted. Strenuous physical exercise, periods of physical growth, pregnancy, lactation and infection are stresses that quickly deplete vitamin A stores. Children with measles rapidly use up vitamin A, which can result in seizures or irreversible blindness.

Women need time to recover from the stress of pregnancy and to rebuild vitamin stores, especially stores of vitamin A. Dr. Price reported that throughout the South Seas and Africa, the villagers considered it shameful to have a child more than once every three years. This belief finds validation in modern science. In a study that gathered research from over two million pregnancies in eighteen different countries, researchers found that both mothers and their offspring had better health outcomes when births were spaced three to five years apart.[25]

One aspect of vitamin A that deserves more emphasis is its role in protein utilization. Ironically, high-protein, low-fat diets—the kind promoted by many modern diet gurus—are especially dangerous because protein consumption rapidly depletes vitamin A stores.[26] Children brought up on high-protein, low-fat diets often experience rapid growth. The results—tall, myopic, lanky individuals with crowded teeth and poor posture, a kind of Ichabod Crane syndrome—are a fixture in America.[27] Growing children actually benefit from a diet that contains considerably more calories from fat than from protein. A high-fat diet that is rich in vitamin A will result in steady, even growth, a sturdy physique and high immunity to illness.

High-protein, low-fat diets can even cause blindness, as occurred once in Guatemala where large amounts of instant nonfat dry milk were donated in a food relief program.*[28] Many of the people who consumed the dried milk went blind from vitamin A depletion. Historically, cultures around the world instinctively understood the connection between vitamin A and protein, which is why they never ate lean meat and always consumed the organ meats of the animals that served them for food.[29]

The great discrepancy between what science has discovered about vitamin A and what nutrition writers promote in the popular press contributes to awkward moments. The *New York Times* has been a strong advocate for low-fat diets, even for children, yet a 1992 *New York Times* article on vitamin A noted that vitamin A–rich foods like liver, egg yolk, butter and cream confer resistance to infectious diseases in children and prevent cancer in adults.[30] A 1994 *Washington Post* article hailed vitamin A as "cheap and effective, with wonders still being (re)discovered," noting studies which found that vitamin A supplements help prevent infant mortality in Third World countries, protect measles victims from complications and prevent mother-to-child transmission of the HIV virus.[31] The article lists butter, egg yolks and liver as important sources of vitamin A, but claims, unfortunately, that carotenes from vegetables are "equally important."

Even worse than the claim that plant foods can provide vitamin A are warnings that vitamin A may be toxic in more than the minuscule RDA-recommended amounts. In fact, so great is the propaganda against the vitamin that obstetricians and pediatricians are now warning pregnant women to avoid foods containing vitamin A, like liver.

---

* According to researcher NW Solomans, government reports on blindness from nonfat dry milk were declared secret and stored in a locked file cabinet.

Recently an "expert" panel recommended lowering the RDA (recommended daily allowance) for vitamin A from 5,000 IU daily to about 2,500 IU and has set an upper limit of about 10,000 IUs for women. The panel was headed by Dr. Robert Russell of Tufts University, who warned that intake over the "upper limit" may cause irreversible liver damage and birth defects—a surprising statement in view of the fact that just a few decades ago pregnant women were routinely advised to take cod liver oil daily and eat liver at least one time per week. One tablespoon of cod liver oil contains at least 15,000 IU and one serving of liver can contain up to 40,000 IU vitamin A. Russell epitomizes the establishment view when he insists that vitamin A requirements can be met with one-half cup of carrots daily.[32]

The anti–vitamin A campaign for pregnant women began in 1995 with the publication of a Boston University School of Medicine study in the *New England Journal of Medicine*.[33] "Teratogenicity of High Vitamin A Intake," by Kenneth J. Rothman and his colleagues. The study correlates vitamin A consumption among more than twenty-two thousand pregnant women with birth defects occurring in subsequent offspring. The study received extensive press coverage in the same publications that had earlier extolled the benefits of vitamin A. "Study Links Excess Vitamin A and Birth Defects" by Jane Brody appeared on the front page of the *New York Times* on October 7, 1995; on November 24, 1995, the *Washington Times* reported: "High Doses of Vitamin A Linked to Babies' Brain Defects."

When a single study receives front-page coverage, it's important to take a closer look, especially as earlier research points to the importance of vitamin A in *preventing* birth defects. In fact, the defects listed as increasing with increased vitamin A dosage—cleft lip, cleft palate, hydrocephalus and major heart malformations—are also defects of vitamin A *deficiency*.

In the study, researchers asked over twenty-two thousand women to respond to questionnaires about their eating habits and supplement intake before and during pregnancy. Food questionnaires are notoriously inaccurate, but their responses were used to determine vitamin A status. As reported in the newspapers, researchers found that cranial-neural-crest defects increased with increased dosages of vitamin A; what the papers did not report was the fact that in this study, neural tube defects *decreased* with increased vitamin A consumption, and that no trend was apparent with musculoskeletal, urogenital or other defects. The trend was much less pronounced, and less statistically significant, when cranial-neural-crest defects were correlated with vitamin A consumption from food alone.

The study is compromised by a number of flaws. Vitamin A status was assessed by the inaccurate method of recall and food questionnaires; and no blood tests were taken to determine the actual usable vitamin A status of the mothers. Researchers did not weight birth defects according to severity; thus we do not know whether the defects of babies born to mothers taking high doses of vitamin A were serious or minor compared to those of mothers taking lower amounts.

The most serious flaw was that researchers failed to distinguish between manufactured vitamin A in the form of retinol, found in supplements and added to fabricated foods, and natural vitamin A complex, present with numerous cofactors, from vitamin A–containing foods. Typically, synthetic vitamins are less biologically active, hence less effective, than naturally occurring vitamins. This is especially true of the fat-soluble vitamins like vitamin A, because these tend to be more complex molecules, with numerous double bonds and a multiplicity of forms. Natural vitamin A occurs as a mixture of various isomers, aldehydes, esters, acids and alcohols. Pure retinoic acid, a metabolite of vitamin A used to treat adult acne, is well known to cause birth defects.

The most serious problem with the Rothman study is the fact that it conflicts with other studies on vitamin A during pregnancy. A study carried out in Rome, Italy, found *no* congenital malformations among one hundred twenty infants exposed to more than 50,000 IU of vitamin A per day.[34] A study from Switzerland looked at blood levels of vitamin A in pregnant women and found that a dose of 30,000 IU per day resulted in blood levels that had *no* association with birth defects.[35]

Warnings against vitamin A as a cause of birth defects are aimed at pregnant women; warnings that vitamin A is generally toxic are aimed at other adults. The following statement, posted at the University of Maryland Medical Center website, is typical of this orthodox medical view: "Vitamin A can be very toxic when taken in high-dose supplements for long periods of time and can affect almost every part of the body, including eyes, bones, blood, skin, central nervous system, liver, and genital and urinary tracts. Symptoms include dizziness, nausea, vomiting, headache, skin damage, mental disturbances and, in women, infrequent periods. Severe toxicity can cause blindness and may even be life-threatening. Liver damage can occur in children who take RDA-approved adult levels over prolonged periods of time or in adults who take as little as five times the RDA-approved amount for seven to ten years. In children, chronic overdose can cause fluid on the brain and other symptoms similar to those in adults... High consumption of vitamin A may also increase the risk of gastric cancer and the risk of osteoporosis and fractures in women."[36]

The *Merck Manual* describes vitamin A toxicity in less hysterical terms. Acute vitamin A poisoning can occur in children after taking a single dose of synthetic vitamin A in the range of 300,000 IU or a daily dosage of 60,000 IU for a few weeks. Two fatalities have been reported from acute vitamin A poisoning in children, which manifests as increased intracranial pressure and vomiting. For the vast majority, however, recovery after discontinuation is "spontaneous, with no residual damage."

In adults, according to the *Merck Manual*, vitamin A toxicity has been reported in Arctic explorers who developed drowsiness, irritability, headaches and vomiting, with subsequent peeling of the skin, within a few hours of ingesting several million units of vitamin A from polar bear or seal liver.* Again, these symptoms cleared up with discontinuation of the vitamin A–rich food. Other than this

* Apparently polar bear liver contains a toxin at certain times of the year, so the symptoms reported in Arctic explorers may not be due to large amounts of vitamin A. Nevertheless, all students in university nutrition courses get warnings about the toxicity of polar bear liver.

unusual example, however, only vitamin A from "megavitamin tablets containing vitamin A... when taken for a long time" has induced acute toxicity, that is, 100,000 IU synthetic vitamin A per day taken for many months.

Unless you are an Arctic explorer, it is virtually impossible to develop vitamin A toxicity from food. The putative toxic dose of 100,000 IU per day would be contained in three to six tablespoons of cod liver oil, two-and-one-half 100-gram servings of duck liver, about three 100-gram servings of beef liver, seven pounds of butter or three hundred nine egg yolks. Even synthetic vitamin A is not toxic when given as a single large dose or in small amounts on a daily basis. Children in impoverished areas of the world are routinely given two 100,000-unit doses of retinol per year for infants and two 200,000-unit doses for children over twelve months.

While scientists in America are creating confusion and fear about vitamin A, WHO and UNICEF vitamin A distribution programs in Africa and Asia have been extremely successful in reducing blindness and death among both children and adults. Vitamin A is more cost effective in saving lives and preventing suffering than immunizations and drugs, and it can be administered with two-cent capsules. The program does not undermine traditional cultures or foodways and is easily carried out on the village level. By some estimates, vitamin A supplementation programs in Third World countries save one million lives per year.[37]

The tragedy is that misplaced concern about vitamin A toxicity has led doctors to advise pregnant women to avoid foods containing vitamin A, and parents to avoid giving cod liver oil and liver to their babies. Yet early books on the dietary needs of pregnant women and infants recommended generous doses of cod liver oil and frequent liver consumption for pregnant women and two teaspoons of cod liver oil per day for babies three months and older.

Research on vitamin A is ongoing and the list of vitamin A miracles continues to grow: vitamin A supplements help children in Africa and Asia grow faster and attain better iron status; and vitamin A supplements have reduced the incidence of malaria in Papua New Guinea. Vitamin A plays a vital regulating role in the immune system; vitamin A deficiency leads to a loss of ciliated cells in the lung, an important first-line defense against pathogens; vitamin A promotes mucin secretion and microvilli formation by mucosa, including the gastrointestinal tract mucosa; vitamin A regulates T-cell production (needed for immunity) and apoptosis (programmed cell death).[38]

A study in Malawi, Africa, found that mothers with the highest levels of vitamin A had an HIV transmission rate of just 7.2 percent[39]; treatment with megadoses of vitamin A (100,000 IU per day) resulted in a 92 percent cure rate of menorrhagia (excessive menstrual bleeding) at Johannesburg General Hospital in South Africa[40]; vitamin A can be helpful in the treatment of psoriasis[41]; and in stroke victims, those with high levels of vitamin A (and E) are more likely to recover without damage.[42]

Vitamin A protects against lung and bladder cancers in men[43]; fourteen out of twenty patients with prostate cancer achieved total remission and five achieved partial remission using vitamin A as part of a natural cancer therapy in Germany[44]; vitamin A was used successfully to combat tropical ulcers in Uganda[45]; vitamin A has also been used successfully to treat a skin condition called Kyrle's disease[46]; and elderly persons who consume adequate vitamin A are less prone to leg ulcers.[47]

The list continues: vitamin A inhibits the effects of phytic acid and increases absorption of iron from whole wheat (which is why it is a good idea to put butter on your bread)[48]; vitamin A supplementation increases absorption of iron and folic acid in women in Bangladesh[49]; use of vitamin A supplements reduces the risk of cataracts[50]; and a study of healthy centenarians found that these long-lived peoples were characterized by high levels of vitamins A and E in the bloodstream.[51]

In 2010, researchers discovered that vitamin A plays a role in the synthesis of ATP, the fuel in the mitochondria of our cells. When vitamin A is deficient, energy production reduces by 30 percent. "These results illuminate a hitherto unsuspected role of vitamin A in mitochondrial bioenergetics of mammals, acting as a nutritional sensor," said the researchers. "As such, retinol is of fundamental importance for energy homeostasis. The data provide a mechanistic explanation to the nearly one-hundred-year-old question of why vitamin A deficiency causes so many pathologies that are independent of retinoic acid action."[52]

Vitamin A not only supports good vision, but also good hearing. For example, a French study from as early as 1823 found that hearing levels were better among those who consumed the most vitamin A and also vitamin B_{12} from various foods, including red meat. A 1984 European study reported a five-to-fifteen-decibel improvement in patients with age-related hearing loss when given vitamins A and E. Other researchers reported that vitamin A deficiency results in a decline in the number of sensory cells in the nose, tongue and inner ear. A 1993 study reported in *Science* found that vitamin A can stimulate the regeneration of mammalian auditory hair cells. In 2009, Japanese researchers found that adults with the highest blood serum levels of vitamin A and carotenoids have the lowest risk for hearing loss. And, in 2014, researchers determined that vitamin A deficiency during pregnancy, especially during the early stages of fetal development, "may predispose offspring to inner ear malformations and sensorial hearing loss."[53]

Vitamin A is critical for normal reproduction in both males and females. In vitamin A deficiency, the male reproductive organs develop pathological tissue and sperm don't develop; and in severely vitamin A–deficient female rats, embryos do not form.[54] Fertility clinics in the United States are filled with couples desperate to get pregnant. How many of them receive advice to consume a vitamin A–rich diet before trying more expensive and invasive measures?

Finally, vitamin A plays an important role in setting the body's circadian rhythm and preventing insomnia. Light helps vitamin A bind to proteins in the rods and cones of the eye, thus allowing sight. It also helps vitamin A bind to a protein called melanopsin, needed for the conversion of serotonin to melatonin, the hormone that helps us get to sleep and sleep soundly throughout the night.[55]

As in America, British consumers get the same mixed messages about vitamin A. Researchers at Cardiff University looked at the effect of cod liver oil on cartilage health in thirty-one patients on a National Health Service waiting list for total knee joint replacement surgery. Half were given high-vitamin cod liver oil providing about 2,400 IU of vitamin A daily. At the time of surgery, samples of cartilage and joint tissue were taken from the knee joint and subjected to analysis. Markers for cartilage damage were significantly reduced in those taking cod liver oil. According to the researchers, "The data suggests that cod liver oil has a dual mode of action, potentially slowing down the cartilage degeneration inherent in osteoarthritis and also reducing factors that cause pain and inflammation."[56]

Meanwhile, other British officials are warning against vitamin A overdose, claiming that vitamin A from foods like liver can weaken the bones. Surveys found that many Britons get "too much" vitamin A by eating liver. A single 100-gram serving of liver can contain up to 32,000 IU vitamin A, a dose that exceeds the puny 2,400 IU maximum recommended amount by as much as fifteen-fold. Yet today we eat far less liver than in former times, and pregnant women were formerly encouraged to eat liver several times per week. The confusion has led health officials to consider whether to issue an advisory against eating liver to the general public—pregnant women already get warned by their doctors against eating this highly nutritious superfood.[57]

A frequent warning against vitamin A correlates vitamin A consumption with weak bones. Establishment nutritionists can indeed cite studies showing a connection between levels of vitamin A in the bloodstream and the risk of fractured bones. For example, a study of more than twenty-three hundred middle-aged Swedish men found that risk of any type of fracture was 64 percent higher in those with the most vitamin A in the blood. For hip fractures, the risk was increased by 147 percent.[58] But the total number of fractures over thirty years was only two hundred sixty-six—about three fractures per thousand men per year—so the differences in fracture occurrence for various groups are actually very small. These figures may simply reflect the fact that people who consume lots of vitamin A are more physically active and more likely to end up in situations in which fractures occur—such as skiing. A study of more appropriate design looked at eighty healthy men ages eighteen to fifty-eight years who were randomly assigned to receive 25,000 IU per day of vitamin A or a placebo for six weeks. Compared with the placebo group, there was no significant change in the vitamin A group in various markers of bone formation and resorption.[59] A 2005 study of elderly women found no evidence of any skeletal harm associated with vitamin A intake.[60] In animal studies only enormous doses of vitamin A—equivalent to 7 million IU per day—induce bone disease, whereas amounts on the order of 100,000 IU per day do not affect bone health.

If there is a connection of vitamin A with poor bone health, the explanation lies in the fact that vitamins A and D work together—large doses of vitamin A in diets that provide little vitamin D can lead to further D deficiency with consequent effects on the bones. Fortunately, if you are eating nutrient-dense animal foods, you will be taking in both vitamins—A and D.

With so many miracles from vitamin A, one must question the motivation of those who pepper the Internet with warnings that vitamin A is toxic. Would a population nourishing itself on vitamin A–rich foods be filling hospital beds, populating lucrative nursing homes and swallowing dozens of pharmaceutical pills per day?

IN CONTRAST TO VITAMIN A, vitamin D today stands at the top of the vitamin hit parade, with many practitioners recommending large amounts of vitamin D from supplements—and offering few warnings about toxicity.

As vitamin A is associated with proper eyesight, so vitamin D is associated with bone health. Vitamin D—either from sunlight or food—plus adequate dietary calcium is necessary for prevention of rickets in children and osteomalacia (soft bones) in adults. Scientists consider overt rickets—with its characteristic symptom of bowed legs—a disease of the past in Western countries, solved with the addition of vitamin D to milk; however, subclinical rickets, characterized by easily fractured skull and bones, may be more common than realized, manifesting as shaken baby syndrome.[61]

American researchers Elmer V. McCollum and Marguerite Davis are credited with the discovery of vitamin D. In the early 1920s, the British doctor Edward Mellanby noticed that dogs fed cod liver oil did not develop rickets and thus concluded that vitamin A, or a closely associated factor, could prevent the disease. In 1922, McCollum took the study one step further, testing modified cod liver oil in which the vitamin A had been destroyed.[62] The modified oil cured the sick dogs as well, so McCollum concluded the factor in cod liver oil that cured rickets was distinct from vitamin A. He called it vitamin D, the next letter in line after the discovery of vitamins A, B and C.

In 1925, researchers found that when a cholesterol precursor in the skin (7-dehydrocholesterol) is irradiated with light, a form of vitamin D is produced (now known as D_3). Later researchers discovered that vitamin D has the structure of a sterol, very similar to cholesterol, with four ring structures, but with one of them opened.

In 1923, American biochemist Harry Steenbock at the University of Wisconsin demonstrated that irradiation by ultraviolet light increased the vitamin D content of foods and other organic materials. After irradiating rodent food, Steenbock discovered the rodents were cured of rickets. The form of vitamin D produced by irradiating yeast and other plant materials is D_2.

In 1971–1972, scientists elucidated the further metabolism of vitamin D to its active forms. In the liver, vitamin D is converted to calcidiol, and calcidiol is then converted by the kidneys to calcitriol, the biologically active form of vitamin D. Since then, scientists have cataloged over nine hundred forms of vitamin D.[63] Calcitriol circulates as a hormone in the blood, regulating the concentration of calcium and phosphate in the bloodstream and promoting—among many other roles—the healthy growth and remodeling of bone.

In addition to preventing rickets and osteomalacia, vitamin D seems to protect against many other conditions. These include hypocalcemia (low levels of calcium in the blood); convulsions, tetany and heart failure in newborns; osteoporosis and arthritis; heart disease and high blood pressure; cancer; chronic pain; depression and mental illness; muscular weakness; radiation poisoning; and diabetes and other autoimmune disorders. A systematic review of clinical studies shows a possible association between low vitamin D levels, cognitive impairment and a higher risk of developing Alzheimer's disease.[64] Deficiency has been linked to increased risk of viral infections, including HIV and influenza.[65] Low levels of vitamin D in pregnancy are associated with gestational diabetes, preeclampsia and low-birth-weight babies.[66]

Researchers at the Harvard Medical School have discovered that low vitamin D is associated with an increased risk of heart disease. In one study, people with levels of vitamin D below 15 ng/ml had twice the risk of heart attack, heart failure and stroke compared to those with higher levels.[67] German scientists have discovered that levels of the vitamin are up to 50 percent lower in the blood of patients with chronic heart failure.[68]

In adults, vitamin D leads to mood improvements and protects against depression.[69] Vitamin D may protect against multiple sclerosis.[70] And researchers at Harvard University's School of Public Health found that low intakes of vitamin D were linked with the highest levels of lead accumulation in bones.[71]

Studies like these have propelled vitamin D to the top of the vitamin hit parade and generated enthusiasm among health-conscious consumers. But in reality, the world of vitamin D research is roiling in contradiction and controversy. For example, what is optimal daily vitamin D intake? Recommendations range from the conservative U.S. Institute of Medicine estimate of 200 IU per day for adults under fifty to amounts as high as 10,000 IU. Some leading vitamin D researchers recommend 3,000 to 4,000 IU per day as both necessary and safe.[72] Is vitamin D relatively harmless, or "the most toxic of all vitamins" as some media outlets claim?[73] And what is the optimal serum vitamin D level? Estimates range from 20 ng/ml (National Institutes of Health) to as high as 75 ng/ml.*[74] Another question: what is the best way to get our vitamin D—sunlight, food or supplements?

And then there is the controversy regarding vitamin D_2 or egosterol (made from irradiating yeast with ultraviolet light) versus vitamin D_3 or cholecalciferol (the most common form, mostly found in animal fats). Most textbooks state that these two forms are equivalent. Vitamin D_2 is much easier and less expensive to manufacture than D_3, and the industry can indeed point to studies showing that it has biological effects. For example, a 2008 study showed that administration of vitamin D_2 plus calcium to elderly patients resulted in a 23 percent reduction of the risk of falling.[75] The industry can also point to a number of studies indicating that D_2 is "just as easily absorbed"—just as able to raise serum levels—as D_3. However, research shows that vitamin D_3 is much more effective than vitamin D_2 at raising levels of serum calcidiol—a much more active form of vitamin D.[76]

Synthetic vitamin D_2 is not only less effective than D_3, but it also may be potentially harmful. As early as 1937, scientists expressed concern about the possible toxicity of D_2. In that year, Wayne Brehm presented before the Ohio State Medical Association the results of an experiment comparing the effects of the administration of cod liver oil with that of vitamin D_2 to more than five hundred pregnant women. Vitamin D_2, especially in conjunction with calcium, produced extensive abnormal calcification of the placenta, in one case extending into the uterine wall, and in three cases producing kidney stones within the developing fetus. Cod liver oil, by contrast,

* While many scientists promoting vitamin D supplementation claim that levels of vitamin D [in the form of 25(OH)D] in the blood should be 50 ng/ml or above, the optimum level is probably in the range of 30–35 ng/ml.[a]

produced no more tissue calcification than seen in controls.[77] From these experiments it would seem reasonable to conclude that vitamin D_2 can cause toxic effects while vitamin D from cod liver oil is safe.*

Dr. E.W.H. Cruickshank's 1951 book *Food and Nutrition* describes an important experiment with chicks. Three groups of chicks were fed the same diet. The first group received no vitamin D at all; the second group got D_2; the third group received a natural vitamin D preparation made from cod liver oil. The chicks receiving no vitamin D gained 259 grams; those receiving the synthetic vitamin D_2 gained 346 grams; and those that had the benefit of the natural vitamin D gained 399 grams. The most important finding was this: of the chicks receiving no vitamin D, 60 percent died; of the chicks receiving synthetic vitamin D, 50 percent died; while in the natural vitamin D group, no chicks died.

Giving D_3 as a supplement (not as it naturally occurs in cod liver oil) can cause soft tissue calcification as well. An excess of vitamin D_3 results in abnormally high blood concentrations of calcium, which can cause overcalcification of the bones and also of the soft tissues, such as the heart and kidneys. In addition, it can result in hypertension.[78] Even overexposure to sunlight is associated with a condition linked to too much vitamin D: kidney stones.[79] Other recent papers suggest additional dangers of taking vitamin D. For example, researchers found that vitamin D supplementation can inhibit gene expression and lead to autoimmune disease.[80] "We have found that vitamin D supplementation, even at levels many consider desirable, interferes with recovery in these patients," said J. C. Waterhouse, PhD, executive director of Autoimmunity Research, Inc. Another report blames brain lesions on vitamin D.[81] A recent paper presented data indicating that the bioactivity of natural vitamin D in food is up to five times higher compared to vitamin D_3 from supplements.†[82]

American research dating back to 1937 shows us that vitamin A protects us against vitamin D toxicity.[83] Researchers fed rats various concentrations of vitamin A with toxic doses of vitamin D in various forms. The doses of vitamin D given to the animals were 4,000 IU per day or greater, which is the body-weight-adjusted equivalent of a typical human consuming over 5,000,000 IU per day. The researchers used both synthetic vitamin D_2 and concentrates of the liver oils of tuna, cod, sea bass and halibut. Although vitamin D_2 was most toxic, massive doses of all forms of vitamin D with only low doses of vitamin A decreased growth and bone mineralization and increased calcification of the lungs, heart and kidneys, while vitamin A consistently protected against these effects in proportion to its dose.

Subsequent research has shown that vitamin A provides protection against skeletal defects, bone demineralization and soft tissue calcification induced in rats by large amounts of both vitamin D_2 and D_3.[84]

---

* Recent analyses of cod liver oil indicate that the major form of vitamin D is not actually D_3, but some other—and still obviously natural—form derived from D_3.[a]

† One explanation for the increased effectiveness of vitamin D from food is the matrix in which it occurs. Vitamin D occurs in foods that contain ample amounts of saturated fatty acids. Increasing levels of polyunsaturated and monounsaturated fatty acids in the diet decrease the binding of vitamin D to D-binding proteins, necessary to carry vitamin D in the blood, whereas saturated fatty acids do not have this effect.[a]

It seems that vitamin D requires vitamin A in order to function, and that high doses of vitamin D cause toxicity by depleting vitamin A stores. In 2006, a team of researchers from Spain and Germany published a report showing that 9-cis-retinoic acid, one of the hormonally active forms of vitamin A, is an essential factor for the full functioning of vitamin D.[85]

Vitamin A protects against calcification, so if high doses of vitamin D use up vitamin A, that leaves less vitamin A for other important processes, such as preventing the calcification of the kidneys or arteries. Likewise, taking vitamin A without vitamin D will call on reserves of vitamin D, leading to weakening of the bones. This is another explanation for why studies from Scandinavia—where the "vitamin D winter," the period when it is impossible to get vitamin D from sunlight, is long and where vitamin A is added to common foods like milk and cereal—show a correlation of vitamin A consumption and bone fractures.

The key takeaway is that we get vitamins A and D—two nutrients absolutely critical for good health—from high-fat animal foods. If we are eating a variety of these foods—egg yolks, animal fats and fatty fish for vitamin D, and butter, cream and organ meats for vitamin A—along with modest amounts of cod liver oil to ensure adequate supplies of both, we will have sufficient amounts and the right kind of balance to use vitamins A and D to the maximum effect and without side effects.

"HUMAN BRINGS CANNOT GET ADEQUATE vitamin D from food." This is the assertion of the Vitamin D Council and similar groups who claim that we must get it either from sunlight, from vitamin D added to foods like milk or from supplements. This dogma begs the question of how our preindustrial ancestors obtained this critical nutrient during "vitamin D winters," that is, periods of the year when the angle of the sun is too oblique for vitamin D production to occur, a period that lasts at least six months in temperate and Arctic zones. Even in warm months, humans like to cover themselves with clothing, and seek the shade or stay inside a dwelling during the hot part of the day. The fact is human beings have always obtained some, or even a large portion, of their vitamin D from food, or we would have died off long ago from vitamin D–deficiency diseases.

It is easy for proponents of vitamin D supplementation and fortification claim that we can't get vitamin D from food, because food data tables in fact do not show much vitamin D in food. Typical values given in food composition databases are as follows:

Food	**IU per 100 grams**
Cod liver oil	10,000 (500 per teaspoon)
Oily fish	759
Fortified cereals	333
Egg yolks	218 (37 per yolk)
Caviar	117
Butter	136
Cheese	110
Lard	102
Chicken liver	0

Source: U.S. Department of Agriculture Food Composition Databases

In 2015, the Weston A. Price Foundation had a number of foods tested for vitamin D content by two independent laboratories. One of the labs—which does considerable work for the USDA—gave very similar results (with results for some foods even lower), but the other lab gave significantly higher results:

Food	IU per 100 grams
Cod liver oil	10,000–33,000 (500–5,500 per teaspoon)
Conventional egg yolks	1,400 (77 per yolk)
Organic egg yolks	2,300 (127 per yolk)
Pastured egg yolks	2,700 (150 per yolk)
Caviar	7,000–12,000
Cheese	900–3,100
Chicken liver	5–700
Lard	0
Butter	0

Using a different method, this same lab gave even higher—considerably higher—results on several food samples analyzed in 2009:

Food	IU per 100 grams
Conventional egg yolks	9,240 (513 per yolk)
Pastured egg yolks	69,560 (3,864 per yolk)
Conventional lard	6,040 (857 per tablespoon)
Pastured lard	74,560 (10,500 IU per tablespoon)
Conventional butter	18,800 (2,667 per tablespoon)*
Pastured butter	6,560 (930 per tablespoon)
Caviar	116,480 (16,521 per tablespoon)

How could testing results be so different for the same foods? It turns out that vitamin D testing is very difficult. To get accurate results, the vitamin D must be extracted from the proteins or matrix in which it is bound, and different foods require different extraction methods; if the extraction is not performed with the right method, the resulting values may be low. Furthermore, the testing equipment often does not measure calcidiol, calcitriol and other forms of vitamin D and, if not calibrated correctly, will result in printout charts with overlapping peaks giving an underestimation of total vitamin D. For example, the type of vitamin D in butter is mostly the same type that is carried in the blood—calcidiol—and few if any labs specializing in measuring vitamin levels in food test for calcidiol.

Since government dogma insists that we can't get vitamin D from food, we can't discount the suspicion that lab certification organizations dictate testing procedures to give deliberately low results. What would happen if the public learned that egg yolks, especially egg yolks from pastured chickens, are powerhouses of vitamin D, or that just one tablespoon of lard could meet our vitamin D requirements better than dozens of capsules? Consumption of these foods would soar and sales of industrial substitutes would decline.

Several vitamin D researchers have expressed skepticism about the accuracy of laboratory tests for vitamin D. Esteemed vitamin D expert Hector DeLuca is especially outspoken in condemning laboratory analysis for determining the amount of active vitamin D in foods. Instead, these critics prefer the rat assay or "line" test, in which a vitamin D–containing substance is given to rats from which vitamin D has been withheld to induce rickets, and then after a fixed period, sacrificing the rats to ascertain the degree of healing in the bones. As early as 1929, these tests determined that cod liver oil had the highest antirachitic activity, followed by egg yolk from animals exposed to bright sunlight.† Most interesting, the early

* Higher levels of D in conventional butter (from confinement cows) compared to butter from pastured cows is likely due to the addition of vitamin D to feed rations.

† In 1931, these line tests found that cod liver oil was one hundred times more potent—more able to cure rickets—than vitamin D_2 from irradiated yeast.[a]

studies on vitamin D, which measured the antirachitic of various foods using the line test, found that butter and lard were both effective in curing rickets.[86] This means that these foods carry a form of vitamin D, even though standard food tests find low or nonexistent levels.

TAKING COD LIVER OIL SEEMS old-fashioned, like something from another era. But modern scientific literature provides a surprising number of studies on this ancient superfood—our best source of vitamins A and D—and almost all of them are positive.

Cod liver oil seems particularly beneficial for rheumatoid arthritis. Cod liver oil supplements were better than controls in relieving arthritis pain[87]; cod liver oil allows reduction of nonsteroidal anti-inflammatory drug dosage and improves chief clinical symptoms, reducing pain and morning joint stiffness[88]; and use of cod liver oil decreased occurrence of morning stiffness, swollen joints and pain intensity in patients suffering from rheumatoid arthritis.[89]

For strong bones, cod liver oil protects against greater bone turnover, bone loss and obesity in winter months.[90] One study found that cod liver oil supplementation was associated with a significantly lower risk of any fracture and no evidence to suggest any skeletal harm associated with increased vitamin A intake.[91] Subjects in Norway with food consumption habits that included frequent *mølje* meals (consisting of cod liver and fresh cod liver oil) during the winter sustained satisfactory vitamin D levels in their blood, in spite of the long "vitamin D winter."[92]

Diabetics can benefit from cod liver oil. Cod liver oil treatment in diabetic rats completely prevented endothelial deficiency and partly corrected several biochemical markers for cardiovascular disorders[93]; use of cod liver oil in mice played an important role in the prevention of diabetic nephropathy.[94]

Using data from the Norwegian Women and Cancer cohort study, researchers explored the relationship of supplement use and survival of cancer patients with solid tumors. They found that women who took cod liver oil were 44 percent less likely to die from cancer than those who did not take supplements. (Women who used supplements other than cod liver oil were 30 percent less likely to die.) Use of cod liver oil was also found associated with improved survival rates for patients with breast and colorectal cancer. Overall, consumption of cod liver oil for a year prior to diagnosis was associated with a 23 percent reduction in the risk of death in patients diagnosed with solid cancers.[95]

Cod liver oil offers excellent protection against coronary artery disease as well. One study looked at the effect of cod liver oil on the development and progression of coronary artery disease in swine.[96] The animals were subjected to coronary balloon abrasion and fed an atherogenic diet for eight months. Analysis of coronary artery sections revealed significantly less disease in the animals fed cod liver oil compared to controls. Furthermore, blood markers for heart disease were significantly reduced in the cod liver oil–fed swine. Blood markers were similarly reduced in swine fed cod liver oil according to a subsequent study.[97]

Regular use of cod liver oil is associated with fewer symptoms of depression in the general population[98]—good news to the 10 percent of the population relying on antidepressants to manage the condition.

Pregnant women receive warnings against cod liver oil. But according to one study, women who used liquid cod liver oil in early pregnancy gave birth to heavier (and therefore more robust) babies, even after adjusting for the length of gestation and other confounding factors.[99] Women using cod liver oil had significantly higher levels of docosahexaenoic acid (DHA) and eicosapentaenoic acid (EPA) in their breast milk[100] and maternal use of cod liver oil resulted in higher levels of fat-soluble vitamins in breast milk, especially vitamins E and A.[101] Children born to mothers who took cod liver oil during pregnancy and lactation scored higher on intelligence tests at age four compared with children whose mothers took corn oil.[102]

Cod liver oil is especially important for growing children, as vitamins A and D work together to support healthy, growing bones. And there are many other benefits. Children supplemented with cod liver oil had a decrease in upper respiratory tract infections and pediatric visits over time.[103] Use of cod liver oil in the first year of life was associated with a significantly lower risk of type 1 diabetes. Use of other vitamin D supplements during the first year of life and maternal use of cod liver oil or other vitamin D supplements during pregnancy were not associated with lower risk of type 1 diabetes.[104] Children prone to earaches (otitis media) receiving cod liver oil plus selenium needed lower amounts of antibiotics during supplementation compared to before supplementation.[105] In Arctic climates, supplemental cod liver oil during childhood may be protective against multiple sclerosis later in life.[106] Reduced breast cancer risks were associated with increasing sun exposure and cod liver oil use from ages ten to nineteen.[107]

Newspaper articles on long-lived people usually credit "good genes," as they did in a recent story on a family of eight brothers and sisters, ages seventy-nine to ninety-six, who have no history of heart attack, stroke, dementia or other diseases associated with getting old. Not one of them needs a cane. But is it good genes—or cod liver oil? "I don't even remember having a medicine cabinet. No, we didn't," says Helen Hurlburt. "Just molasses on bread and cod liver oil. That's about it," says her sister Agnes. "We never had junk food. We always cooked, and we ate together in the evening," says Helen.[108]

Miriam Tyler, of Timperley, UK, age one hundred, credits her longevity to "a spoonful of cod liver oil once a day, washed down with maluca honey."[109,*]

Cod liver oil plus real food starting in childhood and continuing into adulthood looks like the formula for optimal gene expression, meaning that we all have good genes, but often suboptimal expression of those genes due to poor nutrition.

IN 1945, DR. WESTON A. Price described "a new vitamin-like activator" needed to assimilate minerals, protect against tooth decay, support growth and development, optimize fertility, protect against heart disease and support brain function. Using a chemical test, he determined that this compound—which he called Activator X—occurred in the butterfat, organs and fat of animals consuming rapidly growing green grass, and also in certain seafood, such as fish eggs. Most importantly, he found the combination of cod liver oil and butter high in Activator X superior to that of cod liver oil alone. It turns out that Price's Activator X is vitamin K_2, produced by animal tissues, including the mammary glands, from

* How many other centenarians got cod liver oil early in life? It's a question researchers usually fail to ask.

vitamin K_1, which occurs in rapidly growing green plants.*[110]

A growing body of published research confirms Dr. Price's discoveries, namely that vitamin K_2 is important for the utilization of minerals, protects against tooth decay, supports growth and development, is involved in normal reproduction, protects against calcification of the arteries leading to heart disease, and is a major component of the brain.

Just as true vitamin A from animal foods is vastly superior to carotenes from plant foods, and vitamin D from animal foods is superior to the vegetarian form of vitamin D, vitamin K_2 from animal foods is manyfold more active in humans than the plant form, vitamin K_1. Animals are "step-up transformers," so to speak, converting plant forms of these important nutrients into more potent forms for humans, so humans do not have to use their own "disk space" to do it for themselves.

Originally, the medical community considered vitamins K_1 and K_2 as different forms of the same vitamin. The role of vitamin K_2 in skeletal metabolism was not discovered until 1978 and it was not until 1997, nearly twenty years later, that scientists realized that vitamin K was "not just for clotting anymore."[111]

Since the amount of vitamin K_1 in typical diets is ten times greater than that of vitamin K_2,[112] researchers initially considered K_2's contribution to nutritional status insignificant. Yet over the last few years, a growing body of research is demonstrating that vitamins K_1 and K_2 are not simply different forms of the same vitamin, but in reality are two different vitamins: whereas K_1 activates blood-clotting proteins, the main role of K_2 is to place calcium where it belongs, in the bones and teeth, and prevent it from going where it does not belong, in the soft tissues, such as the arteries and kidneys.[113]

Plants contain vitamin K_1 in a complex that is tied to both chlorophyll and beta-carotene. It plays a direct role in photosynthesis, and helps determine the richness in the green color of grass, its rate of growth and its brix rating (which measures the density of organic material produced by the plant). Animals grazing on grass will accumulate vitamin K_2 in their tissues in direct proportion to the amount of vitamin K_1 in their diet. The beta-carotene associated with vitamin K_1 gives a yellow or orange color to butterfat; the richness of this color therefore indirectly indicates the amount of both vitamins K_1 and K_2 in the butter.

Weston A. Price demonstrated the synergy of Activator X with vitamins A and D. When put on a deficiency diet, chickens voluntarily consumed more butter and died more slowly when the butter was high in both vitamin A and Activator X than when it was high in vitamin A alone. Cod liver oil, which is high in both vitamins A and D, partially corrected growth retardation and weak legs in turkeys fed a deficiency diet, but the combination of cod liver oil and butter high in Activator X was twice as effective. Likewise, Price found that the combination of cod liver oil and a high-Activator X butter oil concentrate was more effective than cod liver oil alone in treating his patients for dental caries and other problems.

We now know that vitamin K_2 works together with vitamins A and D—serving as the "activator" for vitamin A- and vitamin

* Much credit for solving the mystery about which nutrient corresponds to Activator X goes to Chris Masterjohn, PhD, who also has described all the research on the benefits of vitamin K_2.

D-dependent proteins. While vitamins A and D act as signaling molecules, telling cells to make certain proteins, vitamin K_2 activates these proteins by conferring upon them the physical ability to bind with calcium. In some cases these proteins directly coordinate the movement or organization of calcium; in other cases the calcium acts as a glue to hold the protein in a certain shape.[114] In all such cases, the proteins are only functional after activation by vitamin K_2. While vitamins A and D contribute to growth by stimulating growth factors and promoting the absorption of minerals, vitamin K_2 makes an equal contribution to growth by preventing the premature calcification of the cartilaginous growth zones of bones.* [115]

Dr. Price's main focus was the teeth. In his travels to remote corners of the globe, he found fourteen isolated groups that exhibited excellent dental health; they had very few cavities and all had broad faces and naturally straight teeth. At the same time, they exhibited "splendid physical development": they had strong bones and exhibited excellent growth, good posture and good musculature. His research convinced him that rich dietary sources of vitamins A and D, along with Activator X, were responsible for this optimal development and freedom from dental caries.

Research into vitamins A, D and K_2 now gives us the scientific explanation for Dr. Price's findings. A child grows until the growth plates at the end of his bones calcify. It is vitamin K_2 that prevents that calcification until the child reaches maturity. At the same time, the triumvirate of fat-soluble vitamins, along with adequate calcium, phosphorus and other minerals, ensures that the bones are densely formed and strong. A mineral-rich diet containing lots of fat-soluble activators from animal fats will ensure that the child grows not only tall, but also strong.†

There are also growth plates in the face, on either side of the maxilla (upper jaw bone). If these growth plates do not calcify too early, the face will end up wide and the cheekbones high and far apart—the hallmark of beauty. Vitamin K_2 likely prevents calcification of the sides of the maxilla until optimal development is achieved. Set into the maxilla is the upper dental palate, and this will be wide if the maxilla is wide. The mandible (lower jaw bone) will be equally wide and strong with optimal prenatal and postnatal nutrition. A wide dental palate can accommodate all the teeth, even the wisdom teeth, without crowding—and these teeth will be well formed and strong as a result of the same nutrients, that is, abundant minerals and abundant fat-soluble activators.

Price and his colleagues in the 1930s and 1940s considered the teeth as the most accessible indicator of overall health. The mouth is the only interior part of the body that we can see. They reasoned that if the teeth are straight and free of infection, then the whole body is well formed and resistant to disease.

---

* Osteocalcin is a protein responsible for putting calcium and phosphorus in bones and teeth. Cells only produce this protein in the presence of vitamins A and D; it will only accumulate in the extracellular matrix and facilitate the deposition of calcium salts, however, once it has been activated by vitamin K_2. Vitamins A and D regulate the expression of another important protein, called matrix Gla protein (MGP), which is responsible for mineralizing bone and protecting the arteries from calcification; like osteocalcin, however, MGP can only fulfill its function once it has been activated by vitamin K_2.[a]

† We need vitamin A to prevent vitamin D toxicity; vitamin K_2 may also play a role in preventing vitamin D toxicity. Toxic doses of vitamin D can cause anorexia, lethargy, slow growth, bone resorption and soft tissue calcification—very similar to the symptoms of deficiencies in vitamin K. In fact, the synergy of vitamin K_2 with vitamins A and D is exactly the type of synergy that Dr. Price attributed to Activator X.

How does vitamin K_2 prevent dental caries? Price found that the vitamin influences the composition of saliva. When he collected the saliva of individuals immune to dental caries and shook it with powdered bone or tooth meal, phosphorus would move from the saliva to the powder; by contrast, if he conducted the same procedure with the saliva of individuals susceptible to dental caries, the phosphorus would move in the opposite direction from the powder to the saliva. Administration of the Activator X concentrate to his patients consistently changed the chemical behavior of their saliva from phosphorus-accepting to phosphorus-donating. The Activator X concentrate also reduced the bacterial count of their saliva.

Thus, vitamin K in the saliva helps the teeth mineralize and also reduces bacteria that might play a role in causing cavities.* Price used the combination of high-vitamin cod liver oil and high–Activator X butter oil to reverse dental caries. This protocol not only stopped the progression of tooth decay, but completely reversed it without the need for fillings. The procedure caused the dentin to grow and remineralize, sealing what were once active caries. One fourteen-year-old girl completely healed forty-two open cavities in twenty-four teeth by taking capsules of the high-vitamin cod liver oil and Activator X concentrate three times a day for seven months.[116]

Likewise, Price used butter oil concentrate to cure rickets. In a four-year-old boy who suffered from rampant tooth decay, seizures and a tendency to fracture, the combination of a large helping of this concentrate and meals of whole wheat and whole milk rapidly resolved each of these symptoms.

Studies from Japan have shown that vitamin K_2 completely reverses bone loss and in some cases even increases bone mass in populations with osteoporosis.[117] It also reduces the incidence of fractures.[118] Another study found that vitamin K_2 protects against hip fractures and osteoporosis.[119]

Vitamin K_2 protects us from heart disease by preventing calcification of the arteries. The Rotterdam Study, which prospectively followed just over forty-six hundred men ages fifty-five or older in the Netherlands, found that the highest intake of vitamin K_2 was associated with a 52 percent lower risk of severe aortic calcification, a 41 percent lower risk of coronary heart disease (CHD), a 51 percent lower risk of CHD mortality and a 26 percent lower risk of total mortality.[120] The conventional view is that foods rich in cholesterol and saturated fat cause heart disease, but these same foods—butter, aged cheeses, poultry liver and fat—provide vitamin K_2, which strongly helps to prevent heart disease.

Price supplied several anecdotes suggesting that Activator X plays an important role in the nervous system. When he administered a daily meal of nutrient-dense whole foods supplemented with high-vitamin cod liver oil and high–Activator X butter oil to the children of impoverished mill workers who suffered from rampant tooth decay, the treatment not only resolved the tooth decay without the need for fillings, but also cured chronic fatigue in one boy and, according to the school teachers, produced a marked increase in learning capacity in two others.

Price also administered the butter oil concentrate to a four-year-old who suffered from rampant tooth decay, a fractured leg and

* Or the bacteria may just be there to clean up dead and dying tissue. Have we falsely accused bacteria of causing tooth decay just as we have falsely accused cholesterol—the body's repair substance—of causing heart disease?

seizures. A spoonful of the butter oil* served over whole wheat gruel with whole milk once before bed and five times over the course of the following day immediately resolved his seizures. Rapid healing of his fracture and dental caries followed soon after. The fact that these three symptoms appeared together and resolved following the same treatment suggests a common cause for each of them.

Sixty years later, modern research is now elucidating the essential role that vitamin K_2 plays, not only in the dental and skeletal systems, but in the nervous system as well. The brain contains one of the highest concentrations of vitamin K_2 in the body; only the pancreas, salivary glands and the cartilaginous tissue of the sternum contain more. Vitamin K_2 supports the enzymes within the brain that produce an important class of lipids called sulfatides. The levels of vitamin K_2, vitamin K–dependent proteins and sulfatides in the brain decline with age; the decline of these levels is in turn associated with age-related neurological degeneration.[121] Comparisons of human autopsies associate the early stages of Alzheimer's disease with up to 93 percent lower sulfatide levels in the brain.[122] Animals that completely lack the enzymes to make sulfatides and a related class of lipids, cerebrosides, progressively suffer from growth retardation, loss of locomotor activity, weak legs and seizures.[123]

These observations suggest that deficiencies in vitamin K, especially vitamin K_2, could result in fatigue and learning difficulties in humans, and that rare, extreme deficiencies of vitamin K_2 in the brain could result in seizures. If this is the case, it would explain why Price observed tooth decay, bone fracture, learning difficulties and seizures to share a common cause and a common solution.

The highest concentration of vitamin K_2 exists in the salivary glands and the pancreas, which suggests a role in activating digestive enzymes and regulating blood sugar.[124] The testes of male rats also exhibit a high preference for and retention of vitamin K_2,[125] and human sperm possess a vitamin K–dependent protein with an unknown function.[126] The kidneys likewise accumulate large amounts of vitamin K_2[127] and secrete vitamin K–dependent proteins that inhibit the formation of calcium salts. Patients with kidney stones secrete this protein in its inactive form, which is between four and twenty times less effective than its active form at inhibiting the growth of calcium oxalate crystals, suggesting that vitamin K_2 deficiency is a major cause of kidney stones.[128] Again we are seeing the role of K_2 in calcium regulation—putting it in the bones, where it belongs, and preventing the formation of calcium deposits in soft tissues, like the kidneys.

A number of cell experiments have shown that vitamin K_2 helps protect us against cancer.[129] A study from Europe found that an increased intake of vitamin K_2 can reduce the risk of prostate cancer by 35 percent. In addition, the potential benefits of K_2 were more pronounced for advanced prostate cancer, while vitamin K_1 offered no benefits.[130] More recently, in a 2010 study involving over twenty-four thousand subjects, dietary intake of vitamin K_2 was found to protect against cancer. The subjects were free of cancer at

* Butter oil is not the same as ghee. Dr. Price made butter oil by centrifuging clarified butter to obtain an oil (in which the vitamins concentrated) and a very hard fat.

enrollment. On follow-up over ten years later, over seventeen hundred cases of cancer occurred, of which four hundred fifty-eight were fatal. Those with the highest intake of vitamin K_2 had the lowest incidence of cancer, and the lowest cancer mortality, especially in men. The authors made the startling suggestion to consume cheese (a rich source of K_2) as a way to prevent cancer![131]

Most interesting of all is research suggesting that vitamin K plays a role in protecting skin elasticity and may help protect against skin aging and the development of wrinkles.[132]

In the Western diet, the best sources of vitamin K_2 are aged, full-fat cheeses of animals that eat green grass, and the fat and livers of ducks and geese. Cheese is rich in K_2 not only because it occurs in the butterfat, but because more is formed during the aging process.* Why the fat and liver of ducks and geese are good sources remains a mystery—but that doesn't prevent us from enjoying goose liver pâté and potatoes cooked in duck fat. Lesser amounts occur in chicken liver, butter, egg yolks and meat fats—all those "empty calorie" delicacies the food police warn us not to eat.

The bottom line: "Solid fats" like butter, cream, whole milk and cheese, egg yolks, poultry fats and meat fats are not empty foods, but rich sources of vital nutrients—nutrients that contribute to optimal health and happiness, especially when combined with foods from the sea, like fish eggs, fatty fish, shellfish and especially cod liver oil. And the more naturally the animals are raised—outdoors, on green pasture—the more nourishing their fats and organ meats will be.

* Certain forms of vitamin K_2 are produced by fermentation, and small amounts occur in fermented foods like sauerkraut. The best source of vitamin K_2 in the Asian diet is a slimy fermented soy food called natto. Natto is definitely an acquired taste for westerners—most living in America and Europe would prefer to get their vitamin K_2 from delicious animal foods like cheese and pâté.

CHAPTER 7

The Rancid and the Trans

The late 1980s represented a high point for the vegetable oil industry. Thanks to decades of marketing efforts by the industry and the lobbying efforts of their friends at the Center for Science in the Public Interest (CSPI), *trans* fats were everywhere: in cakes, cookies, donuts, salad dressing, imitation dairy products, chips and other snack foods, bread, fried foods, stick margarines and soft spreads, shortening, restaurant and fast- food fries, chicken nuggets, onion rings and even in movie popcorn. When the fast-food industry switched from animal fats to partially hydrogenated vegetable oils for frying, levels of *trans* fats increased 700 percent in a McDonald's "Happy Meal" of Chicken McNuggets, a large order of fries, and a danish or pie.[1] Butter consumption had reached a low of 4 grams per day—less than a teaspoon—and only recent Hispanic immigrants still used lard.

The food industry viewed *trans* fats as benign—even healthy—because they could use them in place of liquid vegetable oils, which they knew caused cancer. Early short-term studies showed that *trans* fats were not acutely toxic. Industry spokesmen claimed that *trans* fats were not even well absorbed through the intestinal wall, but this view gave way to the observation that humans absorb more than 96 percent of *trans* fats ingested, incorporating them into the liver, red blood cell membranes, mitochondria, mammary gland—basically everywhere.[2] One 1976 study found levels of *trans* fats up to 18 percent in human breast milk.[3] Still, in that same year, a paper prepared by the Life Sciences Research Organization of the Federation of American Societies for Experimental Biology (LSRO-FASEB) declared *trans* fats to be safe: "There is no evidence in the available information on [partially] hydrogenated soybean oil that demonstrates or suggests reasonable grounds to suspect a hazard to the public when it is used as a direct or indirect food ingredient at levels that are now current or that might reasonably be expected in the future."[4]

But during the 1970s and 1980s, research showing the harmful effects of *trans* fats began to accumulate. Rats fed *trans* fats had reproductive problems, including lowered testosterone levels in male animals and an increase in abnormal sperm—up to 98 percent by the third generation.[5] One early study presented a chilling finding: second generation rats exposed to *trans* fats in utero and during nursing experienced a greater accumulation of *trans* fats in the various tissues than in those rats placed on *trans* fatty acids after weaning.[6]

The lipids research group at the University of Maryland found that *trans* fatty acids not only alter enzymes the body uses to neutralize carcinogens, and increase enzymes that potentiate carcinogens, but they also depress milk fat production in nursing mothers and decrease insulin binding.[7] In other words, *trans* fatty acids in the diet interfere with the ability of new mothers to nurse successfully and increase their likelihood of developing diabetes. Unpublished work indicated that *trans* fats also contributed to osteoporosis.[8] Hanis, a Czechoslovakian researcher, found that *trans* consumption decreased testosterone, caused the production of abnormal sperm and contributed to altered gestation.[9] Koletzko, a German pediatric researcher, found that excess *trans* consumption in pregnant mothers predisposed them to low-birth-weight babies.[10] *Trans* consumption interferes with the body's use of omega-3 fatty acids found in fish oils, grains and green vegetables, leading to impaired prostaglandin production.[11] George Mann confirmed that *trans* consumption increases the incidence of heart disease.[12] In 1995, European researchers found a positive correlation between breast cancer rates and *trans* consumption.[13]

Until the 1995 breast cancer study, only the disturbing revelations of Dutch researchers Mensink and Katan, in 1990, received front page coverage. Mensink and Katan found that margarine consumption increased risk factors for coronary heart disease.[14] The industry—and the press—responded by promoting tub spreads, which contain reduced amounts of *trans* compared to stick margarine. For the general population, however, these *trans* reductions were offset by changes in the types of fat used by the fast-food industry. In the early 1980s, Center for Science in the Public Interest campaigned against the use of beef tallow for frying potatoes. Before that they campaigned against the use of tallow for frying chicken and fish. Most fast-food restaurants dutifully responded by switching to partially hydrogenated soybean oil for all fried foods—leading to deep-fried offerings that contained almost 50 percent *trans* fat.[15]

Epidemiologist Walter Willett, head of the Harvard School of Public Health and author of over one thousand published papers, studied the relation of dietary fat and disease for many years using flawed databases, which did not identify *trans* fats as a dietary component. He found a correlation with dietary fat consumption and both heart disease and cancer. After his researchers contacted lipid researcher Mary G. Enig at the University of Maryland about the *trans* data, they developed a more valid database, which they used in the analysis of the massive Nurses Study. When Willett's group separated out the *trans* component in their analyses, they were able to confirm greater rates of cancer in those consuming margarine and vegetable shortenings—not butter, eggs, cheese and meat.[16] This correlation of *trans* fat consumption with cancer was never published, but was reported at the Baltimore Data Bank Conference in 1992.[17] A year later, in 1993, Willett's research group found that *trans* contributed to heart disease,[18] and this study was not ignored, but received much fanfare in the press. Willett's first reference in his report was Enig's work on the *trans* content of common foods.

At that time, the industry argued that American *trans* consumption was a low 6 to 8 grams per person per day, not enough to contribute to the modern epidemic of chronic disease. Total per capita consumption of margarine and shortening then hovered around 40 grams per person per day. If these products contained 30 percent *trans* (many shortenings contain more), then average consumption was about 12 grams per person per day. In reality, consumption figures were dramatically higher for some individuals. A 1989 *Washington Post* article documented the diet of a teenage girl who ate twelve donuts and twenty-four cookies over a three-day period. Total *trans* worked out to at least 30 grams per day, and possibly much more. The fat in the chips that teenagers consume in abundance can contain up to 48 percent *trans*, which translates into 45.6 grams of *trans* fat (about 3 tablespoons) in a small 10-ounce bag of snack chips[19]—which a hungry teenager can gobble up in a few minutes. High school sex education classes do not teach American teenage boys that the altered fats in their snack foods could severely compromise their ability to have normal sex; nor do girls learn that *trans* fats may inhibit their ability to conceive, give birth to healthy babies and successfully nurse their infants. The eating habits of young Americans—packaged snacks, fast food, premade meals—meant exposure to *trans* fats at a far greater level than adults using a tablespoon of margarine daily.

Enig and the University of Maryland group were not alone in their efforts to bring their concerns about the effects of partially hydrogenated fats before the public. Fred Kummerow at the University of Illinois, blessed with independent funding and an abundance of patience, carried out a number of studies indicating that the *trans* fats increased risk factors associated with heart disease, and that vegetable-oil-based fabricated foods such as Egg Beaters cannot support life.[20] George Mann, formerly with the Framingham Study, possessed neither funding nor patience—he was, in fact, very angry with what he called the "diet/heart scam." His independent studies of the Maasai in Africa,[21] whose diet is extremely rich in cholesterol and saturated fat, and who are virtually free of heart disease, had convinced him that the lipid hypothesis was "the public health diversion of this century…the greatest scam in the history of medicine."[22]

EARLY STUDIES WITH SWINE FOUND that *trans* fats caused undesirable changes in markers for atherosclerosis. Rats fed *trans* fats accumulated 30 percent more fat in their hearts than rats fed saturated beef tallow, and studies were showing that *trans* fats could not provide the heart with the energy it needed in times of stress. These studies showed that *trans* fats built into the cell membranes altered their properties.

What is interesting about these studies is the finding that undesirable effects on cholesterol levels (increased LDL-cholesterol and decreases HDL-cholesterol) occurred only when the levels of saturated fat in the diet were low. With increasing proportions of saturated fats, the undesirable effects were mitigated, but with increasing proportions of unsaturated fatty acids, the kind in vegetable oils, these effects were enhanced. Swine with the highest level of saturated fats in the diet had the lowest amount of undesirable lipids in their aortas. Thus, partially hydrogenated coconut oil, which contains high levels of saturated fats, had fewer adverse effects than partially hydrogenated soybean oil, which is high in unsaturated fatty acids.[23] According to these findings, an occasional serving of fast-food fries in a diet that contains mostly saturated fats like butter, meat fats and coconut oil would not be as harmful as that same serving of French fries in a diet based on so-called "good" fats like sunflower, canola or safflower oil, or even olive oil.*

In her doctorate thesis, published in 1984—just as CSPI was pushing for the use of partially hydrogenated fat in fast-food fryers, and the same year spokesmen for the Lipid Clinic Research trials declared that animal fats were the proven cause of heart disease—Mary G. Enig presented opposing research, describing how *trans* fats interfere with the cytochrome P450 enzyme system. These enzymes are present in most tissues of the body, and play important roles in the synthesis of sex and steroid hormones, cholesterol formation and vitamin D metabolism. Cytochrome P450 enzymes also function to rid the body of potentially toxic and carcinogenic compounds, including drugs. Thus, these enzymes play a key role in protecting us against cancer—and Enig's work showed that *trans* fats interfere with this system, making us more vulnerable to cancer.[24] Enig's work—which was largely ignored—also explains why *trans* fats interfere with reproduction, lower testosterone production and damage sperm.

Enig and her colleagues then carried out a market-basket survey to determine the levels of *trans* fats in common foods such as margarine, shortening, snack foods and baked goods. Up to that point, the government databases did not list *trans* fats, but lumped them together with saturated fats, calling them all saturated fats. When researchers like Willett used these databases, they came up with positive—but false—correlations between saturated fat consumption and cancer and heart disease.[25]

Reports of adverse effects from *trans* fats continued to accumulate. Many researchers showed that *trans* fats increased markers for heart disease.[26] Other studies showed decreased immune response† and decreased insulin levels or decreased response to insulin, which would lead to type 2 diabetes.[27] *Trans* fats interfere with enzymes needed to convert omega-6 and omega-3 fatty acids into their elongated versions (arachidonic acid and DHA); in studies they also caused adverse changes in the cell membranes, escalated adverse effects of essential fatty acid deficiency and increased free radical formation.[28]

A 1994 study estimated that over thirty thousand heart disease deaths per year in the United States are attributable to the consumption of *trans* fats.[29] By 2006, some researchers were suggesting that *trans* fats caused one hundred thousand deaths per year.[30] A comprehensive review of studies of *trans* fats published in 2006 in the *New England Journal of Medicine* reported a strong and reliable connection between *trans* fat consumption and heart disease, concluding that "On a per-calorie basis, *trans* fats appear to increase the risk of CHD more than any other macronutrient, conferring a substantially increased risk at low levels of consumption."[31]

---

* One researcher reported severe, progressive myocardial inflammation and scarring in rats fed partially hydrogenated fish oil—fish oil being more unsaturated than vegetable oil.[a]

† As early as 1978, researchers recognized the fact that unsaturated fatty acids directly kill white blood cells.[a]

The latest establishment theory on heart disease posits low-grade inflammation in the arteries as a cause, leading to the release of blood clots followed by heart attack—and studies indicate that *trans* fats provoke inflammation. A 2002 study found that consumption of stick margarine in human subjects increased the production of inflammatory prostaglandins associated with atherosclerosis. Neither liquid soy oil nor butter had the same inflammatory effect.[32] In a cross-sectional study of participants in the Nurses' Health Study, researchers found that those with the highest *trans* fat consumption also had higher markers of inflammation. The most significant biomarker, C-reactive protein (CRP), was up 73 percent in those with the highest level of consumption compared to those with the lowest.[33] Scientists believe that high levels of CRP indicate inflammation in the lining of the arteries and endothelial dysfunction, leading to heart disease.

Most seriously, several reports associated *trans* fat consumption with increased risk of cancer. For example, mice fed margarine had more mammary tumors than rats fed butter.[34] One study found that the relative risk of breast cancer associated with fat used for frying was increased with margarine and decreased with butter and vegetable oil,[35] while another noted a positive association between breast cancer risk and "fat from cakes, biscuits and snacks."[36] The most convincing study, published in 1995, found that women with breast cancer had more *trans* fats in their adipose tissue compared to controls.*[37]

Recently, a seven-year European study, published in 2008, which followed almost twenty thousand women, documented three hundred sixty-three cases of breast cancer during the course of the study, and matched these cases to breast cancer–free controls according to age, menopausal status at baseline, date and collection center. Increasing blood levels of *trans* fatty acids were associated with a 75 percent increase in breast cancer risk.[38] And researchers from Harvard have reported that increased intakes of *trans* fatty acids may increase the risk of nonaggressive prostate tumors by about 100 percent.[39]

Trans fats seem to contribute to weight gain as well. A 1993 report indicated that women who consumed more *trans* fats were several kilograms heavier that women who consumed less, even though the caloric intake was the same in both groups.[40] Research on monkeys carried out at the Wake Forest School of Medicine indicates that weight gain is accelerated by consumption of *trans* fats compared to other fats. "Diets rich in *trans* fat cause a redistribution of fat tissue into the abdomen and lead to a higher body weight even when the total dietary calories are controlled," said Lawrence L. Rudel, PhD, head of the Lipid Sciences Research Program. "What it says is that *trans* fat is worse than anticipated. I was surprised." Monkeys given *trans* fats rather than monounsaturated fat deposited 30 percent more fat in their abdomen, even though both diets contained the same amount of calories.[41]

When Mary G. Enig and her colleagues studied *trans* fats in the late 1970s, they noticed that rats fed *trans* fats seemed more aggressive than controls; lack of funding prevented them from following up on this observation, but in 2012, researchers found a

* This 1995 study seems to have disappeared from the PubMed database.

strong relation between *trans* fat consumption and self-reported behavioral aggression and irritability.[42]

In short, *trans* fats mess with your body, they mess with your moods—and they mess with your mind. In a 2015 article, researchers reanalyzing results from the 1999–2005 UCSD Statin Study found that greater dietary *trans* fatty acid consumption "is linked to worse word memory in adults during years of high productivity," that is, in adults under the age of forty-five.[43]

It was this accumulation of evidence—only some of which was covered in the mainstream media—that led the FDA to require mandatory *trans* fat labeling, effective January 2006. That same year, the National Academy of Sciences (NAS) concluded that there is no safe level of *trans* fat consumption, quoting a 2006 *New England Journal of Medicine* (NEJM) scientific review, which stated, "From a nutritional standpoint, the consumption of *trans* fatty acids results in considerable potential harm but no apparent benefit."[44]

THESE REVELATIONS HAVE BEEN EMBARRASSING for organizations like the American Heart Association, which for many years assured the public that industrial *trans* fats were a benign substitute for saturated fats like butter* and lard. The organization's new spin is that yes, *trans* fats are bad, but so are saturated fats.

"Americans' Knowledge of Fats Growing, Still Insufficient" was the title of an American Heart Association (AHA) press release issued October 9, 2007, which describes an AHA survey showing that "consumer awareness of the 'bad' fats—*trans* fats and saturated fat—is at an all-time high. But consumers still need key information to improve how they eat." The survey found that "awareness of the link between the bad fats and increased heart disease risk is up from 63 percent in 2006 to 73 percent in 2007 for *trans* fat, and from 73 percent to 77 percent for saturated fat." However, "only" 21 percent of consumers could name three food sources of *trans* fats, and only 30 percent could name three food sources of saturated fat on their own—that is, without prompting from AHA propagandists. "We're encouraged to see that consumer awareness of saturated and *trans* fats is higher than ever and that more people understand the link between these fats and increased heart disease risk," said Robert H. Eckel, MD, past president of the AHA, chair of its *trans* fat task force and professor of medicine at the University of Colorado at Denver Health Sciences Center. "But it's clear consumers need to know which foods contain what [sic] fats to minimize both saturated and *trans* fats, and make heart-healthier food choices. Food labels help, but it goes far beyond that, in knowing more about the food products without labels we purchase in the grocery or when eating out."

The American Heart Association states clearly that the bad fats are saturated fats found in beef, pork, chicken, butter, cheese and the tropical oils. According to the AHA, *trans* fats are "just as bad" as saturated fats. Yet science supports the fact that saturated fats have *opposite* effects from the *trans* fats. For example, *trans* fats cause or encourage inflammation, whereas saturated fats suppress inflammation; *trans* fats are associated with more cancer, especially breast cancer, while stable saturated fats protect against breast cancer.

* The fat of ruminant animals, like butter and tallow, contains a small amount of natural *trans* fats that are beneficial, not harmful.

Saturated versus *Trans* Fats[45]

	Saturated Fats	*Trans* Fats
Cell membranes	Essential for healthy function	Interfere with healthy function
Hormones	Enhance hormone production	Interfere with hormone production
Inflammation	Suppress	Encourage
Heart disease	Lower Lp(a), raise "good" cholesterol	Raise Lp(a), lower "good" cholesterol
Omega-3	Put in tissues and conserve	Reduce levels in tissues
Diabetes	Help insulin receptors	Inhibit insulin receptors
Immune system	Enhance	Depress
Prostagandins	Encourage production and balance	Depress production; cause imbalances
Cancer	Provide protection	Encourage

All of this bad news about *trans* fats has sent manufacturers scrambling to find substitutes for the ubiquitous, *trans*-laden partially hydrogenated oils used in their products. Bayer CropScience, a German firm, teamed with Cargill of the United States to develop a hybrid rapeseed with "desirable oil traits" for producing high-oleic rapeseed oil. Archer Daniels Midland launched a line of *trans*-free and low-*trans* oils using enzymatic interesterification technology (discussed in Chapter 2). U.S. firms Dow AgroSciences, Bunge and DuPont have all launched their own brands of zero- or low-*trans* oils.

By and large, these efforts to remove *trans* fatty acids from the food supply have succeeded.[46] You'll still get them if you use margarine, eat certain brands of crackers and pastries or eat large amounts of almost any processed food or industrial oil, but in many products, the industry has successfully replaced *trans* fats with monounsaturated or polyunsaturated fatty acids and—ironically—with saturated fats from fully hydrogenated oils.

UNFORTUNATELY, THE FOOD INDUSTRY AND influential groups like the American Heart Association (AHA) have sent Americans from the frying pan of *trans* fatty acids to the fire of polyunsaturated oils—this in spite of all that scientists have uncovered on the dangers of liquid vegetable oils.

If *trans* fats are bad, liquid oils are even worse. Early studies (up to the 1980s) showed that because polyunsaturates are highly subject to rancidity, they increase the body's need for vitamin E and other antioxidants. Excess consumption of vegetable oils is especially damaging to the reproductive organs and the lungs—both of which are sites experiencing huge increases in cancer in the United States. In test animals, diets high in polyunsaturates from vegetable oils inhibit the ability to learn, especially under conditions of stress; they are toxic to the liver; they compromise the integrity of the immune system; they increase levels of uric acid in the blood; they cause abnormal fatty acid profiles in the adipose tissues; they have been linked to mental decline and chromosomal damage; they accelerate aging—one study found that women who consumed mostly vegetable oils had far more wrinkles than those who used traditional animal fats. Polyunsaturates turn to a varnish-like substance in the intestines. Excess consumption of polyunsaturates is associated with increasing rates of cancer, heart disease and weight gain; excess use of commercial vegetable oils interferes with the production of prostaglandins, leading to an array of complaints ranging from autoimmune disease to PMS. Disruption of prostaglandin production leads to an increased tendency to form blood clots, and hence myocardial infarction, which has not retreated from epidemic levels in America, in spite of relentless anti–saturated fat propaganda.[47]

As early as 1957, in a letter to *The Lancet*, Denham Harman, a founder of the hypothesis that free radicals cause aging, warned of the negative effects of oxidation products (the creation of free radicals) in polyunsaturated oils. He noted that many important enzymes and vitamins are easily oxidized and warned that increasing the amount of easily oxidized polyunsaturated oils in the diet could "actually increase the severity of atherosclerosis." The present enthusiasm for these unsaturated oils should "be curbed," he wrote, and called for additional study on the possible adverse health effects that could be expected with this dietary change.[48]

Those who have most actively promoted the use of polyunsaturated vegetable oils as part of the Prudent Diet were well aware of their dangers. In 1971, William B. Kannel, former director of the Framingham Study, warned against including too many polyunsaturates in the diet. A year earlier, Dr. William Connor of the American Heart Association issued a similar warning, and Frederick Stare reviewed an article which reported that the use of polyunsaturated oils caused an increase in breast tumors. As far back as 1969, researchers discovered that the use of corn oil caused an increase in atherosclerosis.[49]

As reported by Nina Teicholz in *The Big Fat Surprise*, at a symposium on the topic attended by industry scientists in 1972, teams of food chemists from Japan reported that heated soybean oil produced compounds that were "highly toxic" to mice. A pathologist from Columbia University also reported that rats fed "mildly oxidized" oils suffered liver damage and heart lesions, compared to rats fed tallow, lard, dairy fats and chicken fat, which caused no such damage.[50]

A Finnish study found that children who consumed lots of vegetable oils were more prone to allergies.[51] Researchers in Australia discovered that consumption of vegetable oils is associated with increased rates of asthma.[52] Another study found that mice fed excessive corn oil had increased caloric intake and obesity.[53] Researchers have also found that high vegetable oil consumption is associated with increased rates of macular degeneration, the leading cause of irreversible blindness in adults.[54] These are just several of hundreds of studies indicating that modern vegetable oils are bad news indeed—they'll make you prone to allergies, asthma and weight gain, and possibly give you cancer and make you blind as well.

Such research rarely receives media coverage, and when it does, it often gets spin doctored. For example, in a 2010 study, mice fed a standard rat chow diet plus 10 percent corn oil exhibited increased body weight, total body fat mass and abdominal fat mass along with reduced bone mineral density compared to controls on rat chow alone. The title of the study describes the corn oil diet as a "high-fat" rather than a "high-oil" diet.[55] When a diet high in corn oil but low in fiber, vitamin D and calcium triggered inflammation in the mouse colon, Peter Holt, one of the study authors, stated that the study lent support to the hypothesis that "red meat, processed meat and alcohol can increase the risk of colorectal cancer."[56] But the study did not look at red meat, processed meat and alcohol; it looked at corn oil!

Monounsaturated fatty acids, found in olive oil and canola oil, are the current darling of the research establishment, but researchers at Lund University in Sweden really got tongue-tied when a recent study showed that olive oil and a "new type of canola and flaxseed oil" raised cholesterol levels more than butter. According to a spokesperson for the university, the short- and medium-chain fatty acids in butter are stored preferentially in the intestinal cells. "However, butter leads to a slightly higher content of free fatty acids in the blood, which is a burden on the body... Olive oil is good, to be sure, but our findings indicate that different food fats can have different advantages."[57]

Modern diets can contain as much as 30 percent of calories as polyunsaturated oils, an amount that is far too high. The best evidence indicates that our intake of polyunsaturates should not be much greater than 4 percent of the caloric total, in approximate proportions of 1.5 percent omega-3 linolenic acid and 2.5 percent omega-6 linoleic acid.[58] EFA consumption in this range is found in native populations in temperate and tropical regions whose intake of polyunsaturated oils comes from the small amounts in legumes, grains, nuts, green vegetables, fish, olive oil and animal fats, but not from commercial vegetable oils.

We know polyunsaturated oils are bad; we've known that for a long time. But the dietary gurus have fallen back to recommending them as "heart healthy," more so today now that we know the truth about *trans* fats. In fact, in 2015 for the first time, the USDA Dietary Guideline Committee recommended *increasing* polyunsaturated oil consumption. Up until then, the guidelines had stressed carbohydrates over fats of any kind.

IT CANNOT BE STRESSED ENOUGH that polyunsaturated oils degrade into dangerous oxidation products such as free radicals. These breakdown products can include aldehydes, including formaldehyde—that's right, formaldehyde, the same chemical used to preserve dead bodies. In one analysis, a total of one hundred thirty volatile compounds were isolated from one piece of chicken fried in vegetable oil.[59]

As revealed in the research of Nina Teicholz, of particular concern is the fact that fast-food chains and manufacturers of donuts and potato chips are now frying in liquid vegetable oils. The breakdown products of liquid oils heated to frying temperatures are particularly toxic.* The residue that accumulates in the bottom of the fryers is a thick gunk, like paint shellac—formed because the unsaturated fatty acids polymerize—that is, they join together to make varnish. The gunk comes off the fryers and settles on surfaces throughout the restaurant, creating a thriving business for industrial cleaning companies. Uniforms on which the gunk settles sometimes catch fire, even after the clothes have been cleaned.

Remember that fast-food workers are breathing this stuff in! A report published in 2010 by the International Agency for Research on Cancer (IARC), which is part of the World Health Organization, determined that emissions from frying oils at the temperatures

* Actually, these aldehydes occur in vegetable oils at temperatures well below those regularly used for frying and long before the oils start to smoke or smell.

typically used in restaurants are "probably" carcinogenic to humans.[60]

In a 1991 review, the Austrian biochemist Hermann Esterbauer summarized the evidence that aldehydes cause "rapid cell death," interfere with DNA and RNA, and disturb the basic functions of the cell. Aldehydes cause extreme oxidative stress to every kind of tissue, with a "great diversity of deleterious effects" to health. Aldehydes cause LDL-cholesterol to oxidize, and it is oxidized cholesterol that initiates the process of atherosclerosis.[61] Considerable evidence implicates aldehydes in the development of Alzheimer's and other neurodegenerative diseases.[62]

In one experiment mice were fed a type of aldehyde called acrolein, named for its acrid smell when produced by overheated oils. (It is also present in cigarette smoke.) The mice suffered injuries to their gastrointestinal tracts as well as a whole-body response called "acute phase response," an attempt by the body to avoid septic shock. Markers of inflammation and other signs of acute infection also went up dramatically—sometimes by a hundredfold—and this at a dose equivalent to what humans can typically consume in one day, even if they are not eating fried foods.[63]

The industry is hoping that new interesterified blends will not have the negative health effects of *trans* fats or of liquid polyunsaturated oils. These blends typically contain some saturated fatty acids created from vegetable oils through full hydrogenation. But a 2007 study gives great cause for concern. The researchers compared *trans*-rich and interesterified fats with saturated fat for their relative impact on blood lipids and blood sugar levels. Thirty human volunteers participated in the study, which strictly controlled total fat and fatty acid composition in the subjects' diet. Each subject consumed all three diets in random rotation during the four-week diet periods. HDL-cholesterol dropped slightly with both the *trans* fat and interesterified blends but the real problem concerned blood glucose and insulin levels. Insulin levels dropped 10 percent on the partially hydrogenated soybean oil diet but dropped more than twice as much on the interesterified fat diet, causing blood sugar to rise by an alarming 20 percent.[64] Thus it seems that these interesterified blends affect the production of insulin by the pancreas rather than the receptors for insulin in the cell membranes.

The trade-off of type 2 diabetes from *trans* fats for type 1 diabetes from interesterified vegetable oils does not seem like a good one. There seems to be no trade-off whatsoever in the switch from stick margarine loaded with *trans* fats to soft spreads loaded with toxic vegetable oils in preventing cancer, heart disease and other chronic ailments. And all this comes from research on adults. What happens to children fed *trans* fats and rancid vegetable oils is the subject of the next chapter.

CHAPTER 8

Remember the Little Ones: Why Children Need Animal Fats

Three weeks after a baby is conceived—when the embryo is smaller than a peppercorn—the heart begins to form. By week four, the primitive fetal heart is pumping blood and the neural tube along the back is closing. Basic facial features then appear, including passageways that become the inner ears and arches that become the jaw. Small buds will soon grow into arms and legs.

These changes are the result of a process called differentiation. The embryo begins as a collection of undifferentiated cells—called stem cells—which are cells that can be changed or differentiated into cells that have specialized purposes. Very early in the process of fetal growth, certain stem cells receive a signal to become heart cells, thus initiating the process of forming the heart. Soon after, the stem cells get signals to form cells for the other systems and organs—the nervous system, the lungs, the skeleton, the organs, the skin, the muscles. But what gives that signal?

The specific compound that directs the differentiation of the embryonic stem cells into the heart and other organs is vitamin A. Vitamin A is the concert master of fetal development, necessary for the differentiation and patterning of all cells, tissues and organs within the developing body. It is especially important for the development of communication systems between the sense organs and the brain.[1]

It was in 2010 that researchers at the Keck School of Medicine of the University of Southern California pinpointed the mechanism that guides embryonic heart tissue formation: retinoic acid, an isomer of vitamin A. "This exciting research shows how retinoic acid, a vitamin A derivative, acts to guide cells in the embryo to form parts of the heart and the major blood vessels that emerge from it," said a spokesman for the research. "Defects in this developmental pathway can result in serious congenital malformations in the heart in the fetus and newborns, that may be fatal if not corrected surgically."[2]

The heart begins to form often before the mother knows she is pregnant. Upon realizing she's with child, a mother begins to think about nutrition for her developing baby—but if she is deficient in vitamin A at the time of conception, the heart may not form properly—or at all. The same goes for other organs, which are forming at a rapid pace.[3] When Weston A. Price studied so-called "primitive peoples" during the 1930s and 1940s, he noted that all these groups valued one or more "sacred" foods considered important for men and women to consume at least six months before conception, for women during pregnancy and lactation, and for children during growth. In Switzerland, that food was a deep yellow nutrient-dense butter from cows eating rapidly growing spring grass; in the Outer Hebrides, the sacred food was fish heads stuffed with oats and chopped cod's liver; for many groups the sacred food was fish eggs; for others it was liver. South Sea Islanders of both sexes consumed the oil from fermented shark livers for a period before conception. When Dr. Price asked the various groups why they consumed that particular food, the answer was always the same: "So we can have healthy babies."

The sacred foods had this in common: they were nutrient-dense animal foods with particularly high levels of the fat-soluble vitamins A, D and K_2—and especially vitamin A. By consuming them before conception, fathers would produce healthy sperm and mothers would have plenty of vitamin A in storage to meet the demands of the rapidly differentiating embryo.

Price described his early work on vitamin A deficiency during pregnancy and during the preconception period in *Nutrition and Physical Degeneration*. He noted that in diverse species of laboratory animals, a vitamin A deficiency produced spontaneous abortion, prolonged labor, death of the mother and her offspring during labor; eye defects including the complete absence of eyes, defects of the snout, dental arches and lips; displacement of internal organs including the kidneys, ovaries and testes; and deafness due to degeneration of the nervous system.[4]

Even mild vitamin A deficiency compromises the number of functional units in the kidneys (called nephrons), which could predispose a person to poor kidney function later in life. The number of cells in the kidneys is highly dependent on vitamin A status during embryonic and fetal development.[5]

Vitamin A is critical for lung formation as well.[6] Nepalese children whose mothers received vitamin A supplementation during pregnancy had better lung function compared to those who received a placebo. Children whose mothers received plant-based beta-carotene supplements did not experience any benefits.[7] The researchers explained: "The greater bio-efficacy of preformed vitamin A as compared with beta-carotene may stem from differences in absorption and metabolism."*

Vitamin A is necessary during fetal development and also throughout adult life, as it helps to maintain the presence of cells lining the lungs, which are covered in hairlike projections called cilia.[8] These hairs sweep away debris and foreign material, protecting the lungs from pollutants and infections. During and after the formation of all these systems, vitamin A supports their continued growth.

Dr. Price noted that vitamin A, along with the other fat-soluble vitamins, was critical for normal facial development, wide features, high cheekbones and large dental palates ensuring straight and even teeth—the hallmarks of attractiveness. Children born to parents who consumed "the displacing foods of modern commerce" tended to have narrower faces and crowded teeth—which he called "dental deformities."

---

* While warning American mothers to avoid vitamin A, health officials admit that vitamin A deficiency is a public health problem in more than half of all countries in the world, especially in Africa and Southeast Asia, where it results in half a million cases of blindness each year.[a]

Attractive facial features are symmetrical, and vitamin A holds the key to what scientists call the "holy grail" puzzle of developmental biology: the existence of a mechanism to ensure that the exterior of our bodies is symmetrical while the inner organs are arranged asymmetrically. Researchers at the Salk Institute for Biological Studies have found that vitamin A provides the signal that buffers the influences of asymmetric cues in the early stages of development and allows these cells to develop symmetrically. In the absence of vitamin A, the exterior of our bodies would develop asymmetrically—our right side would be shorter than the left side, and the face misshapen.[9]

We do not have exact figures for the vitamin A content of the preconception and pregnancy diets used by the groups that Price studied, but they were certainly higher than the RDA of 2,600 IU per day. These groups prized organ meats, especially liver, and used them on a regular basis—one serving of liver contains up to 32,000 IU vitamin A.

When discussing the scourge of tuberculosis that plagued mankind during the 1930s, Price speculated that the same factors that resulted in underdevelopment of the face also caused the underdevelopment of the lungs. New research suggests the validity of Price's theory. Researchers at Columbia University Medical Center have found evidence that prenatal vitamin A deficiency results in postnatal airway hyperresponsiveness, a hallmark of asthma. The study, conducted in mice, shows that a short-term deficit of vitamin A while the lung is forming can cause profound changes in the smooth muscle that surrounds the airways, causing the adult lungs to respond to environmental or pharmacological stimuli with excessive narrowing of the airways.[10] "Researchers have long wondered what makes some people more susceptible than others to developing asthma symptoms when exposed to the same stimulus," said Dr. Cardoso, senior author. "Our study suggests that the presence of structural and functional abnormalities in the lungs due to vitamin A deficiency during development is an important and underappreciated factor in this susceptibility. More generally, our findings highlight a point often overlooked in adult medicine, which is that adverse fetal exposures that cause subtle changes in developing organs can have lifelong consequences."

A 2007 European study confirms the importance of adequate vitamin A. The study found that one-third of women with short birth intervals or multiple births had borderline deficiencies in retinol. "If the vitamin A supply of the mother is inadequate," they warned, "her supply to the fetus will also be inadequate, as will later be her milk. These inadequacies cannot be compensated by postnatal supplementation."*[11] Moms need to put sufficient time between births in order to rebuild vitamin A stores.

Vitamin D from fatty animal food plays an equally important role in fetal development. For example, in the late third trimester, the fetal skeleton enters a period of rapid growth that requires calcium, phosphorus and

* The researchers noted that "pregnant women or those considering becoming pregnant are generally advised to avoid the intake of vitamin A–rich liver and liver foods, based upon unsupported scientific findings," and go on to recommend sources of beta-carotene, rather than true vitamin A. As discussed in Chapter 6, plant sources of beta-carotene cannot supply adequate vitamin A, especially for pregnant women and developing children.

vitamin D. An infant born six weeks prematurely has laid down only half the calcium into its bones as an infant carried to term.

Like vitamin A, vitamin D plays a role in lung development,[12] and it probably plays a much larger role in fetal development in general due to vitamin D's interaction with vitamin A—both are needed for optimal effects.

At birth, the infant's blood level of vitamin D is closely correlated to that of the mother.[13] Adequate levels of vitamin D protect the newborn from tetany, convulsions and heart failure.[14] The rapid skeletal growth that occurs in late pregnancy taxes the vitamin D supply of the mother and her blood levels drop over the course of the third trimester. One study conducted in Britain showed that 36 percent of new mothers and 32 percent of newborn infants had no detectable vitamin D in their blood; another showed that 60 percent of infants born to white mothers in the spring and summer had levels under 8 nanograms per milliliter (ng/mL), a level that is extremely deficient.[15]

Vitamin D plays a role in pancreatic function. Although no studies have directly assessed the use of this dose during pregnancy, a study of over ten thousand infants in Norway conducted between 1966 and 1997 showed that direct supplementation of 2,000 IU per day to infants in the first year of life virtually eradicated the risk of type 1 diabetes over the next thirty years.*[16]

Compared to vitamins A and D, very little is known about the role of vitamin K_2 in embryonic and fetal development. The enzyme that uses vitamin K_2 to activate vitamin K–dependent proteins first shows up in the skeletal and nervous tissue of the embryo.[17] Two vitamin K–dependent proteins are present in the first trimester.[18] These proteins help lay down calcium in bone tissue and keep calcium out of the soft tissues, where it does not belong. Indirect evidence indicates that vitamin K plays a crucial role in facial development, ensuring a wide face and high cheekbones that will bless the child with capacious sinus cavities and overall good looks.

Another critical nutrient for the developing fetus is DHA. The fetus hoards DHA from the mother and incorporates it into its brain at ten times the rate at which it can synthesize it.[19] (Maternal loss of DHA may be a contributing factor to postpartum depression.[20]) DHA can be obtained primarily from cod liver oil and fatty fish and in small amounts from organ meats and animal fats. Newborns of mothers with high DHA during the last three months of pregnancy exhibited healthier sleep patterns than others.[21]

Fetal brain development depends on adequate choline, which is especially important for the formation of cholinergic neurons (neurons that use the neurotransmitter acetylcholine). This process takes place from day fifty-six of pregnancy through three months postpartum. Choline is needed for the formation of synapses, the connections between these neurons, which form at a high rate through the fourth year of life. Rats fed three times the normal choline requirement during pregnancy gave birth to offspring with very

* Only cod liver oil was associated with the reduction in diabetes, not vitamin D alone. The researchers conjectured that it was the omega-3 fatty acids in cod liver oil that provided protection; but the likely explanation is that the vitamin A in cod liver oil supports the action of vitamin D.

resilient nervous systems. These offspring had a lifelong 30 percent increase in visuospatial and auditory memory; they grew old without developing any age-related senility; they were protected against the assaults of neurotoxins; they had an enhanced ability to focus on several things at once; and they had a much lower rate of interference memory.[22]

In addition, choline protects the fetus from chronic stress-related illness later in life. When Mom is under stress during pregnancy, the levels of stress hormones in baby also rise, leading to reduced ability to deal with stress after birth.[23] Extra choline during the third trimester protects against this unfortunate outcome.[24] The best sources of choline are liver, egg yolks and full-fat grass-fed dairy foods.

THIS CURSORY LOOK AT THE nutrients needed for optimal fetal development and the subsequent development of the child throws a spotlight on the glaring disconnect between what the science tells us and what passes for conventional nutritional advice for pregnant and lactating women, and young children. Science tells us that those "empty" saturated fats—animal fats and the nutrients they contain—are essential for conception, development and growth; that women need to consume egg yolks, liver, butter, whole milk, cheese, seafood, cod liver oil, meat fats and poultry fats prior to conception and during pregnancy. Science validates the practices of traditional peoples who consumed fatty nutrient-dense animal foods in order to have healthy babies. Yet today, our government and medical establishment warn pregnant women *not* to eat these nutrient-rich foods.

Modern expectant mothers are faced with so much conflicting information and advice—including studies purporting to show that saturated fat is bad for the pregnant woman and her developing baby. These studies have pushed many an expectant mother toward a nutrient-poor diet based on polyunsaturated vegetable oils, or toward a diet severely lacking in vital fats.

The foods Mom needs while pregnant also ensure that she has healthy breast milk. A common myth about breastfeeding is that a woman's diet has little effect on nutrient levels in her breast milk. Yet all breast milk composition is not the same—levels of vitamins, minerals and key fatty acids can vary widely from mother to mother. When investigators in Iceland looked at levels of the all-important fat-soluble vitamins in breast milk, they found that women who took cod liver oil had higher levels of vitamins A, D and E in their milk. Supplementation with cod liver oil supplying about 5,000 IU vitamin A and 130 IU vitamin D per day resulted in breast milk that met the recommended intake of vitamin A for infants but fell short of the recommended intake for vitamin D.[25] The cod liver oil used was very low in vitamin D—the result of modern processing techniques. It would be interesting to repeat the study using high-vitamin cod liver oil to supply at least 500 IU vitamin D per day.

Low vitamin D levels in mother's milk can also cause breastfed infants to develop rickets. Adequate intake of vitamin D can increase breast milk concentrations to 400 IU per liter. Dr. Catherine Gordon of Boston Children's Hospital recommends regular supplementation of vitamin D to nursing mothers after finding widespread deficiency in mothers and cases of rickets in their breastfed infants.[26] But vitamin D–rich foods with their cofactor of vitamin A continue to provide a better way to nourish the breastfed infant than supplements alone.

A 1992 study carried out in Indonesia found that mothers who received vitamin A supplementation had higher levels in their blood and milk than those who received a placebo, and that the infants of the supplemented group were less likely to be vitamin A deficient.[27] Deficiency was measured by the presence of conjunctivitis in the eyes. Incidence of conjunctivitis fell in infants nursing from mothers taking a vitamin A supplement. The authors noted that vitamin A status was lowest in women who were thin and who already had given birth to many babies.

Many theories have attempted to explain the mysterious tragedy of crib death or sudden infant death syndrome (SIDS)—vaccinations, milk allergies, permapress linens, and pesticides or formaldehyde outgassing from plastic mattress covers. A study published in Sweden points to another possible cause—deficiency in vitamin A. Researchers found that SIDS was much more common among children who had not received the supplementation of vitamins A and D that is customary in Norway and Sweden. This effect was statistically significant in Norway and Sweden, but not in Denmark, where babies get vitamin D supplementation alone, without vitamin A. The odds ratios remained significant in Sweden when an adjustment was made for confounding factors, including socioeconomic status. The researchers explained: "We found an association between increased risk of sudden infant death syndrome and infants not being given vitamin supplementation during their first year of life. This was highly significant in Sweden, and the effect is possibly connected with vitamin A deficiency."[28]

Levels of choline in a mother's milk depend on her dietary intake.[29] Choline is essential for the development of the brain and nervous system in the fetus, infant and child. The best dietary sources are egg yolks and liver. Liver is usually the first weaning food among primitive peoples; in Asian folk tradition, egg yolks are fed to infants so they will grow up smart. Liver and egg yolks should be the weaning foods for all infants, but in the United States, babies get rice cereal. Not long ago you could buy canned liver, meat and egg yolks for your baby, which manufacturers advertised as promoting good health and good growth. These have disappeared, replaced with canned fruits and vegetables, and strange concoctions containing lean chicken meat and quinoa. Infant formula is based on powdered skim milk and vegetable oils and popular weaning foods like canned squash and applesauce hardly supply the infant with the complete range of building materials they need for a healthy body and brain.

A mother's diet has a significant influence on the fat content of her milk as well. Traditional dietary fat in Mom's diet increases milk fat as well as the enzymes lipase, esterase and alkaline phosphatase—all necessary for her baby's optimal assimilation and digestion.[30] *Trans* fats found in processed and commercial fried foods will lower the fat content of mother's milk, a discovery made in research on mice.[31] In humans, margarine containing *trans* fat reduces milk fat in lean women, whereas butter consumption increases the levels of antimicrobial short- and medium-chain fatty acids as well as cholesterol in breast milk.[32] Cholesterol is so important to a developing infant that mother's milk contains special enzymes to ensure that baby absorbs 100 percent of it.[33] Cholesterol is critical to the formation of the brain and nervous system, as well as the "second brain"—the digestive tract.

Mother's milk contains AA and DHA, the long-chain polyunsaturated fatty acids that babies need for the development of their nervous systems. These special fats accumulate in the brain and retina and likely protect the infant from learning disabilities and reduced visual acuity. The presence of AA and DHA in the tissues of a growing infant is largely determined by the levels in the milk the baby consumes.[34] These fatty acids are vital for an infant's optimal development, a fact so important that even commercial formula makers now include AA and DHA in their products. What is less well known is the fact that the levels of AA and DHA in human breast milk greatly depend on the mother's diet. An important 1997 study compared the fatty acid composition of breast milk of mothers in two Chinese provinces with that of Canadian mothers.[35] Mothers in the traditional province of Chongqing had higher levels of milk fat than those from westernized Hong Kong, and higher levels of AA, due to a period of special feeding, during which Chongqing mothers consume up to *ten* eggs per day and large amounts of chicken and pork for the first four weeks after the birth. The diet of Hong Kong mothers was much lower in fat and calories, but because of high fish consumption, their levels of DHA were as high as those of Chongqing mothers. But breast milk levels of AA and DHA in both provinces were much higher than those of Canadian mothers eating a Westernized diet.

Arachidonic acid is critical to early neurological development. In one study, funded by the U.S. National Institute of Child Health and Human Development, infants (eighteen months of age) given supplemental arachidonic acid for seventeen weeks demonstrated significant improvements in intelligence, as measured by the Mental Development Index.[36] This effect is further enhanced by the simultaneous supplementation of DHA with AA. According to one study, babies born to vegetarian women have lower levels of DHA and AA in their blood.[37]

Expectant mothers today receive advice that is conflicting and often wrong. In this atmosphere of confusion, we can do no better than reevaluate the dietary choices of isolated, so-called primitive peoples—the practices described by Dr. Weston A. Price—which emphasized foods rich in cholesterol; in vitamins A, D and K_2; and in AA and DHA for optimal health in newborns and indeed throughout life. Modern science completely validates these traditional practices.

IDEAL BREAST MILK CONTAINS HIGH levels of saturated fat as well. Saturated fats in mother's milk stimulate her baby's immune system and work synergistically with DHA and AA to maintain them in the tissues where they belong.[38] Levels of fat in a mother's milk will decrease with each baby unless she takes special care to consume high levels of nutrient-dense fats between pregnancies, during pregnancy and during each lactation.[39]

Nearly half the fatty acids in human breast milk are saturated, suggesting that dietary saturated fats are critical to the development of infants and young children.[40] Saturated fats are so important during these critical stages of development that their abundant presence in breast milk is universal among mammals. The biochemical reason is clear: saturated fats make up nearly half of our cell membranes, where they anchor proteins to specific locations, participate in signaling activities and transport cellular components. They also form an important source of energy and, of course, carry the all-important fat-soluble vitamins. Most importantly, they support the formation of sex hormones, needed for conception and created in copious quantities during pregnancy.

It would therefore seem illogical to insist that a diet rich in saturated fats is harmful to either an expectant mother or her unborn child, yet many scientists in recent years have claimed to show just that. One recent study, for example, claimed that a "high-saturated-fat diet" fed to pregnant and lactating rat dams caused obesity and brain inflammation in the dams and their pups.[41] What media reports never mention, however, is the fact that the fat used in these diets was only about one-third saturated. Another third was monounsaturated, and the remaining third was polyunsaturated, meaning these diets were much lower in saturated fat and six times richer in polyunsaturated fat than breast milk. The fat, moreover, was provided in the context of a diet based on purified sugar, starch and milk protein, with added supplements of vitamins and minerals—not diets of whole foods. In this study, negative effects likely result from the refined ingredients rather than from their modest content of saturated fat.

Several human studies have also attempted to blame problems that occur in pregnancy on saturated fat. One retrospective study found that mothers who gave birth to children with congenital heart defects ate more saturated fat than other mothers, but the difference was only 1 gram per day, which amounts to less than one-quarter teaspoon of butter.[42] These same mothers also had lower intakes of niacin and riboflavin, and the authors provided no compelling reason to blame the extra gram of saturated fat in their diets.

One randomized trial examined the effect of advising pregnant and breastfeeding mothers to eat a diet that "targeted excessive saturated fat and low fiber consumption." The aim was to reduce the blood levels of an unusual form of insulin in their infants, one that predicts the risk of future metabolic disorders. The diet was successful, but unfortunately the authors did not describe the actual diet in great enough detail to make any important conclusions.[43]

A final study was a randomized trial testing the effect of a "low-cholesterol, low-saturated fat diet" on pregnancy complications. The diet reduced the risk of premature delivery by tenfold[44] and improved indices of blood vessel function in the umbilical artery.[45] The diet, however, was not simply low in cholesterol and saturated fat. It restricted coffee and was high in fatty fish, whole grains, fruits, vegetables, legumes, olive oil, nuts, olives, seeds, vitamin C, vitamin E, vitamin D and magnesium. With these many changes, why should we blame saturated fat or cholesterol, compounds we know to be essential to a developing human being because they are so abundant in breast milk?

Ultimately, the totality of the evidence provided by these studies suggests that pregnant and breastfeeding mothers should eat a diet based on nutrient-dense whole foods. Such a diet inevitably provides a healthy amount of saturated fat and cholesterol along with plenty of vitamins and minerals needed to keep a mother strong and produce a healthy baby.

HOW ARE ANIMAL FATS LIKE SEX? It's a question I often ask the audience at seminars. The answer is that they are both needed for reproduction, and for that reason we have very strong instincts to indulge in both. Suppress these instincts—tell growing girls that sex is unnatural and evil, or that animal fats are unnatural and evil—and they are often shunted into unhealthy sexual expression and eating disorders.

Researchers faced an embarrassing dilemma when a recent study showed that full-fat milk products may help women conceive. Over a period of eight years, Jorge E. Chavarro of the Harvard School of Public Health in Boston assessed the diets of over eighteen thousand married women without a history of infertility who attempted to get pregnant or who became pregnant. During the study, over two thousand women were examined medically for infertility and four hundred thirty-eight were found to be infertile due to lack of ovulation. The researchers found that women who ate two or more servings of low-fat dairy foods per day, particularly skim milk and yogurt, increased their risk of ovulation-related infertility by more than 85 percent compared with women who ate less than one serving of low-fat dairy food per week.[46] Chavarro's advice to women wanting to conceive: consume high-fat dairy foods like whole milk and ice cream, "while at the same time maintaining their normal calorie intake and limiting their overall intake of saturated fats in order to maintain good general health." Once a woman becomes pregnant, says Chavarro, "she should probably switch back to low-fat dairy foods." If we need full-fat dairy foods to conceive, the logical conclusion is that the body needs the same kind of foods to carry a baby to term.*

BACK WHEN NUTRITION WAS A new science, doctors consistently recommended foods like butter, eggs, liver and cod liver oil for pregnancy and proper growth of the developing baby. Liver once a week was commonplace advice for pregnant women, and cod liver oil was a standard supplement up to the Second World War. Much of this advice stemmed from the work of American biochemist Elmer V. McCollum. His diet studies with rats and pigs—both omnivores like humans—convinced him that the healthiest diets for humans contained milk, eggs, butter, organ meats and leafy greens because these foods supported healthy growth and reproduction for the omnivorous animal. Rats on vegetarian diets had low fertility and difficulty raising their young. "They grew fairly well for a time," he noted, "but became stunted when they reached a weight of about 60 percent normal adult size. They lived 555 days, whereas omnivores had an average span of life of 1,020 days. The vegetarians grew to be approximately half as large, and lived half as long as did their fellows which received animal food."[47]

During the 1920s and 1930s Nobel Prize–winning nutritionist Sir John Boyd Orr compared the diets of impoverished Britons to those who were well off. His studies showed that providing milk to poor schoolchildren improved their health and helped them grow.

* No one has looked at the effect of low-fat dairy on fertility, starting at age two, as government agencies recommend. The odds are that infertility due to lifelong fat starvation—which is what most girls today engage in—will not be so easily reversed by a temporary return to high-fat dairy foods.

To alleviate poverty and ill health, he and others in the British Medical Association recommended that the British people drink 80 percent more milk (whole milk, of course) and eat 55 percent more eggs, 40 percent more butter and 30 percent more meat—that was the advice given to the British people in 1938. The government introduced free school milk—full-fat milk—and later worked to provide eggs to all. As a consequence, child deaths from diphtheria, measles, scarlet fever and whooping cough fell dramatically—well before the introduction of antibiotics and widespread immunization. Rickets also declined precipitously. Other factors helped, but the most important factor was the better nutrition that gave children a higher resistance to disease and infection. These recommendations shaped the British diet for nearly fifty years and helped achieve a life expectancy that is now among the highest in the world. Now we are told these same foods are shortening our lives—killing us with coronary heart disease.[48]

These dietary principles continued in Britain until after the Second World War. Food rationing ensured eggs, cod liver oil and orange juice for all children, and schools provided full-fat milk. Even up to the 1980s, full-fat milk, butter and eggs were the norm for pregnant women and growing children. Then came Dean Ornish and other high-profile promoters of a low-fat vegan or vegetarian diet. Ornish condemned what he called the "Group Five" foods—red meat, liver, butter, cream and egg yolks—which he considered worse than "Group Four" foods—doughnuts, fried pastries, cakes, cookies and pies. High-fat diets made people impotent, he pontificated. This is a strange claim considering the fact that early promoters of the same low-fat, plant-based, high-fiber diet had already attempted to take the moral high ground, claiming that red meat and high-fat foods encouraged lust and "natural urges." Sylvester Graham (1794–1851), one of the founders of the American Vegetarian Society, preached that excessive sexual desire caused disease. He advocated a whole grain, vegetarian diet to promote chastity and curb lust. Graham advised parents never to hug and kiss their children, in order to avoid prompting sexual feelings. Boys were to sleep on hard beds to promote manliness and discourage masturbation. John Harvey Kellogg (1852–1943) promoted a high-fiber, vegetarian diet to combat the twin evils of constipation and "natural urges." He railed against sexual activity, even in marriage. His treatment for masturbation: sewing the foreskin shut with silver wire. If that didn't work, then circumcision without anesthesia. Carbolic acid to burn the clitoris for women and girls who showed sexual tendencies.

Today we recognize the dangers of demonizing our natural urges, but the low-fat diet advocated by these nutcases is enshrined as national policy. At first, the target was people "at risk" for heart disease, but children were soon drawn into the net of low-fat dogma. In the 1920s, German scientists performing autopsies on children found fatty streaks and lesions, which they claimed were indicative of atherosclerosis, and without further research, children became the target of the low-fat school of nutrition.[49] In the 1960s, the National Heart, Lung, and Blood Institute began putting children as young as four years old on cholesterol-lowering drugs—but did not follow them into adulthood to see what the long-term effects would be.[50]

Published in 1992, a popular vegetarian cookbook by Frances Moore Lappé, *Diet for a Small Planet*, suggested that a meat-free diet, low in saturated fat and cholesterol, would reduce the risk of obesity, heart disease and cancer. Lappé found another moral reason to justify a vegetarian way of life—it would reduce world hunger, energy costs and the environmental impacts of agriculture.

Many studies at that time cataloged nutrient deficiencies, especially deficiencies in vitamin A, caused by plant-based diets in the Third World. But the dietary gurus in America urged parents to throw out "cholesterol-laden high-fat foods" and give their kids a Third World vegan diet. T. Colin Campbell, director of the Cornell China Study, reported that the healthiest people are those who eat no meat or dairy products at all.*[51] A vegan diet for children would protect them from heart disease and cancer later on, he claimed. The proof, he says, is that the eighty-year-old Dr. Benjamin Spock felt "much better" when he switched to a vegan diet.† Charlotte Gerson, daughter of the late Max Gerson and director of the Gerson Institute, lauded Campbell's work and claimed that her father's remarkable results with cancer patients were due to a vegan diet.[52] She seemed to have forgotten that the main component of the Gerson diet was raw liver juice. Not to be outdone, Dr. Neal Barnard, president of the Physicians Committee for Responsible Medicine (PCRM), filed a lawsuit against the U.S. Department of Agriculture, asserting that the dietary guidelines did not promote a diet "low enough in fat and rich enough in plant products to reduce the higher rates of hypertension, diabetes and prostate cancer among minorities."‡

As pointed out by Nina Teicholz, for many years, the American Academy of Pediatrics refused to bow to NHLBI and AHA pressure. A 1986 editorial in the AAP journal *Pediatrics* noted that a fat-restricted diet "would affect consumption of foods currently providing high quality protein, iron, calcium and other minerals essential for growth."[53] In 1989, pediatrician Fima Lifshitz published a paper describing several cases where, following a diagnosis of heart disease, a parent had significantly reduced dietary fat and cholesterol for the whole family. Lifshitz found that the "overzealous application of a low-fat, low-cholesterol diet" led to "nutritional dwarfing," low weight gain, delayed puberty and serious vitamin deficiencies.[54]

In that same year, Dutch epidemiologist P. C. Dagnelie published a paper describing the nutritional status of children in the Netherlands raised on a macrobiotic regime. The diet of cereal porridges, vegetables, sesame seeds and pulses, with little or no animal foods, would certainly win AHA approval. However, the children were seriously deficient in iron, riboflavin, vitamin B_{12}, vitamin D and calcium. He suggested supplementing the diet with "fat, fatty fish and dairy products."[55] Follow-up papers noted a high prevalence of rickets in the children, slow growth, fat and muscle wasting, and slower psychomotor

* His study did not find any benefits from a largely plant-based diet.[a]

† Maybe so, but Dr. Spock's mind became so addled that he began recommending a vegan diet for growing children.

‡ Restriction of animal protein and fat in children's diets will reduce these adult diseases in one way only—by preventing them from reaching adulthood at all.

development.[56] Children who had increased consumption of fatty fish, dairy products or both grew more rapidly in height than children who remained on the restricted diet.

Undaunted, in 1991, the bureaucrats who administered the National Cholesterol Education Program added children over age two to the list of those receiving "dietary advice." Since that time, parents taking their children in for their two-year-old check-up receive the same scripted lecture: give your child reduced-fat milk; avoid butter, eggs and meat fats; use margarine or tub spreads. Or as restated in 2005: "The general dietary recommendations of the AHA for those aged 2 years and older stress a diet that primarily relies on fruits and vegetables, whole grains, low-fat and nonfat dairy products, beans, fish, and lean meat."[57] Studies referenced for these recommendations abound in praise for their cholesterol-lowering effects, but none look at overall health outcomes as these children grow—such as height and weight; intellectual development; musculature; motor skills; freedom from asthma, allergies and digestive disorders; and reduced fertility.

It was in 1998 that the American Academy of Pediatrics fell in with the American Heart Association to target children with a starvation diet guaranteed to saddle them with health and behavioral problems as they enter adulthood. Clothed in platitudes—"breast feed through the first year," "skip calorie-packed, low-nutrient foods," "delay introducing juice until at least six months of age"—the new guidelines dictated withholding foods that growing children need most, namely animal fats and salt. "Diet changes that lower fat, saturated fat, and cholesterol intake in children and adolescents can be applied safely and acceptably," insisted the AAP's Committee on Nutrition.[58]

Since then parents are advised to feed their children lean meats, skinless chicken, "low-mercury" fish and fat-free milk. In this scheme, children don't even get the small amount of fat in low-fat milk—it must be fat free. And they don't get butter either, but vegetable oils and soft margarine. Plenty of whole grains (including extruded, sugar-laden, whole grain breakfast cereals) mean lots of stress on the developing intestinal tract, and salt restriction guarantees suboptimal intellectual development.*

Not to be outdone, Dr. Daniel Steinberg of the American Heart Association called for "more aggressive cholesterol control" in children by instituting a low-saturated-fat, low-cholesterol diet at *seven months.* Basically this means depriving growing children of eggs, butter, cheese, whole milk, liver and red meat, which supply, among many other nutrients, choline and arachidonic acid, necessary for brain development. And how do these guardians of the nation's health propose to implement such a goal? The language in the report is chilling: "It would, of course, take generations to achieve and would require an all-out commitment of money and manpower to reeducate and modify the behavior of the nation. Is this impossible? No. We have already shown that even a frankly addictive behavior like cigarette smoking can be overcome (eventually) with the right combination of *education, peer pressure, and legislation* [emphasis ours]."[59]

---

* Salt is essential for growth and intellectual development in children—a subject beyond the scope of this book.

For decades the USDA has promoted a low-fat, high-fiber, mostly plant-based diet for the general population, schematically presented in the form of a pyramid. Then in 2007, the USDA came up with My Pyramid for Moms, enshrining the same low-fat suggestions in stone for pregnant women. The guidelines urged expectant moms to eat lean meat, skinless chicken breasts, nonfat milk and dairy products, vegetables and fruits, lots of grains and pasta—and to avoid butter—while carrying their developing child. The same diet is recommended for breastfeeding also. It is impossible to find words harsh enough to describe this evil, baseless plan—one guaranteed to result in more low-birth-weight babies, more birth defects, more miscarriages, more health problems, more behavior disorders, more learning problems and more suffering for both children and parents than ever before—especially with the big promotion it received from columnists like Sally Squires of the *Washington Post*'s Lean Plate Club, who described the new plan as "a savvy way to be a healthier new mom."[60]

In 2011, the USDA replaced their food pyramid with a new schematic: MyPlate. But the diet is not much different than that of the Pyramid, featuring lean meat, low-fat dairy products and plenty of grains. The main difference is higher levels of polyunsaturated oils—namely soy and canola oils. The 2008 publication *MyPlate for Moms, How to Feed Yourself & Your Family Better*, by Elizabeth M. Ward, MS, RD, continues to demonize saturated fats while promoting tub spreads and polyunsaturated oils. The recipes shun all animal fats—not a dab of butter is allowed for growing children. Low-fat cheese, skim milk, low-fat sour cream, low-fat yogurt, lean meat and skinless chicken breasts feature in the recipes. "Lower-fat animal and plant foods should dominate your protein choices," says Ward, "no matter what your age or stage in life."[61]

AND WHAT IS THE RESULT of these "prudent" low-fat dietary choices for our children? News reports from a variety of sources paint an ominous picture of their health, from infancy through adolescence. While scientists and nutritionists are still studying the link between low-fat diets and childhood illness and disability, the array of correlating research is telling.

Starting with the growing problem of premature birth, one baby in eight is now born before thirty-seven weeks, according to a recent report by the Institute of Medicine,[62] a rate that has increased more than 30 percent in the last twenty years—and surveys indicate that preterm births correlate with more processed food in the mother's diet.[63] Most hospitals have invested in expanded premie wards—which are always full and which provide a significant source of revenue for these institutions.

Childhood learning disabilities and emotional problems have also reached epidemic proportions. A report from the 2003 National Survey of Children's Health found that one child in two hundred was autistic and about 20 percent of all children had learning disabilities or attention deficit disorder.[64] Today the number is much higher—one child in sixty is autistic with a rate of one in two predicted within a couple of decades. The consequences for these children and their families can be life altering. "Children with developmental problems had lower self-esteem, more depression and anxiety, more problems with learning, more missed school, and were less involved in sports and other community activities. Their families experienced more difficulty in the areas of childcare, employment, parent-child relationships and caregiver burden."[65]

Other news reports describe children lining up for morning medications while at summer camp—including medication for depression and a host of medications for attention deficit disorder[66]; and bans on games of tag, touch football and soccer at elementary schools because children are getting injured too easily.[67] The latest U.S. census has found that one in every twelve U.S. children and teenagers—more than five million—has a physical or intellectual disability. The figures, which cover children ages five to twenty, are the first collected on childhood disability in the census in more than a century. Special education enrollment has risen twice as fast as overall school enrollment in the past decade, and a growing number of children receive federal Social Security payments because they suffer from serious disabilities.[68]

Meanwhile, reports trickle in about the importance of cholesterol and animal fats for the proper development and overall health of our children. A study by Dutch scientists found that daily consumption of whole milk and butter was linked with significantly reduced rates of asthma and wheezing.[69] Another study found that a high-fat diet protects brain cells in children who have seizures (a condition that affects one in every twenty-five children and 1 percent of adults[70]). And children whose mothers took cod liver oil during pregnancy and lactation scored higher on intelligence tests.[71] And finally, an unpublished report on holoprosencephaly, a birth defect associated with cognitive impairment and facial deformity, found that the condition occurs in infants whose mothers have low levels of cholesterol. Regarding these findings, Judith Hall, professor of pediatrics and medical genetics at the Children and Women's Health Center of British Columbia in Vancouver, stated: "One of the concerns beginning to emerge is that our fad for low-cholesterol may be good for heart disease that affects adults later in life, but may be bad for the embryo and the fetus."[72] With our children's health at risk, we need to express this more strongly: the fad for low-fat, low-cholesterol diets is bad enough for adults, but for children it has been an absolute disaster.

WORRY ABOUT OBESITY IS A big factor in getting moms to conform to low-fat dietary guidelines. The premise is that saturated fat—but not unsaturated fats and not carbohydrates—cause obesity. Not even babies are safe from intervention. Traditional wisdom deems a chubby baby a healthy baby, a joy to behold, a baby asking to be cuddled—a well-nourished child will turn that baby fat into muscle, as it is easier for the child to make muscle out of fat than out of nothing. Now officials are claiming obesity starts in the womb. Intensely worried parents have even gone as far as putting their babies on special diets. In one extreme case, a Washington State couple was found guilty of starving their baby by putting laxatives in her bottle so she wouldn't gain weight.[73] Some parents simply restrict food choices for their infants, especially those containing healthy fats. How can parents be blamed when they get such mixed messages from the so-called experts? "We need to stop the notion that fat, cuddly, cute babies are a good thing," says Dr. Jatinder Bhatia, chairman of the nutrition committee of the American Academy of Pediatrics. But then Bhatia moans, "I have seen parents putting their infant and one-year-old on diets because of history [of obesity] of one parent or another." The experts have lots of suggestions, including breastfeeding, frequent checkups at the pediatrician, and withholding the bottle when baby cries—everything but what growing infants really need, that is, nutrient-dense foods to support the optimal development of the endocrine system and ensure a complete supply of nutrients so that overeating becomes unnecessary.[74]

The premise that saturated fats, rather than unsaturated fats, cause obesity does not hold up to scientific scrutiny. Baby fat is normal and healthy, but signs of obesity often appear somewhat later, in childhood. Researchers in Southampton, UK, found that mothers who have higher levels of omega-6 polyunsaturated fatty acids in their bloodstream during pregnancy have fatter children.[75] Additionally, new results from experiments using animal models show that a high intake of omega-6 from vegetable oils leads to overproduction of signaling compounds that stimulate the appetite, with the result that the animals ate more and developed obesity.[76]

The notion that saturated fats cause obesity has led to draconian policies in schools and day-care centers. Children are no longer allowed full-fat milk at lunch—their choices are reduced-fat milk or "flavored" beverages made with skim milk powder and sweeteners.* The result is more obesity, not less, as discovered in a 2006 Swedish study, which looked at two hundred thirty families in Göteborg, Sweden. Almost all of the children were breastfed until five months and 85 percent had parents who were university educated. Seventeen percent were classified as overweight, and a higher body mass index (BMI) was associated with a *lower* fat intake—and those on lower fat diets consumed more sugar. A lower fat intake was also associated with high insulin resistance.[77]

The 2010 Nutrition Guidelines went further than ever before. Previously, the recommendation for children over the age of two was reduced-fat milk (usually 2 percent milk), yet the new guidelines stipulated fat-free milk for this age group. A mother whose son was in the Dickinson College Children's Center (DCCC), a day-care center in Carlisle, Pennsylvania, received the following letter: "Dear DCCC Families: On October 3, 2011, in order to meet the recommendations of the 2010 Dietary Guidelines of Americans, the Child and Adult Care Food Program (CACFP) is requiring its Centers to serve fat-free milk to children ages two and up. Because we participate in this program for morning and afternoon snack, in order for our snacks to be reimbursed by the CACFP, we will be required to make the change from 2% to fat-free milk."

Such policies can only lead to more obesity. Researchers from the Division of Pediatric Endocrinology at the University of Virginia School of Medicine found that after adjusting for ethnic and economic factors, children who drank skim or 1 percent milk had higher body mass index scores that those who drank whole or 2 percent milk. "We found that among pre-schoolers, consumption of 1 percent skim milk was associated with overweight and obesity," concluded the authors.[78] Many children

* These flavored dairy beverages often contain more sugar than sodas!

compensate for fat deprivation by bingeing on ice cream, which with its load of sugar is bound to contribute to weight gain.

In a recent study, one hundred fifty girls ages eight to ten were put on low-fat diets to "reduce elevated cholesterol levels" while a similar group consumed a normal diet. After five years, the average estrogen and progesterone levels were almost one-third lower in the group assigned to the low-fat diet.[79] (Similar studies in adults show a drop in estrogen in women and a decline in testosterone in men on low-fat diets.) Rather than issue a warning on these alarming results—how can these girls expect normal reproduction with lowered hormone levels?—the researchers proposed that the reduced hormonal output might protect them from breast cancer later in life! This speculation emerged as headlines stating "Eat Less Fat and Stave Off Breast Cancer" in some newspapers.

IN ADDITION TO AVOIDING HEART disease and obesity, the other reason given for restricting fats in children older than two years is the assumption that neurological development is complete by that age. We now know that neurological development continues well into adulthood; indeed we are always growing new neurons, and the brain and nervous system need appropriate nourishment throughout life.

Physicians have always blamed the surge of hormones at puberty for reckless adolescent behavior, but neuroscientists have come up with a different explanation. Beginning around age eleven, the area of the brain associated with social behavior and impulse control actually sprouts a tangle of nerve cells. After puberty, this thicket of nerve sprouts is "pruned." About half the new nerve fibers are cut away to create an efficient network of circuits. The new wiring allows the adult to manage "executive functions" such as goal setting, priority setting, planning, organization and impulse inhibition.[80] Now consider the fact that most American children are denied the kind of fats the brain needs when they are put on low-fat milk and tub spreads at the age of two. How does the brain get fed during this period of delicate rewiring? The answer is that many teenagers enter adulthood not fully wired, and unable to participate in those kinds of activities that give pleasure and a sense of meaning to adults—goal-oriented behavior, priority setting, planning, organization and the kind of patient follow-through that requires impulse inhibition.

Researchers in Kenya have published findings that should give pause to those promoting low-fat vegetarianism in children. The study looked at four groups of children. One group received a plant-based stew with added meat, one group got stew without meat plus whole milk, one group got the stew with added oil, and the fourth group served as a control. Students got the special meals for five consecutive terms. Those getting the stew plus meat showed significantly greater improvements in test scores than those in all the other groups, while those getting the stew plus milk outperformed those getting the stew with oil and the control group. The researchers credited increased folate, iron, vitamin B_{12}, zinc and riboflavin as nutrients that contributed to better cognitive function, but the saturated fats in the meat and whole milk certainly played an important role.[81]

A provocative new study suggests that human intelligence is on the decline, and in fact indicates that Westerners have lost fourteen IQ points since the Victorian era. The researchers looked at studies on visual reaction times—how long it takes to press a button in response to seeing stimulus. Reaction time reflects a person's mental processing speed, and so is considered an indication of general intelligence. Since the late nineteenth century, visual reaction times have increased from an average of 194 milliseconds to 275.[82] According to the head researcher, Dr. Jan te Nijenhuis, the decline is due to the fact that women of intelligence are having fewer children; in fact, he says, the decline may be even greater than what the study results suggest because of environmental factors, "such as better education, hygiene and nutrition." These factors may mask the true, steeper decline in "genetically inherited intelligence in the Western world."[83] No one is considering the possibility that nutrition is a bigger factor than genetics when it comes to intelligence, and that in fact, our nutrition is getting worse. How can we expect anything but decline when our babies and growing children are deprived of the very things they need to develop normal brains: cholesterol and saturated fat.

Not all countries are as zealous about restricting fats as our own. In a major departure, new Canadian guidelines say parents should be offering their six-month-old infants puréed meat, fish and poultry two or three times a day. (Unfortunately, they also allow "meat alternatives" for baby.) According to the guidelines, these iron-rich foods should be the first that babies consume—not cereal and vegetables. "Traditionally, we've been telling parents that meat is the last food to introduce," said Daina Kalnins, manager of clinical dietetics at the Hospital for Sick Children. "But when you look at why, there is no reason to do that." Iron is critical for a baby's growth and cognitive development. By about six months, a baby's iron stores start to diminish; those solely fed breast milk will not meet their iron requirements and are in danger of becoming anemic or iron-deficient. According to Kalnins, iron deficiency during infancy and childhood may affect proper brain development. Interestingly, the guidelines mention that meat and fish have been traditional first foods for some aboriginal groups. Parents are urged to make baby's food, puréeing meat and fish with water. Unfortunately, they recommend leaving out salt. Still, the recommendation to introduce meat early is a real step forward in baby care.[84]

One of the dangers of a cholesterol-lowering diet for children is anemia. Without meat to supply iron, and without organ meats and animal fats to supply vitamin A (needed for iron assimilation), children are at great risk of deficiency. In addition to lowered IQ, anemia in young children manifests as follows: "Infants with chronic, severe iron deficiency have been observed to display increased fearfulness, unhappiness, fatigue, low activity, wariness, solemnity, and proximity to the mother during free play, developmental testing and at home. In a recent preventative trial in Chile, ratings after thirty to forty-five minutes of developmental testing showed that, compared with infants who received iron supplementation, a greater percentage of unsupplemented infants never smiled, never interacted socially, and never showed social referencing."[85]

Anemia is a major health concern for children in developing countries. In a study of children in Bangladesh, vitamin A supplementation proved to be the most successful micronutrient intervention for treating the debilitating condition.[86] The researchers noted that no sign of improvement appears with iron supplementation programs. While American medical personnel are hell-bent on demonizing vitamin A—and frightening parents away from giving their children sources of vitamin A like butter, liver and cod liver oil—researchers in other parts of the world are developing a grudging appreciation for the role of vitamin A in mineral metabolism.

Reasons for taking cod liver oil—and giving it to children—just keep piling up. A recent clinical trial found that supplementation with a multivitamin containing selenium together with cod liver oil can reduce rates of ear infections in children.[87] In the study, five of seven children who had experienced frequent ear infections had none while taking the supplements. The study authors also found that children suffering from ear infections had lower levels of vitamin A, selenium and EPA compared to healthy adults. Cod liver oil provides EPA and vitamin A—and probably helps in the absorption of selenium also.

RAMPANT TOOTH DECAY IS EMERGING as a serious problem in children, even as young as two years of age. Dentists regularly see preschoolers with ten cavities at a time; according to an American Dental Association spokesman, the problem is "so severe that they often recommend using general anesthesia because young children are unlikely to sit through such extensive procedures while they are awake."[88] While dentists rightly warn parents about feeding sweets and fruit juice to children, their only real solution to the problem is drill and fill. The notion that teeth can heal themselves is completely foreign to the dental profession. Yet as far back as 1928, Julian D. Boyd, MD, and C. L. Drain, DDS, of Iowa City reported "numerous instances of definite arrest of caries in children. Teeth containing large cavities, which ordinarily would have an area of softened dentin surrounding the zone of destruction, were found instead to be very dense." The doctors made the fascinating observation that all the children with cavities that reversed and healed were diabetics who had been put on a high-fat, low-carb diet for blood sugar control. The regimen consisted of "milk, cream, butter, eggs, meat, cod liver oil, bulky vegetables and fruits. The daily menu was designed to include approximately one quart of milk and cream daily." Levels of vitamins and minerals in the diet were high. The doctors concluded that oral hygiene had little to do with dental health, and that resistance to dental decay was due mainly to a nutrient-dense diet during the period of growth.[89]

Cheese is one of the victims of modern diet theories—if cheese is allowed at all, it must be low-fat, say the pundits. Researchers have found that babies born to women who consume cheese during pregnancy are likely to have better dental health than babies born to non–cheese consumers. Surprisingly, this research took place at the Fukuoka University, University of Tokyo and Osaka City University. The researchers looked at the long-term effects of prenatal cheese and dairy consumption on an infant's tooth development, tracking three hundred fifteen Japanese mother-and-child pairs, recording prenatal diets and performing dental examinations of children between forty-one and fifty months of age. The study found a strong connection between cheese consumption during pregnancy and decreased risk of childhood dental caries, such as tooth decay and cavities.[90] Ironically, the results were not related to calcium intake. "Components of cheese other than calcium might be responsible for the protective effects of maternal cheese intake against dental caries in children," the researchers said. In fact, cheese is a perfect food for developing strong teeth (and bones) with its content of vitamins A, D and K_2, along with calcium, phosphorus and other minerals—as long as it is full-fat cheese. There was no evident relationship between maternal milk intake and the risk of childhood dental caries, suggesting that cheese from pasteurized milk is a better choice for pregnant moms than pasteurized milk.

Margo Wootan, nutrition policy director for the Center for Science in the Public Interest, one of the organizations responsible for replacing healthy saturated fats with toxic *trans* fats in the American food supply, objects to local food for school lunches because the children might end up eating "full-fat cheese from a local farmer, and it's still going to clog your arteries and give you heart disease."[91]

UNFORTUNATELY, THE FOOD POLICE SEEM more determined than ever to remove the last scrap of animal fat from children's diets. In an article on obesity in the October 2010 issue of the *Journal of the American Dietetic Association*, authors Jill Reedy and Susan M. Krebs-Smith bemoan the fact that, "Nearly 40 percent of total calories consumed by 2–18 year olds were in the form of empty calories from solid fat and from added sugars. Half of empty calories came from six foods." And which are the foods contributing to "empty" calories? Soda, fruit drinks, dairy desserts, grain desserts, pizza…and whole milk."[92] Dairy desserts (that is, conventional ice cream), pizza, and conventional whole milk, while not optimal, at least provide desperately needed saturated fats in the diets of growing children. The proposed solution: a starvation diet of fruits, vegetables, whole grains, nonfat milk and lean meat.

Describing her family's eating habits as a "bacon-and-eggs" diet when her husband first took office, Michelle Obama then took a wrong turn and used her influence to promote a lean diet based largely on fruits and non-starchy vegetables for schoolchildren. Under the three-billion-dollar National School Lunch Program, participating schools can provide only one serving of meat or other protein (more well-off children can buy a second portion each day with their own dime). There's no butter for the dry brown bread (which the children do not like), and no whole or even 2 percent milk. Worst of all, there's a calorie cap of 850 calories for high schoolers, 700 for middle schoolers and a mere 650 calories for kids in elementary schools—so even potatoes are limited to a single small serving and ketchup packets are rationed to one per student. Parents complain that their kids are starving, and the kids say the food "tastes like vomit." Across the country, some wealthier suburban school districts are simply backing out of the program, although doing so means giving up a six-figure annual subsidy from the federal government.[93] Last year the New York City school system dropped out after the students complained of starvation, and an Illinois school district dumped the guidelines before even fully implementing them.[94]

A 2007 USDA survey found that almost 90 percent of Americans "are still choosing diets out of sync with dietary guidance."[95] Proposals to induce compliance include use of prepaid cards in grocery stores and schools that prohibit purchase of "unhealthy" foods; encouragement of online food ordering with less "tempting" options; and more restrictions on food stamp and school meal programs.[96] The Arizona health director has issued an edict forbidding participants in the WIC (Women, Infants and Children) program from using their coupons to purchase whole milk. They must buy low-fat, skim or soy milk. And only 16 ounces of cheese is allowed per month.[97] The program has also cut back on eggs, allowing only one dozen per month. Similar guidelines are now in place in many other states. Even during the austerity of the Second World War, British rationing regulations allowed one egg per child per day.

Schoolchildren are not only targets for manipulation via diet; they also find themselves in the headlights of the pharmaceutical industry. If we need any proof that our culture has completely sacrificed the health and well-being of future generations to financial interests, consider the 2008 recommendations for "wider cholesterol screening for children and more aggressive use of cholesterol-lowering drugs, starting as early as the age of eight."[98] Why do we need these draconian measures? In "hopes" of preventing adult heart problems. Since cholesterol-lowering measures have not stemmed the tide of heart disease, the hope of preventing heart disease using the same measures in children is a vain hope indeed. The new guidelines come from the American Academy of Pediatrics (AAP), which admits that there is not "a whole lot of data" on pediatric use of cholesterol-lowering drugs but that the drugs are "generally safe for children."[99]

Taking things one step further, the pharmaceutical industry is targeting children with a chewable cholesterol-lowering product! In 2010, Pfizer, Inc., announced that the European Commission had approved a chewable form of Lipitor for use in children over the age of ten. Pfizer's Lipitor is the best-selling medicine worldwide, with sales of over eleven billion dollars in 2009. But revenues are steadily dropping so children are the natural targets for boosting lagging sales.[100]

FDA lists statins in category X for pregnancy, along with thalidomide and Accutane—meaning that they should *never* be taken by pregnant women.[101] They are teratogens, with the potential to cause horrible birth defects. For this reason, the March of Dimes has opposed over-the-counter statin sales—women might respond to advertising for the drugs and take them during the early stages of pregnancy. But researchers at New York's Hospital for Special Surgery have pregnant women in their sights. They tested statins on mice with a condition called antiphospholipid syndrome (APS), which can cause miscarriages, and found that biochemical markers indicative of better pregnancy outcome improved. Now they are claiming that statins should be given to women with APS-induced pregnancy complications. Guillermina Girardi, PhD, lead author of the study, claims that statins are perfectly safe for pregnant women and that a trial involving pregnant women is needed.[102] Even if birth defects do not manifest, low cholesterol during pregnancy is tied to premature birth.[103]

According to a recent study carried out at the University of Rome, low cholesterol levels in children are also associated with an increased risk for attentional impulsivity with mood symptoms. "Impulsivity is directly mentioned in the...diagnostic criteria for several disorders and is implied in the criteria for others, including attention-deficit hyperactivity disorder, personality disorders, mania, and substance abuse/dependence," writes study author Alfonso Troisi in the journal *Psychiatry Research*. Troisi notes that "evidence linking impulsivity and cholesterol levels to suicide risk attests to the clinical relevance of studying the relationship between cholesterol levels and impulsivity." In the study of three hundred one patients in psychiatric institutions, after accounting for factors such as age, gender, diagnosis and current mood symptoms, the researchers found that lower total cholesterol levels were significantly associated with increased attentional impulsivity, particularly among patients with levels below 165 mg/dl. Troisi concludes: "The current study adds to the growing body of evidence pointing to the association between serum cholesterol and mental health...Considering that attentional/cognitive impulsivity is a demonstrated risk factor for suicide, patients presenting with low cholesterol and mood symptoms may warrant increased clinical attention and surveillance."[104] If low cholesterol is associated with increased impulsivity in adults, it makes sense that low cholesterol in children curses them with the same effects.

A GREAT BODY OF RESEARCH shows us that animal foods rich in cholesterol and saturated fat are fundamental to normal growth, development and behavior in children. Many years in the future we will look back on this benighted age as one professing to love children while feeding them in a way that results in their profound unhappiness. But the epidemic of poor health in our children today is not without a silver lining; many parents are waking up to the need for nutrient-dense, high-fat animal foods starting before conception and continuing throughout the years of growth. While scientists have yet to formally study these children, reports from their parents uniformly record optimal growth, straight teeth, keen intelligence and good disposition in their offspring.[105] Perhaps the day will come when all young people will learn the principles of good nutrition before conception, and when all health professionals will support prospective parents with the knowledge they need to produce optimally healthy babies.

CHAPTER 9

Animal Fats for the Mind

Smith-Lemli-Opitz Syndrome (SLOS) is a genetic disorder that prevents the body from manufacturing all the cholesterol it needs. Symptoms include intellectual disability, hyperactivity, irritability, poor attention span and tendency toward aggressive and self-injuring behavior. The most common treatment for SLOS is a cholesterol supplement, which leads to improvement in many of the symptoms found in SLOS patients—including hyperactivity, irritability, attention span, muscle tone, endocrine function, resistance to infection and gastrointestinal problems.

Twenty-five percent of the body's cholesterol resides in the brain—an organ that provides only 2–3 percent of the body's total weight. Cholesterol is so critical to the brain and all its functions, that it manufactures cholesterol on-site.[1] Most of this manufacture occurs at night, during sleep, which is one of the reasons a good night's sleep is so important to mental function.

Until recently, scientists held that cholesterol in the bloodstream could not get past the blood-brain barrier and that, as a consequence, the brain made all its own cholesterol. But the fact that cholesterol supplements uniformly help those suffering from SLOS indicates that at least some cholesterol from the bloodstream does pass into the brain. In 2010, scientists confirmed the fact that the brain is not a "closed circuit," but that it can take cholesterol from the bloodstream as needed.[2] In the elderly, eggs improve memory,[3] again indicating that dietary cholesterol can be sequestered into the brain.

To better understand the role cholesterol plays, it's important to look at the way the brain functions. Two types of cells populate the brain. First are the neurons, cells specialized to pass signals to other neurons or to other target cells. These signals—which can be electrical or chemical—pass across structures called synapses. All mental function—thoughts, memories, reasoning and learning—depends on the formation of synapses.

The other main type of cell in the brain and nervous system are the glial cells—from the Greek word for glue. These are nonneuronal cells that maintain homeostasis and provide support and protection for neurons in the central and peripheral nervous systems.

During sleep, the genes in the glial cells

needed for the synthesis and maintenance of myelin become active. It is the glial cells that form myelin—a kind of electrical insulation material around the neurons, allowing them to send electrical impulses in a quick and orderly way. The myelin is especially rich in cholesterol. Multiple sclerosis is an illness in which the myelin sheaths are inadequate or disintegrating—yet typical advice for MS sufferers is to avoid saturated fat and full-fat dairy foods on the false premise that saturated fats cause inflammation. Butter, egg yolks, liver and saturated animal fats are some of our best sources of cholesterol, the essential building material of myelin, and the saturated fats they contain help resolve inflammation; they would seem to be the logical first treatment for this dreadful degenerative disease.

For over a century, investigators believed that the glial cells did not play any role in neurotransmission. However, we now know that the glial cells assist the neurons to form connections across the synapses.[4] Early research discovered an unidentified compound made by glial cells that was responsible for the ability of neurons to form synapses. Without this "glial factor," neurons formed few synapses, and the synapses they did form were inefficient and poorly functioning. In the presence of glial cells, which secrete the unknown factor, neurons formed many highly efficient synapses.

It was in 2001 that researchers identified the mysterious glial factor—it was cholesterol! The glial cells release the cholesterol in a carrier called apolipoprotein E (apoE). At first, the investigators thought that apoE was the glial factor itself, but neurons treated with apoE did not show any increased synapse formation. The apoE carries a number of compounds, including phosphatidylcholine, sphingomyelin and cholesterol. Yet only cholesterol increased synapse formation when applied to the neurons—in fact, a solution of cholesterol increased synapse formation twelvefold. The other compounds had little effect and actually inhibited synapse formation at high doses.[5]

The investigators then used the cholesterol-lowering drug mevastatin to reduce cholesterol secretion by the glial cells. The reduced-cholesterol glial secretion had a strongly diminished effect on synapse formation. When they added cholesterol back to the low-cholesterol secretion, synapse formation was fully restored.

The authors identified cholesterol as a limiting factor of synapse formation. In other words, low availability of cholesterol can directly limit the ability to form synapses.

CHOLESTEROL DOES MORE THAN HELP fire the synapses; it also helps the brain's neurons grow and connect. Neurons have many tentacles or arms, which connect the neurons with other neurons, or with muscles across synapses. These arms are called neurites: those that send impulses away from the cell are called axons and those that receive impulses are called dendrites.

The synapses in our brains, where axons and dendrites meet, are constantly breaking and re-forming. The neurites grow toward other neurites in response to a stimulus given by a signaling protein in the membranes of neurons. These signaling proteins rely on cholesterol-rich lipid rafts (see Chapter 4), where long-chain saturated fatty acids secure some of the proteins. A 2004 study found that when investigators removed some of the cholesterol from the lipid rafts in the neuron membrane, the neurons could not find the signaling proteins.[6]

Because one of the characteristics of Alzheimer's is a cholesterol by-product in the brain, the dietary gurus promote low-fat,

Neurons and Glial Cells

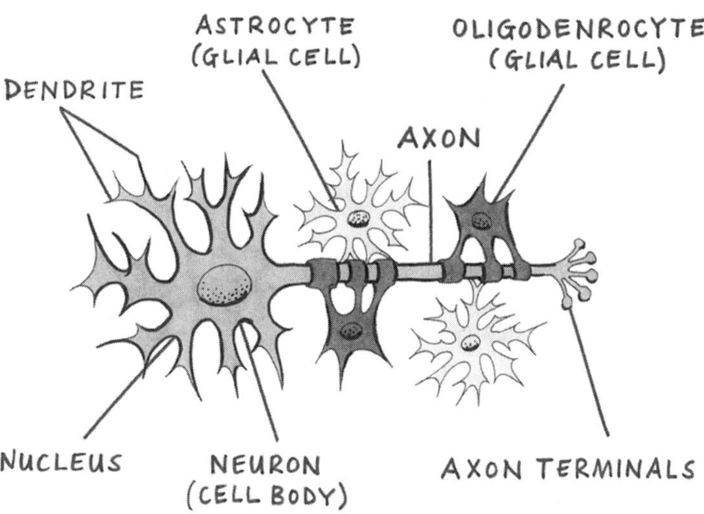

Glial cells attached to the neurons use cholesterol to support synapse formation.

low-cholesterol foods as brain-healthy and a way to prevent Alzheimer's. But what the current research shows us is that the brain is completely dependent on cholesterol to function properly—for all thought processes and all memory—for reading, reasoning and relationships.

The traditional view of human brain development is that babies are born with all the brain cells they will ever have, and that neurological development occurs through the connection of these cells in the early years. We now know that from birth through late adolescence, the brain adds billions of new cells, constructing its circuits out of freshly made neurons as children and teenagers interact with their environments. In adulthood, the process of adding new cells slows down but does not stop. Mature brain circuits appear to be maintained by new cell growth well into old age.[7] In addition, the neurites are constantly seeking new connections, and the synapses fire millions of times per second.

These discoveries reveal why everyone benefits from high-cholesterol foods. For infants and growing children, who don't make all the cholesterol they need, these foods are essential for optimal intellectual growth. For adults, these foods may be the critical input to protect against degenerative diseases like Alzheimer's and even just annoying conditions like short-term memory loss.

High levels of cholesterol in the blood provide protection against mental decline. A 2005 Swedish study analyzed data from three hundred ninety-two men and women in Göteborg, Sweden, over an eighteen-year period. Researchers found that high total cholesterol at ages seventy, seventy-five and seventy-nine was associated with a reduced risk of dementia between ages seventy-nine and eighty-eight.[8] American researchers found that in the elderly, the best memory function was observed in those with the highest levels of cholesterol. Low cholesterol was associated with an increased risk for depression and even death.[9]

These discoveries also show the increased risk of taking cholesterol-lowering statin drugs, which are so often associated with mental decline, amnesia and neurological disorders like Parkinson's disease. But scientists wedded to the cholesterol theory of heart disease dare not make so bold a statement. Referring to the Swedish study, Michelle M. Mielke of the Center on Aging and Health at Johns Hopkins Bloomberg School of Public Health stated: "These findings raise more questions than they give answers. Therefore, we strongly urge that consumers not make changes in their diet or medication without consulting with their doctors first." Rachel Whitmer, a research scientist specializing in cognitive aging at Kaiser Permanente Northern California Division of Research, also danced around the issue: "Lingering questions were not put to rest, but new exciting ones are raised... This study is another example of the importance of timing in terms of when one measures a risk factor, and the need to consider risk factors for dementia over the entire life course."[10]

A 2005 follow-up to the famous Framingham Heart Study, published in *Psychosomatic Medicine*, found that lower naturally occurring total cholesterol levels were associated with poorer performance on cognitive measures such as abstract reasoning, attention, concentration, word fluency and executive functioning. Once again, double-talk was necessary: "Competing risks must always be taken into consideration," said the researchers. "Lower cholesterol values may have modestly detrimental effects on cognitive function for the individual but, depending on the patient's risk profile, may have beneficial effects with respect to cardiovascular morbidity and mortality."[11]

It seems that cholesterol is important for neuromotor reactions as well. In 2009, the military funded a study to find out which foods are best for pilots. Since the military has a lot invested in pilots, they wanted to know which kind of diet supported them the best. University of North Dakota researchers found that forty-five pilots who ate the fattiest foods, such as butter or gravy, had the quickest response times in mental tests and made fewer mistakes when flying in tricky cloud conditions.*[12]

A growing body of research supports the idea that diets rich in animal fats improve and protect brain function in many ways. Animal fats supply much-needed cholesterol—cholesterol for the brain forming in utero, cholesterol for the brain that is growing and maturing in the infant and child, and cholesterol for the mature brain of the adult. In principle, an adult can make all the cholesterol he or she needs, but why not give the complex cholesterol-production mechanism relief by supplying as much cholesterol as possible from the diet, through sources like chicken liver, beef liver, chicken and turkey giblets, meat fats, egg yolks and butter? These foods nourish the brain in many other ways as well.

AT AGE TEN, BILLY (NOT his real name) could not speak. His parents suspected that he could read, but since he could not communicate with them, they were not sure. The diagnosis: autism. Standardized IQ tests indicated moderate intellectual disability.

His pediatrician, Dr. Mary Megson of Richmond, Virginia, had noticed that night blindness and thyroid conditions—both signs of vitamin A deficiency—were common in family members of autistic children. Billy's

* Surprisingly, after those on the high-fat diet, pilots on the high-carbohydrate diet performed best, with the worst performance from pilots on the high-protein diet.

mother had a thyroid condition and also suffered from dry eyes (another sign of vitamin A deficiency) and gluten intolerance.[13]

Megson began giving Billy cod liver oil, supplying the boy with 2,500 IU vitamin A twice daily. After one week, his behavior began to change—he began to sit farther from the television and to notice paintings on the walls at home. He started running across the grass from the front door to the school bus—while before he had carefully followed the sidewalk and driveway to the bus. After three weeks, Megson gave Billy a small dose of a pharmaceutical version of choline, called Urocholine. Thirty minutes later, Billy swung his feet over the side of the chair, pointed to a glass candy jar on the shelf and spoke his first words in eight years: "May I have the red Jolly Rancher, please?" His parents now had proof that he could read.*

Megson and his mother took him outside. "The leaves, the leaves on the trees are green!" he said. "I see, I see!" When Megson asked to take his picture, he looked at the camera, smiled and waved. When he left the office, Megson said, "See you later," to which he responded, "What time?"

As Dr. Megson explains, in genetically predisposed children, autism is linked to a G-alpha protein defect. G-alpha proteins form one of the most prevalent signaling systems in our cells, regulating processes as diverse as cell growth, hormonal regulation and sensory perception—like seeing. The defect may be triggered by a variety of factors, especially when the child is already deficient in vitamin A, and cause the separation of the G-alpha protein from retinoid receptors. Vitamin A helps reconnect the retinoid receptors.

Children like Billy do not see the way people with normal vision do. Dr. Megson explains: "These children live in a 'magic-eye puzzle:' you've probably seen these puzzles at the mall. You stare at a cluster of shapes and colors, and eventually an image will pop out. These children, because of the blocked pathway affecting their vision, can't see like most people do. The blocked pathway has caused the rods in their eyes to not function correctly. They must compensate for the rod dysfunction the best way they can. They 'see' the world around them as though it's in a 3-D box. They have such a limited visual field that everything that doesn't fit in their box blurs and is perceived as color and shape alone. And, the most incredible thing is that they actually have to piece together each 'box' that they see in order to see a complete shape."

According to Megson, the blocked visual pathways explain why children on the autism spectrum "melt down" when objects are moved or when you clean up their lines or piles of toys sorted by color. They work hard to piece together their world; it frightens and overwhelms them when the world as they are able to see it changes. It also might explain why children on the autism spectrum spend time organizing things so carefully. It's the only way they can "see" what's out there.

Megson claims that their main issue is a visual problem. They typically look at things sideways—including at parents telling them to "look at me." They turn their eye so that the light reflected off the parent's face lands on the edge of the fovea or the lateral retina, where they have some rod function remaining. The fovea is the area in the back of the eye where the cones are closest together. When you force the child to look directly at you, you are actually

---

* For many reasons, the artificially colored red candy would not be a good food for Billy.

forcing them to look away from you because their only good field of vision is off to one side.*

With vitamin A from cod liver oil, Megson has witnessed improved rod function—vitamin A is not called retinol for nothing. She's seen the sideways glance, so typical of an autistic child, disappear in front of her. Megson believes that Vitamin A—along with the jolt of pharmaceutical choline—made the connections that facilitated Billy's speech as well. The retinoid receptors are critical not only for vision but for sensory perception, language processing and attention.†

What's interesting is that Dr. Megson feels that the retinol form of vitamin A is absorbed best—retinol being the form found in butter and in the livers of animals and fish. Most vitamin supplements and infant formula contain vitamin A palmitate, which is not effective in connecting the G-alpha proteins to the retinoid receptors. Of all the food sources of retinol vitamin A, fish liver oil is the only source of a form of vitamin A called 14-hydroxy-retro-retinol (14-HRR). G-protein defects can block the conversion of vitamin A into this 14-HRR.

Urocholine is a prescription drug that stimulates the release of acetylcholine at nerve endings, and acts like an artificial acetylcholine. (Bethanechol is the generic name for Urecholine.) It stimulates gastric motility, increases gastric tone and often restores impaired rhythmic peristalsis of the intestines. It also increases bile and pancreatic secretions and indirectly stimulates the vitamin A receptors in the brain's hippocampus.‡

In Billy's case, he continued to improve as long as he faithfully took his cod liver oil and small doses of Urecholine. When he did not take it, he quickly regressed.

Megson's work with Billy and other patients on the autism spectrum is supported in studies of mice. Researchers at the Salk Institute for Biological Studies found that removing vitamin A from the mouse diet diminishes chemical changes in the brain considered the hallmarks of learning and memory. Lack of vitamin A interferes with optimal function of the hippocampus. Earlier work indicated that mice born without receptors for vitamin A in the hippocampus performed under par in standardized learning tests. When vitamin A is added back to the diets of the mice, the impairment is reversed. Said the researchers, "These data suggest a major mental consequence for the hundreds of millions of adults and children who are vitamin A deficient."[14]

Billy's case, and others like it, indicate that vitamin A from animal fats like butter and cod liver oil can have profound effects on mental function and behavior. We need more of these old-fashioned foods to protect our young people from modern diseases.

SHAPED LIKE A SEAHORSE, THE hippocampus resides deep in the brain, halfway

* Physicians and psychologists often blame this tendency for children to look sideways or away on "cold parenting"—especially laying blame on mothers who may appear "emotionally remote" or "cruel." But these parents usually love their children very much. The tendency to look away results from a flaw in the retina, not faulty parenting techniques.

† Vitamin A is also extremely important for the maintenance of healthy intestinal flora—remember that Billy's mother was gluten intolerant, a sign of disrupted gut bacteria.

‡ Megson also stresses the importance of salt for autistic children. If there is a G-protein defect, three of the channels that remove calcium from the cells are blocked. The only other major means of removing calcium is with salt. If there isn't enough salt in the diet, there is the danger of brain cell calcification.

between the ears and the midpoint of the skull. Considered the seat of memory—humans in whom the hippocampus is damaged or removed cannot form memories of near-term experiences—the current view holds that the organ plays a key role in learning. The hippocampus also seems to play a role in spatial memory and navigation, impulse control and even olfaction—the sense of smell. In Billy's case, vitamin A helped support hippocampus function as vitamin A is required to support neuroplasticity in the hippocampus; this is one reason that vitamin A deficiency will depress learning and memory.[15] And if a lack of vitamin A results in impaired function of the hippocampus, so does a lack of vitamin D.

Aging rodents—one pictures rats in slippers and bathrobes—have helped researchers define the relationship between vitamin D and cognitive decline. Using middle-aged rats, scientists found that rats with high levels of vitamin D in their blood outperformed low and medium groups in an activity called maze reversal, a particularly challenging task for the aging rodent, one that detects subtle changes in memory. Their explanation was that vitamin D optimizes gene expression in the hippocampus—improving the "likelihood of successful brain aging," an outcome desirable for both aging rats and aging humans.[16]

The discovery of vitamin D, its activating enzyme and vitamin D receptors in the brain has the research community aglow with enthusiasm about the role of vitamin D in neurological function. It seems that vitamin D is critical for brain development, brain protection (through programmed cell death), nerve growth throughout life, maintenance of glial cells and normal brain function. Vitamin D deficiency is associated with cognitive impairment, dementia, Parkinson's disease, multiple sclerosis, epilepsy and schizophrenia.[17]

Vitamin D has also shown neuroprotective effects, including the clearance of amyloid plaques, a hallmark of Alzheimer's disease.[18] Associations of low vitamin D with Alzheimer's disease and dementia emerged in an important European study, published in 2005.[19] Researchers found that the risk of cognitive impairment was up to four times greater in severely deficient elders.[20] Vitamin D seems to protect against stroke,[21] and two large prospective studies indicate that low vitamin D concentrations may increase the risk of cognitive decline.[22]

However, study results on vitamin D and brain health are not uniform. Two studies, conducted in an older middle-aged healthy population who were participating in the Atherosclerosis Risk in Communities (ARIC) Brain MRI Study, failed to find significant associations between lower levels of vitamin D and lower cognitive test scores, dementia risk or the development of brain pathologies.[23]

But the link between low vitamin D and dementia was clear in a 2014 study, which found that participants who were severely vitamin D deficient were more than twice as likely to develop dementia and Alzheimer's disease.[24] Adults in the study who were moderately deficient in vitamin D had a 53 percent increased risk of developing dementia of any kind, and the risk increased to 125 percent in those who were severely deficient. Similar results were recorded for Alzheimer's disease, with the moderately deficient group 69 percent more likely to develop this type of dementia, jumping to a 122 percent increased risk for those severely deficient.

A COMMON CHARGE LEVELED AGAINST vitamin A is the accusation that it causes depression. The main argument for this is the observed side effect of Accutane—a synthetic type of vitamin A used to treat acne—namely, depression and suicide.

But Accutane is not vitamin A; in fact, evidence indicates that it can cause vitamin A deficiency. When newborn mice receive treatment with dexamethasone, a drug that damages lung tissue, natural vitamin A helps treat the condition while the active ingredient of Accutane has no effect and may even make it worse.[25] Accutane can cause night blindness, a traditional sign of vitamin A deficiency, whereas vitamin A supplementation is the treatment that cures night blindness.[26] In rats, the active ingredient of Accutane accumulates in the eyes and interferes with vitamin A recycling; rats receiving it at high doses took fifty times longer to recover from exposure to intense light than controls.[27]

Natural vitamin A can actually resolve depression—this is the conclusion of a physician who had two patients who developed depression while taking Accutane[28]; when the physician took them off the drug and supplemented them with 10,000–12,000 IU of vitamin A for seven to ten days, the depression resolved.*

Researchers have not examined the relationship between vitamin A status and depression, but it appears that the physical ailments associated with such mental illnesses can be associated with vitamin A deficiency. For example, the incidence and severity of Crohn's disease and ulcerative colitis, the two most common forms of inflammatory bowel disease, and the incidence and severity of asthma in children, are all associated with deficient blood levels of vitamin A.[29] These findings imply that vitamin A might be involved in preventing depression or anxiety as these conditions often have depression as a side effect.

Looking at the evidence carefully, one can conclude that natural vitamin A might not cause depression, but actually chases away the blues.† While research has yet to confirm a direct link, the evidence is building. However, owing to vitamin A's low status in the vitamin hierarchy, most scientists still stand behind the idea that vitamin A causes depression.[30]

THE ESKIMOS ARE A HAPPY people. This is the observation of many anthropologists who have lived with this resourceful population. The exception is a kind of hysteria called *pibloktoq*, a disorder where the victim becomes irritable and withdrawn, and then, in a sudden excitation, leaves the camp and engages in irrational and dangerous behavior. After that come convulsive seizures and a twelve-hour period of coma or stuporous sleep. Only after this train of events does the afflicted person's behavior become normal again.

In the first paper to describe *pibloktoq*, published 1985, vitamin A got the blame.[31] The researcher noted that the Eskimos consider polar bear liver, which is the richest source of vitamin A, to be toxic. Explorers who ate polar bear liver out of necessity experienced drowsiness, irritability, headaches and nausea within

* The physician then put them back on Accutane to treat their acne. Surely a better solution is to have them keep taking the natural vitamin A.

† I knew of a woman who was able to get off her antidepressants by taking cod liver oil; when she reported the happy news to her psychiatrist, however, he warned her vehemently against this old-fashioned remedy, claiming that it would destroy her liver. She dutifully stopped taking it and soon after needed to go on antidepressants again.

hours of consuming it. Case reports of vitamin A toxicity describe irritability, drowsiness, double vision and anorexia.

Pibloktoq proved perplexing for researchers, however. The Eskimos consumed a diet rich in vitamin A throughout the year, while the specific symptoms of *pibloktoq* occurred in Arctic latitudes only in late winter and early spring. Furthermore, they consider polar bear liver safe as long as the membrane is removed. And they eat seal liver, which is also high in vitamin A, in unlimited quantities. How is vitamin A toxicity to blame?

A better theory ties *pibloktoq* to tetany, which is characterized by involuntary muscle contractions and caused by severe deficiencies of calcium and vitamin D. The muscle contractions occur because the peripheral nerves cannot regulate their impulses without calcium. Other symptoms of tetany include "emotional and cognitive disorganization" and convulsive seizures, probably resulting from the absence of calcium in the central nervous system. As with *pibloktoq*, episodes are acute and sporadic.

The primary source of vitamin D and calcium in the Eskimo diet is fish, and in the late winter and early spring, when stores of dried fish may become depleted, vitamin D and calcium deficiencies may occur.* These two nutrients are critical for the production of endocannabinoids—and one of the roles of these calming chemicals is the prevention of seizures.

VITAMIN K_2—THE THIRD IN OUR triumvirate of fat-soluble vitamins—supports cognitive processes in a variety of ways. The brain contains one of the highest concentrations of vitamin K_2 in the body; only the pancreas, the salivary glands and the cartilaginous tissue of the sternum contain more.† Vitamin K_2 supports the formation of compounds called sphingolipids in both the neurons and the glial cells, and in this way vitamin K_2 is critical to optimal myelination of the nerve cells. Also, there is growing evidence that the most prevalent vitamin K_2 isomer has anti-inflammatory activity and offers protection against oxidative stress.

In addition to supporting sphingolipid function, vitamin K_2 supports the enzymes within the brain that produce an important class of fats called sulfatides, two fatty acids—again, saturated fatty acids—attached to, among other things, a sulfur molecule. The levels of vitamin K_2, vitamin K–dependent proteins and sulfatides in the brain decline with age; and low levels are associated with neurological degeneration in the elderly.[32] Alzheimer's patients have up to 93 percent lower sulfatide levels in the brain.[33] Animals that completely lack the enzymes to make sulfatides progressively suffer from growth retardation, loss of locomotor activity, weak legs and seizures.[34]

ANIMAL FATS PROVIDE NOT ONLY vitamins A, D and K_2 for our brains but other nutrients as well. One of these is choline. Choline is involved in the process of brain cells making connections with each other. In humans, higher dietary choline is related to better cognitive performance and sharper memory—in other words, those who ignore conventional dietary advice and eat plenty of egg yolks and liver, our best sources of choline,

* A major source of calcium in the Eskimo diet is fermented fish bones.

† It is interesting to ponder the reason for this reservoir of vitamin K_2, right in the middle of the body.

have a better chance of keeping all their marbles into old age.

Want smart children? Then Mom needs to consume an abundance of food containing choline while pregnant, and give lots of choline-rich foods—egg yolks and pureed liver—to baby, especially during the critical first two years when a large portion of the nerve connections are made. Brain function in baby rats was enhanced by feeding extra choline during the equivalent of the third trimester of pregnancy, according to a 1998 study at Duke University Medical Center. The offspring performed significantly better on memory tests than those of mothers with the normal intake of choline. Researchers found that choline enhanced a brain function responsible for paving the path between nerve cells, allowing electrical messages to travel more easily. The improved brain wiring persisted in the rats through early adulthood.[35]

And then we have our fatty acid brothers, DHA and AA, found primarily in certain nutrient-dense animal foods—DHA in seafoods like oily fish, cod liver oil, shellfish and fish eggs, and AA in butter, animal fats and organ meats. Together, these two fatty acids make up 20 percent of the fats in the brain.

DHA is essential for the growth and functional development of the brain in infants and for maintenance of normal brain function in adults. The inclusion of plentiful DHA in the diet improves learning ability, whereas deficiencies of DHA are associated with deficits in learning.[36] DHA is taken up by the brain in preference to other fatty acids. The turnover of DHA in the brain is rapid, although saturated fats ensure that DHA stays in the tissues as long as possible.

DHA deficiencies are associated with fetal alcohol syndrome, attention deficit hyperactivity disorder, cystic fibrosis, phenylketonuria, unipolar depression, aggressive hostility and a degenerative disease called adrenoleukodystrophy.[37] Higher DHA levels in middle-aged adults are related to better performance on tests of nonverbal reasoning and mental flexibility, working memory and vocabulary.[38] DHA deficiency is associated with cognitive decline,[39] and DHA levels are reduced in the brain tissue of severely depressed patients.[40]

AA seems to play roles similar to those of its DHA brother. For example, low AA contributes to neurological disorders such as Alzheimer's disease and bipolar disorder.[41]

However, study results for both DHA and AA are mixed, probably because many researchers use the algae-derived, synthetic forms of these nutrients, rather than natural forms in whole foods like cod liver oil, liver and butter. These natural foods also supply vitamins A and D, which help regulate the actions of these important fatty acids. For example, calcium supports the conversion of AA to other compounds in the cells, and we need vitamin D to properly maintain the proper levels of calcium in the blood and tissues. Vitamin A works with vitamin D in many ways and also helps us synthesize AA from omega-6 fatty acids in plant foods.[42] In nature, the fatty acid twins occur in the same foods that provide us with vitamins A and D; scientists giving supplements of algae-derived DHA and AA to patients lacking vitamins A and D should not expect beneficial results.

CANNABINOIDS, OPIATES (SUCH AS heroin and morphine), and cocaine come from plants. One of the great discoveries of modern science is the finding that our bodies can manufacture the same feel-good compounds. Moreover, we have receptors for these compounds, especially in the brain and the nervous system, and also in surprising places like the pancreas and the liver. Endorphins (from "endogenous morphine") like serotonin and dopamine are produced by the central nervous system and the pituitary gland, while endocannabinoids are formed during neurotransmission.*

The earliest clear description of the use of opium as a recreational drug comes from China, where opium was promoted as increasing masculinity and vigor. Opium became popular during the eighteenth century as a remedy for nervous disorders. Recognizing its sedative and tranquilizing properties, physicians gave it to those with psychosis or insomnia, and to help treat people considered insane. But the dark side of "God's Own Medicine," as it was called, soon emerged. Doctors noted that in cases of psychosis, opium could cause anger, and that the drug's euphoric effects often gave way to depression.

In the nineteenth century, the most common use of opium was for the treatment of "female problems," usually to relieve menstrual pain. Unfortunately, the treatment was addictive. Up to two hundred thousand opiate addicts lived in the United States in the late nineteenth century, and between two-thirds and three-quarters of these addicts were women.[43]

Cocaine acts by inhibiting the reuptake of the endorphins serotonin and dopamine. This results in greater concentrations of these neurotransmitters in the brain, with a stimulating and feel-good effect. Cocaine increases alertness, feelings of well-being and euphoria, energy and motor activity, and feelings of competence and sexuality. Unfortunately, after the high comes the body's reaction—which is lower-than-normal levels of serotonin and dopamine in the brain, leading to anxiety, restlessness and depression.

Along with endogenous cannabinoids and opiates, scientists have discovered a neuropeptide and neurotransmitter called CART, which elicits behavior in animals similar to that of cocaine and amphetamine. CART is found at the same locations where cocaine and methamphetamine act in the brain, leading to speculation that CART serves as an "endogenous cocaine."[44]

A KEY FACTOR IN LEADING a successful life is the ability to deal with stress. Everybody encounters stress. Those who use this stress as a springboard for action can accomplish many good things; those who are paralyzed by stress can disappear down the rabbit hole of depression and anxiety.

One of the potential reactions to stress is the fight-or-flight response. The adrenal glands produce the hormone cortisol, which raises blood sugar, increases muscle tension and strength, and prepares us for the kind of extreme reactions needed in situations of danger or urgency. However, the body is not designed to be in a fight-or-flight mode all the time. If we react to the minor stresses in our daily lives with the fight-or-flight response, we develop chronic disease or burn out.

The endocannabinoids are key regulators of cortisol production. Do we chill out or freak out with minor stresses? Our internal marijuana production may determine the outcome.†

* New evidence indicates that gut flora can produce a variety of endorphins, including serotonin.[a]

† Chris Masterjohn, PhD, has described the relationship of fat-soluble nutrients with our moods and emotions in his brilliant article "The Pursuit of Happiness."[a]

Researchers can create a stress reaction in rats by physically restraining them for thirty minutes. The rats become terrified and their blood levels of fight-or-fight hormones increase sevenfold. When they are given a drug that raises the level of natural endocannabinoids in the brain, however, these hormones only rise two- to threefold.[45]

Scientists can study the reaction of rats to stress in another way, using the "elevated zero maze." Rats are placed in a maze held high off the ground and are given the opportunity to stay in closed spaces or explore open spaces—the freaked-out, fearful rat will stay in an enclosed space; the chilled-out rat will be curious and explore. Rats on an ordinary lab chow diet spend only 20 percent of the time in open spaces, but rats given a drug that raises the level of natural endocannabinoids spend about half the time in the open spaces.[46] This finding suggests that the levels of endocannabinoids in the brain determine whether our behavior is cool and productive, or fearful and stressed.

Endocannabinoids made within the body activate the same receptors as THC, the active component of marijuana, but without the undesirable effects. While the study of endocannabinoids is in its infancy, we already know that this system of multipurpose chemicals plays many roles, including balancing short-term and long-term memory; developing nerve cells in the hippocampus; regulating appetite, hunger, taste perception and the pleasure value of food; modulating the stress response—or as scientists would put it, regulating "the organism's overall sense of arousal during novel situations"; reducing pain; determining the receptivity of the uterus to embryonic implantation; regulating intestinal motility for normal digestion and elimination; and protecting against diabetes, cardiovascular disease and multiple sclerosis. In other words, wherever researchers have looked, they have found the family of endocannabinoids playing critical roles in helping us feel well and helping the body to work normally.

Do animal fats play a role in helping us produce these feel-good chemicals? Yes, they do! Arachidonic acid—that magical omega-6 fatty acid we get from animal fats—is the direct precursor to the endocannabinoids; and a brain cell will convert arachidonic acid into endocannabinoids only in response to a rapid influx of calcium into the cell—which means that vitamin D is intimately involved in this process.*[47] If calcium is not present, due to deficiency of either calcium or vitamin D, there will be no influx of calcium into the cell to initiate the conversion of arachidonic acid to endocannabinoids.

If our internal cannabinoids are not working, or if we can't make them due to a lack of AA and vitamin D—and also vitamins A and K_2 and saturated fats, because all these compounds work together—we feel terrible. A diet without sufficient animal fat, and sufficiently nutrient-dense animal fat, leaves your cannabinoids lacking. We feel chronically depressed, anxious and tense. Enter marijuana to give a temporary high—a temporary sense of *feeling normal*—followed by its unfortunate aftereffects, which make you feel worse than before.

ENDORPHINS—NATURAL HEROIN COMPOUNDS LIKE SEROTONIN and dopamine,

* This influx is tightly controlled: the cell deliberately keeps the concentration of calcium outside its boundaries ten-thousand-fold higher than the concentration of calcium within its boundaries; only when told to do so by another chemical signal will the cell open the calcium channels that will let this mineral come flooding in.[a]

along with their binding proteins and receptors—also occur throughout the body. Like the endocannabinoids, they are involved in multiple processes, not just helping us feel good, but making sure the body functions properly. Derived from the amino acid tryptophan, serotonin is produced primarily in the intestinal tract, where it regulates intestinal movement; the rest is produced in the central nervous system, where its functions include regulation of mood, appetite and sleep; support of memory and learning, and direct brain development in the womb.

The blood platelets store serotonin, and when these platelets bind to form a clot, they release serotonin, which helps vasoconstriction and works to prevent both excessive clotting and bleeding. Serotonin also plays a role in wound healing. When humans smell food, the release of dopamine increases appetite; serotonin works to decrease appetite. Low levels of serotonin receptors are associated with increased weight gain. If irritants are present in food, the gut releases more serotonin to make digestion move faster, resulting in diarrhea to empty the gut of the offending substance. If serotonin is released into the blood faster than the platelets can absorb it, serotonin receptors are activated to induce vomiting.

In humans, serotonin controls the release of insulin (which regulates blood sugar levels) and also of insulin-like growth factor (IGF) (which regulates growth). Does that mean that happy children achieve optimal growth and happy adults enjoy stable blood sugar? Something to consider.

Serotonin also regulates executive function and social behavior—low levels are associated with attention deficit/hyperactivity disorder, bipolar disorder, schizophrenia and impulsive behavior.[48]

A key role of this happy-making chemical is to reduce aggression. Those lacking one type of serotonin receptor are at double the risk of suicide.[49] Serotonin in the brain is recycled, and anxiety-related personality disorders are common in those whose recycling mechanisms are faulty.[50] Genetically altered mice lacking one type of serotonin receptor show increased aggressiveness and lack of maternal care for their young.[51] Alcohol consumption leads to a reduction of tryptophan and a resulting decrease in serotonin. The impulsive behavior associated with drunkenness can be partially explained by this decrease in serotonin.[52]

"The life of the body is a heart at peace, but envy rots the bones" (Proverbs 14:30). Research on serotonin tells us why. Adequate levels of serotonin in the blood are a sign of good bone health—low levels are associated with low bone density. The bones have three different receptors for serotonin, and can even manufacture it.[53]

Depletion of serotonin can lead to obsessive-compulsive disorder, depression and anxiety.[54] Surprisingly, depletion of serotonin can occur in people who have recently fallen in love—an explanation for the lack of appetite or obsessive behavior in the early stages of a relationship.[55] Cupid's arrow has its sting! As do insects. Wasps, hornets and scorpions have serotonin in their venom, and it is one of the chemicals responsible for the feeling of pain after a bite.

Antidepressants called serotonin selective reuptake inhibitors (SSRIs) keep serotonin longer in the nerve synapses, thus increasing levels in the brain. However, the benefits may decline over time as overall serotonin levels tend to fall in reaction to the drug. Side effects include repressed libido, erectile dysfunction, difficulty achieving orgasm, fatigue, weight loss or weight gain, apathy, insomnia, headaches and birth defects.[56] SSRIs can also cause suicidal thoughts and actions, especially in teenagers. None of this is good. Another way to treat depression and anxiety might exist without the difficult side effects—supporting the body's serotonin system with good nutrition, including plenty of animal fats.

How do animal fats affect our production and use of serotonin? One important factor is cholesterol—the serotonin receptors need adequate cholesterol to work properly, and many studies have linked low cholesterol with violent and aggressive behavior, in dogs and monkeys as well as in humans. People with low cholesterol levels are more likely to be violent when drunk; prisoners with low cholesterol levels are more likely to be aggressive; and dogs with low cholesterol are more likely to be vicious.[57]

A growing body of evidence suggests that vitamin D regulates the enzyme that converts the amino acid tryptophan into serotonin, and vitamin D activates genes that release serotonin. This may explain why sunbathing—or fatty foods—gives our moods a boost. Vitamin K_2 may also play a role in supporting an active and curious outlook on life. In rats, vitamin K_2 deficiency causes lack of exploratory behavior and reduced physical activity.[58]

ENDOCANNABINOIDS AND ENDORPHINS WORK TOGETHER to make us feel good. For example, endocannabinoids regulate dopamine production in the brain—dopamine is an endorphin, like serotonin, that helps with mood.

Far from causing depression, vitamin A supports the production of arachidonic acid, leading to the production of feel-good dopamine. Vitamin A also helps stimulate the production of dopamine receptors, and certain proteins support the cellular response to dopamine.[59] Dopamine concentrations ordinarily increase in response to novel or pleasurable experiences, such as food and sex, but this increase can be completely abolished by feeding rats a drug that blocks the cannabinoid receptor.[60]

Dopamine plays many roles in the human biochemistry—often balancing the actions of serotonin. In the bloodstream, dopamine acts as a vasodilator; in the kidneys it increases sodium excretion and urine output (it makes you pee more); in the pancreas it reduces insulin production; in the digestive system it reduces motility (slows down digestion) and protects the intestinal mucosa; in the immune system, it reduces the activities of lymphocytes. If serotonin revs things up, dopamine dampens them down. In the brain, dopamine plays important roles in motor control (dopamine depletion is associated with Parkinson's disease), motivation, arousal, cognitive control, reinforcement and reward—as well as lactation and sexual gratification.

We even have dopamine-secreting neurons in the eye. Dopamine enhances activity of the cone cells and suppresses activity of the rod cells, allowing increased sensitivity to color and contrast when the light is bright, at the expense of reduced sensitivity when the light is dim.

Dopamine is like family—we need it, but not too much. When we have an overproduction or overexpression of dopamine, we are revved up, unfocused. Too little has the opposite effect—we are lethargic and unable to function. Too much dopamine can result in schizophrenia[61]; too little is associated with depression.[62] The treatment for attention deficit hyperactivity disorder (ADHD) is drugs that stimulate dopamine, while antipsychotic drugs act by suppressing the effects of dopamine.

Dopamine plays a role in dampening pain*—decreased levels of dopamine often manifest as painful conditions like burning mouth syndrome, fibromyalgia and restless legs syndrome.

The conventional view of dopamine is that it serves as a "reward" stimulus, as most types of reward increase the level of dopamine in the brain. But a more accurate description is that dopamine increases the effects of motivators, of what is called "seeking" behavior. In test animals, dopamine-stimulating drugs like cocaine and methamphetamine increase seeking behaviors, but do not increase expressions of pleasure, while opiate drugs like heroin and morphine produce increases in expressions of pleasure, but do not increase seeking behaviors.

One way scientists study the behavior of rats is by making them do work—like pushing levers—to obtain a food they like. If the rats are depleted of dopamine, either through surgery or drugs, they will stop doing the work. At first the researchers concluded that without dopamine, food is no longer pleasurable. But after many more lever pushes, another conclusion emerged. It seems that rats with low dopamine levels are less oriented to the future and only willing to do work that will provide an immediate reward.[63] When no lever pressing is required, rats still chose a pleasurable food, whether or not their dopamine levels were low. When dopamine-depleted rats have to push a lever for a short time—even a lever that has weights on it—they will do so to get the food they prefer. But the low-dopamine rats can't seem to go the distance. If they have to push a lever many times to get a food they enjoy, they just give up. But rats with normal dopamine levels will keep pushing that lever—even hundreds of times—to get their reward. What all these lever-pushing rats teach us is that the endorphin dopamine helps us look to the future, helps us sustain effort over time toward a goal.

It is the endocannabinoids that regulate dopamine production in the brain. Normally, new or pleasurable experiences cause dopamine to increase. But when rats receive a drug that blocks cannabinoid receptors, no dopamine increase occurs.[64]

Chris Masterjohn, PhD, explains it so well: "Endocannabinoids regulate the adrenal response to stress, mediated primarily by the hormone cortisol, which is responsible for the "fight-or-flight" response; they also regulate the production of dopamine in the brain, which is responsible for the motivation to sustain goal-oriented effort over time. By curbing the excess production of cortisol and supporting adequate production of dopamine, endocannabinoids help prevent excess tension, anxiety, burnout and feelings of self-defeat, and help support the confrontation of challenges with the attitudes necessary for success... Endocannabinoids thus not only prevent the anxiety and feeling of

* Feeling pain? Eat a banana! Bananas contain 40–50 parts per million of dopamine. Other fruits and vegetables come in at much lower values, around 1 part per million. Unfortunately, ingested dopamine does not get past the blood-brain barrier but it might ameliorate a pain in your knee or elbow.

self-defeat that leads us to run from challenges rather than confronting them, but also help support the future-oriented maintenance of sustained effort that is necessary for personal financial and career success and a prosperous society."[65]

To summarize: arachidonic acid (from animal fats) is the precursor of the endocannabinoids; vitamin D (from animal fats) regulates calcium needed for this conversion; vitamin A (from animal fats) is needed for the production of arachidonic acid and supports the dopamine system more directly by stimulating the production of dopamine receptors; vitamin K_2 (from animal fats) supports neurological function in many ways; cholesterol (from animal fats) supports all receptors in the brain and saturated fat (also from animal fats) supports all hormonal conversions. For thinking, remembering, adjusting, planning, enjoying, learning and loving, animal fats are our best friends.

BEING HIGH IS THE NATURAL state of a well-nourished brain. Taken as a whole, modern research points to the conclusion that animal fats, rich in cholesterol, fat-soluble vitamins, arachidonic acid and many other components, not only help us avoid mental illnesses such as depression and anxiety, but also give us the curiosity, courage and stick-to-it-iveness to act positively and accomplish goals in a challenging world—activities that create the foundation of real happiness. Multiple studies have shown the link between achieving long-term goals and changes in subjective well-being; most research shows that achieving goals that hold personal meaning to an individual increases feelings of contentment.[66]

No wonder so many people are struggling with depression, chronic pain and even addiction in our fat-phobic world! Almost 50 percent of Americans suffer psychiatric disorders for at least one period of time during their lives. Those born after the Second World War—when processed foods based on vegetable oils entered the American diet—experience depression, anxiety, lack of impulse control and substance abuse at twice the rate as those born before. The proportion of Americans diagnosed with three or more disorders has more than tripled during the last sixty-five years.[67]

The addict is not degenerate or perverse, but someone who takes drugs to *feel normal*, to feel the way human beings should feel every day, even during times of difficulty and challenge.

The foods that protect us against depression and help us engage in future-oriented activities are the same foods that traditional cultures valued for good health. They provide fat-soluble vitamins. They contain cholesterol and arachidonic acid in abundance—along with other factors that support the lipid components, such as calcium, magnesium and B vitamins. By and large—with the exception of cod liver oil—these foods are satisfying and delicious: creamy pâté, aged cheeses, caviar with sour cream, full-cream milk, homemade ice cream made with real cream and egg yolks, eggs and bacon, omelets and quiche, cream-based soups, potatoes cooked in goose fat, oysters on the half shell, crab cakes and shrimp, lobster with (real) drawn butter, and in fact anything at all with butter, lots of butter—including potatoes, bread, fish, meat and vegetables.

CHAPTER 10

The Queen of Fats: Why Butter Is Better

"Eat butter. Scientists labeled fat the enemy. Why they were wrong." This was the *Time* Magazine cover article on June 23, 2014.* Five days earlier, on June 18, the *Washington Post* declared: "Butter Is the Big Fat Winner." The article noted that butter consumption was at its highest level in thirty years, at just over five pounds per person per year. The shocking admission: all the science condemning butter was wrong. On June 25, two days after the *Time* cover story appeared, the *Wall Street Journal* published an article entitled, "Butter Makes Comeback as Margarine Loses Favor," crediting celebrity chefs and cooking shows for butter's increasing popularity. Since the *Wall Street Journal* is a business publication, it contained a key financial fact: in 2013, Americans spent more than 2 billion dollars on butter compared with 1.8 billion dollars on spreads and margarines. With so many studies exonerating saturated fats, and butter in particular, the media had to take notice.

Still, we've got a long way to go. Butter consumption was almost nineteen pounds per person per year as late as 1934, and very few consumers will read or understand these articles and immediately abandon their deep fear of butter. Advertising for "heart-healthy" spreads continues unabated. There's still no butter or whole milk in school lunches, mandated by ironclad regulations—a standard that remains difficult if not impossible to change. The industrial "edible" oil industry, quick to pick up on trends, will find new ways to demonize nature's perfect fat. Industry insiders like Mike Faherty, a vice president of marketing at Unilever North America, continue the negative campaign: "Consumers believe that butter is a simpler product that feels more natural, without understanding that it's an indulgence made from animal fats." We'll be seeing more subtle messages making Americans feel guilty for "indulging" in butter.

A report in the *Los Angeles Times*, published on January 7, 2014, credits butter's growing popularity with "more understanding about the health hazards of its processed counterparts," namely margarines containing *trans* fats. But the *Los Angeles Times* report

* The material for the *Time* Magazine article mostly came—without attribution—from Nina Teicholz's *The Big Fat Surprise*.

muddied the message, stating as fact that "it's not a health food. In a word, butter is fat—and not the good kind. It's loaded with saturated fat, which has been linked to heart disease." Still, food manufacturers "are working hard to take advantage of [the new] demand by labeling their cookies and frozen pies as 'made with real butter.'" The article pointed out that even "healthier" margarine is struggling to stand out in a nation "increasingly captivated by foodie culture. Butter has become a symbol of America's growing appreciation of authentic cooking."

The battle over butter isn't just an American concern. New Zealanders eat far more butter than Americans do—twenty-four pounds of butter per year, up from a low of fifteen pounds. Representatives from the pro- and anti-butter camps "nearly came to blows" at a debate in New Zealand between Grant Schofield, a cheerleader for high-fat, low-carb diets, and Rod Jackson, the "anti-butter" professor. Professor Jackson says he told Professor Schofield after their Queenstown meeting that "I thought it was both irresponsible and dangerous to encourage the public to eat more saturated fat, given the weight of evidence about saturated fat and coronary heart disease."

An article by Nina Teicholz appeared in the *Wall Street Journal* on October 28, 2014, lambasting the low-fat dietary guidelines as hopelessly outdated and contrary to the current science. She cited a landmark meta-analysis of all the available evidence, which concluded that saturated fats could not, after all, be said to cause heart disease.[1] Even though funded in part by the British Heart Foundation, the authors concluded, "Current evidence does not clearly support cardiovascular guidelines that encourage high consumption of polyunsaturated fatty acids and low consumption of total saturated fats."

An earlier meta-analysis came to the same conclusion.[2] "A meta-analysis of prospective epidemiologic studies showed that there is no significant evidence for concluding that dietary saturated fat is associated with an increased risk of CHD or CVD. More data are needed to elucidate whether CVD risks are likely to be influenced by the specific nutrients used to replace saturated fat." The problem, said the vegetable oil industry, was that consumers were replacing saturated fats with bad fats and carbs in foods like donuts, when we should be eating more polyunsaturated fatty acids in vegetable oils and fish. But the 2014 study cited in the *Wall Street Journal* dispelled any notion that vegetable oils were healthier than saturated fat—a major blow to the oil industry rhetoric.

We should have seen these headlines twenty-five years ago. Way back in 1991, a Medical Research Council survey showed that men eating butter ran half the risk of developing heart disease compared to those eating margarine.[3] And a 1997 report in *Epidemiology* found that butter consumption in men did not predict the incidence of coronary heart disease while those who ate margarine had increased risk.[*4] Yet butter consumption only began to climb many years and many studies later, not until after the turn of the century.

A 2009 industry document in the UK, *The Yellow Fats Report*, noted that consumers are turning away from "active healthy spreads" like cholesterol-lowering margarine to more

* One of the study authors was William Castelli, former director of the Framingham Study.

"balanced diet management and natural ingredients." Or to put it another way, people are eating more butter, especially those over fifty-five years of age. Sales for the "total functional spreads category" in the UK remained flat, complained the manufacturer of the "functional" cholesterol-lowering spread Benecol, in spite of a recent EU health claim ruling, which confirmed the fact that plant stanol esters in the product can lower cholesterol.[*5] While food manufacturers tried to figure out which functional food ingredients "will triumph," consumers were increasingly turning to real foods like butter, which in the UK grew 19 percent in sales in 2009.

Fruits, vegetables, oily fish and whole grains—this remains the mantra of the anti-butter camp, in the teeth of surprising findings from Sweden. Researchers there followed coronary heart disease morbidity and mortality in a group of over seventeen hundred rural men. The men filled out a dietary questionnaire and were then followed for twelve years, during which one hundred thirty-eight were hospitalized or died due to coronary heart disease. Daily intake of fruit and vegetables was associated with a lower risk of coronary heart disease *only* when combined with high dairy fat consumption (which makes them taste so much better), but *not* when combined with a low dairy fat consumption. Eating whole meal bread or fish at least twice a week showed no association with the outcome.[†6]

Dietary questionnaires do not always provide an accurate indication of what people actually eat, so researchers often look at clues in the blood. One study, published in 2013, looked for markers of "dairy fat" in the blood of twenty-eight hundred U.S. adults and correlated the findings with occurrences of heart disease in the same population. Researchers found that participants who self-reported whole-fat dairy and butter intake had the highest occurrence of a minor fifteen-carbon saturated fatty acid found in mostly in butter, but not in other fats. Presence of this fat in the blood was *inversely* associated with the incidence of cardiovascular disease and coronary heart disease. No association of cardiovascular or heart disease was found with saturated palmitic acid (which raises cholesterol slightly in some studies) and a natural *trans* fat, both prevalent in butter.[7] The finding that palmitic acid is not associated with more heart disease is especially interesting because in the absence of dietary saturated fat, the body transforms carbohydrates into saturated palmitic acid. Some advocates of the paleo diet look to this fact as a reason to avoid grains, potatoes and other starchy foods, claiming that palmitic acid causes heart disease.

---

* Phytosterols used in "functional" cholesterol-lowering spreads like Benecol are hormone-like compounds from plants, present in large numbers in the effluent from the wood pulp industry. Water contaminated with phytosterols causes endocrine damage to fish downstream from wood pulp plants. The fish become "sex-inverted" and hermaphroditic; fertility is also reduced. Phytosterols also have the classic estrogenic effect of stimulating the growth of uterine tissues, which may explain their folkloric use as abortifacients. There is a remarkable similarity between the chemical structure of plant sterols and diethylstilbestrol, the synthetic hormone associated with reproductive cancers in women. This is one reason scientists seriously considered them as natural antifertility agents in place of the modern synthetic contraceptive pill. This potential usage was abandoned when phytosterols were found to have harmful side effects. But food manufacturers think it is okay to add them to spreads and margarines.[a]

† Meanwhile, findings from a large European study indicate that animal fats from meat, eggs and dairy products do not increase a woman's risk of breast cancer.[a]

THE FOES OF FULL-FAT DAIRY products like to warn consumers that butterfat and other animal fats will cause weight gain. But two recent studies, both published in 2013, have concluded that the consumption of whole-fat dairy products is actually linked to *reduced body fat*. In one paper, middle-aged men who consumed high-fat milk, butter and cream were significantly less likely to become obese over a period of twelve years, when compared to men who never or rarely ate high-fat dairy.[8] The second study was a meta-analysis of sixteen observational studies aimed at exploring the hypothesis that high-fat dairy foods contribute to obesity and heart disease risk.[9] The researchers concluded that the evidence does not support this hypothesis; in fact, they found that in most of the studies, high-fat dairy consumption was associated with a lower risk of obesity. Scientists are scratching their heads as to the reason—there's the satiety factor in butter, for one, and possibly bioactive components that boost metabolism. Vitamin A and iodine in butter make it a great food for thyroid function, and short-chain fatty acids in butter raise body temperature. But maybe it's because butter is a real food that nourishes the whole body, and does not make us tempted to eat more and more, the way butter substitutes do.

By way of damage control, in October 2015, Harvard University issued a paper that analyzed data already collected from two large studies, the Nurses' Health Study and the Health Professionals Follow-Up study.[10] The data showed that "polyunsaturated fatty acids and/or high-quality carbohydrates can be used to replace saturated fats to reduce CHD risk."

"Butter is not back," said the press release. "Limiting saturated fat is still best for the heart."[11] An analysis by Zoë Harcombe[12] noted that the overall numbers were very small—the chances of any one person in these surveys having a coronary heart disease incident was only about one in four hundred fifty, surprisingly low considering their age. The data actually showed that *higher* intakes of total fat and higher intakes of saturated fat were associated with a *lower* risk of heart disease; and higher intakes of *trans* fat were significantly associated with a higher risk of heart disease. But most importantly, those participants consuming the highest levels of saturated fat were also consuming the highest levels of *trans* fats, meaning that they were eating more processed food. Harcombe notes that according to the 2010 USDA dietary guidelines, "The main sources of saturated fat are processed food, pizza, grain-based desserts, dairy desserts (ice cream), KFC, hot dogs, burgers, tortillas, candy, and potato chips. Butter accounts for 2.9% of saturated fat sources and milk 7.3%." The Harvard analysis did *not* show that butter predisposed a person to heart disease, but butter was the target in the press release headline.

IF YOU COULD DESIGN THE perfect fat, one that would spread at room temperature while remaining resistant to rancidity, one that would supply all the types of fat molecules that human beings need, what kind of fatty acids would it contain? For stability, it would need a large portion of saturated fat, and for fluidity it would need a good fraction of monounsaturated fatty acids.* This perfect

* Fat that contains more than 60 percent long-chain saturated fatty acids is hard and unspreadable, even at room temperature.

fat would contain a small amount of omega-6 and omega-3 essential fatty acids—at less than 1 percent of total fat content—and a ratio of about two parts omega-6 to one part omega-3. For good measure, this fat would contain some short- and medium-chain saturated fatty acids, the same kind you find in coconut oil. And to top it off, this fat would provide some arachidonic acid (AA), a component so important for the production of feel-good chemicals, healthy skin and an impervious digestive tract.

Guess what? This perfect fat already exists. This checklist pretty much describes the fatty acid profile of butter: about 50 percent saturated (a mixture of sixteen-carbon palmitic acid and eighteen-carbon stearic acid), 30 percent monounsaturated (the kind of "healthy" fat in olive oil), 13 percent short- and medium-chain fatty acids, and small amounts of all the rest, including a total of 0.3 percent essential fatty acids at the perfect ratio of two to one. Butter is a source of arachidonic acid as well. The only thing missing is DHA, which we need to get from seafood, cod liver oil and organ meats.

The short- and medium-chain fatty acids—ranging from four to fourteen carbons—in butter are always saturated and they have unique properties. The body uses them directly for energy and never stores them as fat, so they are ideal for weight loss—boosting the metabolism, creating satiety yet never adding pounds. These short- and medium-chain fatty acids in butter stimulate the immune system and support intercellular communication, making them ideal for fighting cancer. Finally, these saturated fatty acids have antimicrobial properties, killing pathogens including candida in the gut. Twelve-carbon lauric acid, a medium-chain fatty acid not found in other animal fats, is highly protective against disease and should be called a conditionally essential fatty acid because it is made only by the mammary gland and not in the liver like other saturated fats.[13] We must obtain it from one of two dietary sources—small amounts in butterfat or large amounts in coconut oil. Four-carbon butyric acid is all but unique to butter. Butyric acid helps increase the number of thyroid hormone receptors on cells, allowing for delivery and utilization of more thyroid hormones.[14] It also has antifungal properties as well as antitumor effects.[15]

Butter is one of the only sources of fourteen-carbon myristic acid in the Western diet, totaling almost 20 percent. The body uses myristic acid in an important process called myristolation, needed in the cell membranes and also within the mitochondria of the cells. Myristoylation is especially important for kidney function.

If you had included "no *trans* fats" in your list of requirements for the perfect fat, butter would not make the grade. That's because butter contains a natural form of *trans* fat called *trans*-vaccenic acid.* The nomenclature comes from the Latin *vacca,* meaning cow, because it occurs predominantly in the butterfat and the adipose fat of cows—but also of other ruminants.†

Ruminants extract the nutrients from plant food by fermenting it in a specialized stomach prior to digestion, then regurgitating and chewing again—this category of animals get their moniker from the Latin *ruminare*, which

* The technical name is (E)-Octadec-11-enoic acid, but we will stick with *trans*-vaccenic acid.

† Kangaroos have the highest levels of *trans*-vaccenic acid in their fat.

means "to chew over again." The one hundred fifty species of ruminants include cattle, goats, sheep, giraffes, yaks, deer, antelope, kangaroos and wallabies—all of them harboring an intestinal flora that does amazing things with the fatty acids in plant foods. Ruminants are able to saturate fatty acids from plants by adding or rearranging hydrogen to create odd fatty acids like *trans*-vaccenic acid—or creating short- and medium-chain fatty acids from carbohydrates.

Discovered in 1928 in animal fats and butter, *trans*-vaccenic acid gave the food manufacturers the argument they needed to defend industrial *trans* fats in margarine and shortening. Natural *trans* fats in butter appeared to do no harm, so they claimed the *trans* fats in industrial fats were likewise innocuous. It would take decades to unravel the difference between natural and industrial *trans* fats. Not surprisingly, the natural *trans* fats in butter turned out to be beneficial, whereas the industrial isomers cause everything from cancer to heart disease to infertility.*

We now know that mammals—including humans—convert *trans*-vaccenic acid into something called conjugated linoleic acid (CLA), a hairpin-like structure. CLA disappears from the fat when cows are fed dry hay or processed feed,[16] a discovery that gave a boost to proponents of pasture-based agriculture. In fact, meat and dairy products from grass-fed animals can produce 300–500 percent more CLA than those of cattle fed the usual diet of 50 percent hay and silage, and 50 percent grain.

Health benefits claimed for CLA include anti-cancer, anti-diabetic, anti-atherosclerosis and anti-osteoporosis effects, as well as protection from weight gain and immune system. The popularity of CLA supplements skyrocketed on the premise that CLA helps build muscle at the expense of fat. These effects appeared in studies with animals and *in vitro* on human cancer cell lines, but studies with humans give mixed results. For example, a 2012 meta-analysis found that CLA has no useful benefit for overweight or obese people as it has no long-term effect on body composition,[17] and a 2010 review found that CLA had no effect on insulin response in humans.[18]

However, a 2014 study found that CLA increases tissue levels of retinol (vitamin A) as well as its carrier protein in the bloodstream.[19] This property could explain the findings that CLA protects against cancer, atherosclerosis and osteoporosis, and supports immune function.

IF BUTTER AS A "SOLID FAT" provides only "empty calories," why are manufacturers adding a manufactured form of vitamin A—vitamin A palmitate—to margarine to mimic butter's vitamin composition? The fact is, when margarine and spreads replaced butter in the food supply, Americans, including children, lost their best source of fat-soluble vitamins—not only vitamin A with its range of isomers, but also vitamins K_2 and even vitamin D. Butter is—or was—America's best source of these important nutrients. In fact, a fascinating early study from the Agricultural Institute in Texas found that vitamin A is more easily absorbed and better utilized from butter than from other sources, including cod liver oil.[20]

No one studied butter more thoroughly than Dr. Weston A. Price. Throughout the 1930s, he analyzed thousands of butter samples shipped to him from all over the world.

* Natural *trans* fats occur in fish oils as well; they are manufactured by marine fungi, which fish consume.

In those days, the test he used was a chemical test—the presence of vitamin A changed the color of a sulfated ammonia compound—not the more perfected gas chromatography that researchers use today. Nevertheless, he was able to chronicle the rise and fall of vitamin A content in butter in different regions of the country and throughout the year.

A similar test—one in which iodine turned purple in the presence of Activator X—allowed him to determine levels of what we now know to be K_2. He found that vitamins A and K_2 in butter rose and fell together according to the season. In warm-weather California, these vitamins reached a maximum early in the year; in temperate regions, they usually showed two peaks—one peak in the spring and another in the fall; and just one peak, in midsummer, in northern latitudes. These peaks paralleled the growth of grass. Dr. Price found that green, rapidly growing grass translated into maximum levels of A and K_2. Such high-vitamin butter is naturally yellow, with no dyes required. And in fact, before industrialization, people judged the quality of the butter by its color—the deeper the yellow, the better the butter.

Dr. Price also looked at the numbers of deaths from heart attack and pneumonia in local hospitals. He found a consistent negative relationship between deaths in local hospitals and vitamin content of local butter. In other words, when levels of the two vitamins were high, deaths from heart attacks and pneumonia went down, and when levels of the two vitamins were low, the deaths went up—these deaths went up not only in winter, as expected, but also in midsummer when the grass was brown or even just not growing quickly.[21]

Other studies convinced him that these two vitamins were critical for reproduction, infant growth, strong bones, prevention of tooth decay, learning capacity, resolution of seizures, and even as a treatment for fatigue. Modern research completely validates these early findings.

When Dr. Price studied isolated traditional peoples around the world, he found that butter was a staple in many of their diets. (He did not find any isolated peoples who consumed polyunsaturated oils.) The groups he studied particularly valued the deep yellow butter produced by cows feeding on rapidly growing green grass. Their natural intuition told them that its life-giving qualities were especially beneficial for children and expectant mothers. When Dr. Price analyzed this deep yellow butter, he found that it was exceptionally high in vitamin A and Activator X (vitamin K_2). Without them, according to Dr. Price, we are not able to utilize the minerals we ingest, no matter how abundant they may be in our diets. It bears repeating that vitamin A, with its cofactors, is especially important in the Western diet because Americans eat a lot of protein. Protein consumption depletes vitamin A because the body needs vitamin A to utilize it properly. In 1970, investigator I. W. Jennings described the typical results of a diet high in protein but low in vitamin A—tall spindly growth, poor posture and poor eyesight—the typical tall, skinny, near-sighted kid.[22] The combination of plentiful vitamin A and adequate complete protein (especially animal protein) is a recipe for growth that optimizes not only height but also strength—that results in "splendid physical specimens," as Dr. Price would say.

USDA GOVERNMENT TABLES LIST BUTTER as a low-vitamin D food, with a mere 136 IU of vitamin D_3 per 100 grams, or about 7 IU per tablespoon. But results for vitamin D_3 in butter from an independent laboratory have ranged from 328–940 IU per tablespoon, making butter a real vitamin D powerhouse, almost on par with cod liver oil.*[23] As discussed in Chapter 6, vitamin D testing is in its infancy, and many factors can influence the results, from extraction methods to the way the chromatograph is calibrated and displayed.

The mammary gland transforms blood into milk—it is perfectly appropriate to refer to milk as "white blood," because it contains all the factors in blood—immuglobulins, neutrophils, lymphocytes and so forth—except for red blood cells. Along with vitamin D_3, blood carries calcidiol [25(OH)D_3], the activated form of D_3. In fact, calcidiol is the primary form of vitamin D in the blood, and therefore likely to be the primary form of vitamin D in butter. But food testing laboratories do not generally test for calcidiol in food, so this type of vitamin D is not going to show up in the food charts. Yet calcidiol is more potent in increasing calcidiol levels in the blood than unactivated vitamin D_3.[24]

It makes sense that the primary form of vitamin D in butter is calcidiol because infants with immature livers may lack the enzymes to make the transformation of D_3 to calcidiol. In fact, there must be vitamin D in butter, including the butterfat in human breast milk, in considerable amounts because this is the only way for the infant to obtain this critical nutrient. Vitamin D supplementation in pregnancy results in higher vitamin D levels in breast milk.[25] Cows in the sunlight or cows given feed containing vitamin D will therefore reflect this dietary intake in their butterfat.†

Vitamin K specialists do not consider butter a particularly good source of this nutrient, but tests carried out by the Weston A. Price Foundation found 10–20 micrograms per 100 grams in butter from various sources, about on par with the levels in lard, but lower than levels in egg yolks (which range from 30 to 40 micrograms).‡ Dr. Price found very high levels of Activator X (vitamin K_2) in butter from cows eating rapidly growing green grass in the spring and fall.

Vitamin E is not exclusive to animal fats, as it occurs in all plant foods and all fats and oils. It plays many roles, one of which is to protect lipids and prevent the oxidation of polyunsaturated fatty acids. In vegetable oils, the levels of vitamin E range from 30 to 150 milligrams per 100 grams, with the highest levels in those oils that contain high levels of fragile omega-3 fatty acids—rapeseed oil and wheat germ oil. (Unfortunately, most vitamin E in vegetable oils is destroyed by processing.) Butter comes in at only 2 milligrams per 100 grams, as we would expect in a fat composed largely of stable saturated and monounsaturated fatty acids.§

And then there is cholesterol. Butter is a

---

* Surprisingly, the higher value in the range came from conventional butter, the lower one from butter produced by cows on pasture. The likely explanation is the fact that vitamin D_3 is added to the feed.

† Cows on pasture get their vitamin D by licking their fur—and the fur of other cows. Sunlight activates the cholesterol-rich lanolin on their coats and transforms it into vitamin D_3.

‡ The real powerhouses of vitamin K_2 in the western diet are the fat and livers of ducks and geese, followed by aged cheese.

§ The scientific term for vitamin E is tocopherol, which comes from the Greek words *tokos*, meaning "offspring," and *phero*, meaning "to bear." Tocopherol literally means "to bear children." The vitamin is so named because it is essential to healthy fertility. A study performed in 1922 showed that rats whose diet was devoid of vitamin E became infertile. Once they were given wheat germ oil (rich in vitamin E) as part of their diet, the rats' fertility was restored.[a]

natural source of cholesterol. Cholesterol is in all mammalian milk fat—along with special lipase enzymes to ensure 100 percent absorption—and it must be there for a reason! The reason is that babies and children lack the necessary enzymes to manufacture their own cholesterol, and cholesterol is vital to growth, especially of the nervous system. Cholesterol is also needed to produce a variety of steroids that protect against cancer, heart disease and mental illness.

Along with cholesterol, butter contains lecithin, a dietary source of choline and related compounds. Lecithin assists in the proper assimilation and metabolization of cholesterol and other fat constituents. Glycosphingolipids in butter play many roles, one of which is to aid digestion.* The list of positive compounds goes on and on.

Many trace minerals are incorporated into the fat globule membrane of butterfat, including manganese, zinc, chromium and iodine. In mountainous areas far from the sea, iodine in butter protects against goiter. Butter is extremely rich in selenium, a trace mineral with antioxidant properties, containing more per gram than herring or wheat germ.

One objection to the consumption of butter and other animal fats is the premise that butterfat accumulates environmental poisons like dioxins. However, the main source of dioxins in Western diets is fatty fish and fish oils; truly grass-fed butter is not likely to be a source of dioxins.[26] Keep buttering that toast!

Fat-soluble poisons may accumulate in fats, but water-soluble poisons such as antibiotics and growth hormones accumulate in the protein fraction of milk and meats. Vegetables and grains also accumulate poisons. The average plant crop receives ten applications of pesticides—from planting to storage—while cows on grass generally graze on pasture that is unsprayed. Aflatoxin, a fungus that grows on grain, is one of the most powerful carcinogens known. It is wise to assume that all conventionally grown food, whether of vegetable or animal origin, may be contaminated. The solution to environmental poisons is not to eliminate animal fats—so essential to growth, reproduction and overall health—but to seek out organic meats and butter from pasture-fed cows, as well as organic vegetables and grains. Animal fats like butter are our best sources of vitamin A, which is key to helping the body deal with dioxins and pesticides. Many effects of dioxins can be reversed by vitamin A supplementation. For example, giving vitamin A enabled 25 percent of rats fed a lethal dose of the dioxin TCDD to survive, while supplementation with vitamin E enabled only 10 percent to survive.[27]

Vitamin E in butterfat, coupled with vitamins A, D and K_2, along with the much-maligned cholesterol, all support fertility in both men and women. Indeed, a 2007 study showed that butterfat supported fertility and ease of conception.[28] As butter consumption in America has declined, infertility and problems with sexual development have increased. In calves, skimmed milk is unable to promote normal growth or ensure the calves reach adulthood.[29] If you want to have grandchildren, give your own children butter!

SHOULD OUR BUTTER BE RAW or pasteurized? The fat-soluble vitamins in butter are fairly stable and persist even after pasteurization—they

* For this reason, children who drink skim milk have diarrhea at rates three to five times greater than children who drink whole milk.[a]

also remain after freezing, even up to a year.[30] But one factor in butter is destroyed by pasteurization, and that is called the Wulzen factor. Discovered by researcher Rosalind Wulzen, a professor at the University of California during the 1920s, the Wulzen factor is a substance in raw cream that protects humans and animals from calcification of the joints—degenerative arthritis. It also protects against hardening of the arteries, cataracts and calcification of the pineal gland.[31] Wulzen showed that guinea pigs fed pasteurized milk or skim milk develop joint stiffness and do not thrive. Their symptoms are reversed when raw butterfat is added to the diet. Pasteurization destroys the Wulzen factor—it is present only in raw butter, cream and whole milk.

The consensus today is that the Wulzen factor is stigmasterol, a plant sterol or phytosterol, a chemical similar to the cholesterol found in butterfat, certain Chinese herbs, and various legumes, nuts, seeds, vegetables and especially in sugar cane. One pharmaceutical company has used stigmasterol as the starting raw material for the synthesis of cortisone,[32] which can be used to treat arthritis.

Stigmasterol is precursor of the anabolic steroid boldenone, which is commonly used in veterinary medicine to induce growth in cattle, but also as a much-abused anabolic steroid in sports. Body builders used to consume a lot of raw butter and cream—surely a better way to put on muscle than taking an anabolic steroid.

So get raw butter if you can—with no worries about food-borne illness as there has never been any illness associated with raw butter. But pasteurized butter is just fine, preferably from grass-fed cows.

"I CAN'T BELIEVE IT'S NOT BUTTER!" and the appropriately named "Country Crock," both Unilever brands, have new formulations for their vegetable oil spreads. Both are popular and extremely profitable products sold in tubs as large as forty-five ounces (almost six cups). The change in ingredients comes in response to "rising consumer preferences for more simple, natural foods." Touted as "Non-GMO Sourced" and "0% Artificial Preservatives," the new "simple recipe" contains just ten ingredients: purified water, soybean oil, palm kernel and palm oil, salt, lecithin (soy), vinegar, natural flavors, vitamin A palmitate, beta-carotene (for color) and vitamin D_3.

But customers are not altogether pleased. "It is the most foul margarine I've ever had the displeasure of eating," reads one customer post on the Unilever site. "When it melts it leaves a hardened film that feels like plastic," complained another. "Literally gagged when I tasted it," was the comment of a third.[33] Another customer complained, "Since the change it doesn't taste buttery anymore. We have stopped using it completely and went back to real butter, which is better. We just use less of it. Really wish ICBINB had the same great taste it used to have, it won't even melt on hot toast or a hot potato. Very disappointed."[34]

The new tasteless versions—lacking artificial flavor—certainly do have a better ingredients list than the original, which included: vegetable oil blend (liquid soybean oil, partially hydrogenated soybean oil, hydrogenated cottonseed oil), water, whey (milk), salt, vegetable mono- and diglycerides, soy lecithin, (potassium sorbate, calcium disodium EDTA, used to protect quality), citric acid, artificial flavor, vitamin A (palmitate), beta-carotene (color).

The manufacturers have replaced *trans* fats in part with saturated palm and palm kernel oils; or added fully hydrogenated saturated fatty acids through the process of interesterification. Interestingly, the new formula provides vitamin D_3—a tacit admission that butter contains vitamin D, even if it doesn't show up in the nutrient tables. But the new "simpler" product contains no cholesterol, no arachidonic acid, no CLA, no glycosphingolipids, no myristic acid, no lauric acid, no butyric acid or other short- and medium-chain fatty acids, only one form each of vitamins A and D, no vitamin K_2, no vitamin E, no minerals, no Wulzen factor—in short, almost none of the life-sustaining components of butter. What it does offer: a package of highly processed soybean oil full of free radicals, polymers, cyclic compounds, ketones, epoxides, aldehydes and residual processing chemicals including hexane. And while revenue from this stuff may be declining, it still amounts to something like one and one-half billion dollars per year worldwide.[35]

Scientists and historians tend to discount the hypothesis that rampant lead poisoning led to the downfall of Rome. But we know that the Romans had plenty of exposure—through lead pipes, in cosmetics, in utensils and in cooking pots, including cooking pots used to boil wine down to a thick syrup, a favorite dish among the upper classes. Analysis of bones from Roman times found lead levels *twenty times higher* than modern recommendations and *two times higher* than the level the WHO considers "very severe lead poisoning."[36] Lead interferes with normal enzyme reactions within the human body and can mimic or replace other essential metals. Lead poisoning manifests as developmental delay, learning difficulties, behavioral problems and mood disorders, fatigue, anemia, hearing loss, infertility and miscarriage.

Are the industrial fats and oils that have replaced animal fats like butter and lard the equivalent of lead pipes in Roman times—slow toxins that enervate the populace and eventually lead to reduced intelligence and population decline? Conspiracy theorists may even assert that industrial fats and oils are a kind of fifth column, designed to destroy Western culture—or even possibly worldwide culture. Bombs and invasions are messy and expensive. Industrial fats and oils are slow and inexorable; they are also immensely profitable, and they leave the infrastructure intact.

It's amazing we fell for the notion that something made in a factory could be healthier than the real thing, could be better for us than the fat that nature uses to nourish all mammalian infants. Fortunately, there is still time to turn back and start eating butter, lots of butter!

POST SCRIPT

FOR IMMEDIATE RELEASE

Cholesterol Theory Wipes Out Human Race

PLANET EARTH, April 9, 2057—A faulty theory about the origin and cause of heart disease, introduced on Planet Earth one hundred years prior to this date, has caused the demise of the human race, according to a Pleiadean delegation report. The theory led to food choices that proved lethal to humans over several generations.

"We were surprised at the rapidity of its effects," said the commission's chairman, "and the tenacity of the theory. Even when infertility and early death became widespread, humans did not question the validity of the basic assumptions."

The delegation, which visits Planet Earth once every fifty earth years on fact-finding missions, estimated the decrease in earthling numbers at almost 99 percent. Only pockets of isolated populations and some descendants of impoverished dairy farmers, too poor to purchase supermarket foods, remained.

Proponents of the cholesterol theory maintained that saturated animal fats and cholesterol from animal foods were the cause of heart disease. Vegetable oils gradually replaced animal fats in the human diet as Earth-dwellers sought to lower their blood cholesterol below the levels needed to produce reproductive hormones. The introduction of imitation foods rich in plant-based estrogens, and of plant sterols into commonly eaten foods, exacerbated the antifertility effects.

Humans were also encouraged to take drugs to lower cholesterol levels, and these had side effects such as cancer, which contributed to the population decline. And heart disease increased, in spite of rigid adherence to cholesterol-lowering regimes. Low cholesterol levels also contributed to an increase in deaths from suicide and violence. In addition, children experienced growth problems and increasing numbers failed to reach sexual maturity. The investigators cited the lack of protective nutrients found in animal fats as a factor exacerbating all these conditions.

Ironically, a few earthling scientists had warned against the effects of diets based on vegetable oils, the commission found. But these souls were either ignored or persecuted. Over time, mental ability declined, with great numbers of children experiencing learning difficulties. Alzheimer's and senility increased among the elderly. Humans could no longer make sense of ancestral dietary traditions or of published studies on the role of animal fats in human nutrition.

The real enemy, according to the report, was fear. "Humans were taught to fear the very foods that had made their existence possible," said the observers. "They were very gullible and believed the advertisements and pronouncements of those who profited from the sale of vegetable oils and cholesterol-lowering drugs."

"Even if earthlings can overcome their fear and return to traditional foods," said the commission, "it will take centuries to repopulate the earth." The delegation expressed regret at the waste of a fine planet.

RECIPES

Cooking with Nourishing Fats

When you give yourself permission to cook with nourishing animal fats, a transformation ensues. Eggs, meat, seafood, vegetables, grains and desserts become scrumptious and satisfying. You will gain the reputation as a wonderful cook, and your meals will be gobbled down by even the harshest of critics—your children!

The following fats and fatty foods deserve a place of honor in your kitchen, supplying many important nutrients:

Butter: The queen of fats, with a perfect fatty acid profile, is the best source of myristic acid in the Western diet; it also provides arachidonic acid (which the body turns into feel-good chemicals), glycosphingolipids and vitamins A, D, E and K_2. Butter contains valuable minerals as well, including selenium, iodine and magnesium. Use butter in a variety of ways—for light sautéing, in hot oatmeal, slathered on bread, melted over meats, fish and vegetables, or as an ingredient in various desserts.

Cream: Velvety fresh cream or tangy sour cream and crème fraîche provide the same nutrients as butter, but with the added bonus of calcium and phosphorus. The fat-soluble vitamins in the fat portion support assimilation of the minerals in the milk portion of cream. Fresh cream can be whipped as a topping for fruit and other desserts, and fresh or cultured cream is delicious added to soups and sauces.

Lard: A stable, healthy fat we should all be proud to use. You can fry just about anything in lard, and the fat won't break down. Lard is an unacknowledged source of vitamin D, with much higher levels in pastured lard. Healthier and less expensive than olive oil, lard can be your number one choice for cooking.

Bacon and bacon fat: Lard on steroids, bacon and bacon fat provide the same benefits as lard, enhanced by irresistible bacon flavor and aroma.

Duck and goose fat: We need to use more of these fats in everyday recipes; they are our best sources of vitamin K_2 and arachidonic acid.

Tallow: The fat of ruminant animals (cows, sheep, goats), tallow is the most common and the best fat for deep frying; it is stable even at high heat.

Egg yolks: A highly desirable source of fat-soluble vitamins, arachidonic acid as well as protein and important minerals like iron. Eggs from pastured chickens are best. Eat as many as you like; they do not contribute to heart disease.

Cheese: The quintessential soul food, full-fat, aged cheese is a complete food, supplying fat-soluble vitamins—especially vitamin K_2—a range of beneficial fatty acids and CLA, an anticancer substance. Cheese abounds in calcium, phosphorus, magnesium and a range of microminerals. If the cheese is made from raw milk, it will be a source of vitamin C as well. And aged cheese made from raw milk is highly probiotic, containing more beneficial microorganisms, and a wider variety of microorganisms, than yogurt.

Liver: The most nutrient-dense food on the planet, providing not only fat-soluble vitamins but also vitamins B_{12}, B_6 and many important minerals, especially iron. Poultry liver has the best balance of vitamins A, D and K_2, with duck and goose liver the clear winners for vitamin K_2. Cook beef and calves liver in lard to provide vitamin D, to balance high levels of vitamin A in ruminant liver. Liver is delicious made into liverwurst, pâté and scrapple—these are ways of making offal taste good!

Bone marrow: Underappreciated and underused, bone marrow contains 90 percent of calories as fat. Primitive peoples knew how to crack open the femur to extract its rope of marrow, which they relished raw. Today we have much more appetizing ways of preparing marrow.

Gizzards: The "mechanical" stomach of the bird, this little muscle is surprisingly rich in vitamin A, as well as vitamin B_{12}, vitamin B_6 and selenium.

Cod liver oil or skate liver oil: Our best dietary source of vitamins A and D, as well as DHA for brain function. Skate liver oil has a better proportion of DHA to the less desirable EPA. Use only products that are processed at low heat and contain their natural vitamins.

Breakfast

Cod Liver Oil Shooter

Serves 1

1 teaspoon cod liver oil
juice of 1 organic orange

Mix together in a small glass. Drink quickly to avoid the cod liver oil taste.

Better than Coffee

Serves 2

1 tablespoon molasses
¼ cup cream
¼ teaspoon powdered ginger
¼ teaspoon powdered licorice root

Place all the ingredients in a large mug and add hot water to fill. Stir well and enjoy.

Scrambled Eggs and Cheese

Vitamin D in egg yolks, vitamin A in cream and butter, and vitamin K_2 in the cheese make this dish the perfect combination of fat-soluble vitamins.

Serves 2

2 pastured eggs
1 pastured egg yolk

1 tablespoon fresh cream or crème fraîche

1 tablespoon butter

⅓ cup grated Cheddar or Jack cheese

1 teaspoon finely chopped chives or parsley (optional)

In a small bowl, whisk the eggs, egg yolk and cream until combined. Melt the butter in a small, well-seasoned cast-iron pan. Add the egg mixture and cook over medium heat, stirring constantly with a wooden spoon. At the last minute, stir in the cheese and chives or parsley. Serve immediately on heated plates.

Bacon Delight

Serves 4

1 pound bacon

2 apples, peeled, cored and sliced or 4 slices pineapple

Place the apple or pineapple slices in a 9-inch by 13-inch glass baking dish and lay the bacon slices over them. Bake at 350 degrees for about 20 minutes or until the bacon starts to crisp. Use tongs or a slotted spoon to serve.

Breakfast Casserole

Serves 6

1 pound Cheddar cheese, grated

1 pound sausage meat, browned and crumbled

1 dozen pastured eggs

1 cup cream

1½ teaspoons sea salt

1 teaspoon freshly ground black pepper

2 tablespoons chopped parsley

Grease a 9-inch by 13-inch glass baking dish using butter or lard. Sprinkle half the cheese on the bottom of the pan, and reserve the rest. Top the cheese with the crumbled sausage.

In a large bowl, whisk together the eggs, cream, salt and pepper. Stir in the parsley. Pour over the sausage meat and sprinkle with the remaining cheese.

Bake at 350 degrees for about 20 minutes. Enjoy while warm. Leftovers may be frozen.

Breakfast Smoothie

Serves 1

2 pastured egg yolks
½ cup ripe fruit, such as bananas or strawberries
½ cup cream
½ cup plain unsweetened whole-milk yogurt
2 tablespoons natural sweetener (such as honey, maple syrup or maple sugar)

Blend all the ingredients in a food processor or blender until smooth.

Note: Raw egg whites are very difficult to digest and should not be consumed.

Appetizers

Steak Tartare with Bacon Butter

Grass-fed beef tends to be lean, but this version of steak tartare is well balanced when eaten on toast spread with delicious bacon butter.

Serves 6–8

1 pound ground grass-fed beef
1 small onion, finely chopped
2 pastured egg yolks
1 tablespoon capers
1 tablespoon finely chopped parsley
1 teaspoon fish sauce (Red Boat brand recommended)
sea salt and pepper to taste
1 stick butter, softened
2 pieces bacon, cut very small and sautéed until crisp
about 24 thin slices of sourdough baguette, lightly toasted

Place the capers in a strainer, rinse well, and pat dry with paper towels. Place the beef, onion, egg yolks, capers, parsley and fish sauce in a medium bowl and mix well with your hands until combined. Season to taste with salt and pepper. Move to a ramekin or crock, cover and chill well.

In a small bowl, mix softened butter with crispy bacon pieces and place is a ramekin. To serve, smear toasted baguettes with bacon butter and top with a scoop of steak tartare.

Cheddar Cheese Spread

Makes about 3 cups

1 pound aged Cheddar cheese, grated
¼ cup butter, softened

¼ cup port wine
¾ cup crème fraîche
⅛ teaspoon cayenne pepper
½ teaspoon fish sauce (preferably Red Boat brand)
crackers or sourdough baguette, for serving

Combine all the ingredients in a food processor until smooth. Transfer to ramekin or a small soufflé dish. Serve at room temperature with crackers or toasted slices of sourdough baguette.

Endive Leaves Stuffed with Bleu Cheese

Makes 24

1 cup crumbled bleu cheese
½ cup crème fraîche or sour cream
about ¼ cup fresh pomegranate seeds
24 endive leaves, separated, rinsed and dried

In a food processor, blend the bleu cheese and crème fraîche or sour cream to a smooth paste. Spread a little of the bleu cheese paste into each endive leaf (or use an icing pipette). Sprinkle each with a few pomegranate seeds and serve.

Caviar Canapes

Makes 12

¾ cup crème fraîche or sour cream
12 slices sourdough baguette, lightly toasted
2 ounces caviar
2 tablespoons very finely diced red onion
1 tablespoon very finely diced parsley

Place a dollop (about 1 tablespoon) of crème fraîche or sour cream on each slice of baguette. Top each slice with 1 teaspoon caviar, then ½ teaspoon diced onion and a pinch of parsley. Serve and enjoy.

Bacon-Wrapped Chicken Livers

Makes about 36

1 pound chicken livers
1 pound bacon (not thick sliced)
1 can water chestnuts, sliced
about 1 cup naturally fermented soy sauce

Trim the chicken livers of any membranes and cut each liver into 3 pieces. Cut the bacon slices in half. Pat the water chestnut slices dry and place a slice on a bacon slice, and top with a piece of liver. Fold up the bacon ends and secure with a toothpick. Dip each bundle in soy sauce and place in a greased glass baking dish. Repeat for the remaining livers and bacon. Let marinate in the refrigerator for an hour or so. Bake at 300 degrees for about ½ hour, turning frequently, until the bacon is crisp. Serve warm.

Soups

Cream of Potato Soup with Bacon

Makes about 3 quarts, serving 6–12

½ pound bacon, cut into small pieces
1 medium onion, chopped
2 leeks, sliced open, washed and chopped into ½-inch pieces
½ cup dry white wine or vermouth
3 baking potatoes, peeled and cut into ½-inch cubes
2 quarts chicken stock or combination stock and water
bouquet garni (parsley sprigs, thyme springs and 1 bay leaf, tied together)
1 cup crème fraîche
salt and freshly ground pepper to taste
2 tablespoons finely chopped chives

In a heavy-bottomed pot, sauté the bacon pieces until crisp. Remove with a slotted spoon and set aside. In the remaining bacon fat, sauté the onion and leeks over low heat, stirring frequently, until soft. Add the wine or vermouth and bring to a boil. Add the potatoes, stock and bouquet garni and bring to a simmer. When the potatoes are soft, remove the bouquet garni and blend the soup with a handheld blender until smooth. Stir in the crème fraîche and season with sea salt and freshly ground pepper.

Serve in heated bowls and garnish with the reserved bacon pieces and chives.

Gizzard Soup

Serves 4–6

½ pound chicken gizzards
about 1 cup unbleached white flour
1 teaspoon sea salt

½ teaspoon freshly ground pepper

4 tablespoons butter or lard

2 medium onions, peeled and chopped

½ cup dry white wine or vermouth

1 quart homemade chicken broth

bouquet garni (parsley sprigs, thyme springs and 1 bay leaf, tied together)

4 medium red potatoes, cut into a ¼-inch dice

1 cup crème fraîche

sea salt and freshly ground pepper to taste

Wash the gizzards, remove any small stones or grit, and peel away any yellow skin. Cut into small pieces. Pat dry and dredge in a mixture of unbleached white flour, sea salt and freshly ground pepper.

Melt the butter or lard in a medium saucepan. Sauté the gizzard pieces in batches over medium-high heat until lightly browned. Remove with a slotted spoon and reserve. Sauté the onion in the remaining fat until golden brown. Add the wine or vermouth and bring to a boil. Add the chicken broth, gizzards and bouquet garni, and bring to a simmer over low heat. Simmer for about 1 hour or until the gizzards are tender. Add the potatoes and simmer for an additional 10 minutes until they are barely cooked through (but not mushy). Remove the bouquet garni and stir in the crème fraîche. Season with sea salt and freshly ground pepper and serve in heated bowls.

Cream of Veal Soup

Serves 4–6

½ pound bacon, cut into small pieces

1 pound ground veal

1 medium onion, peeled and diced

3 medium carrots, peeled and grated

2 sticks celery, diced

½ cup dry white wine or vermouth

1 quart homemade chicken broth

bouquet garni (parsley sprigs, thyme springs and 1 bay leaf, tied together)

about 2 cups greens (such as spinach, chard or radicchio), chopped

1 cup crème fraîche

sea salt and freshly ground pepper to taste

Sauté the bacon in a large saucepan until most of the fat is rendered, about 15 minutes. Add the veal and sauté, stirring frequently, until lightly browned. Add the onions, carrots and celery and sauté for an additional 15 minutes, stirring frequently.

Add the wine or vermouth and bring to a boil. Add the chicken broth, bouquet garni and greens and simmer for 15 minutes. Remove the bouquet garni and stir in the crème fraîche. Season with sea salt and freshly ground pepper to taste and serve in heated bowls.

Sauces

Brown Butter Tarragon Sauce

This versatile sauce is simple to make and can be used on meat, fish, vegetables or pasta.

Makes ½ cup, about 4 servings

1 stick unsalted butter, cut into 8 slices
2 tablespoons tarragon leaves, finely chopped
1 tablespoon chopped shallot
1 clove garlic, peeled and minced (optional)

Heat a heavy skillet on medium-high. When the skillet is hot, add the butter. Once it foams, add the tarragon leaves and turn the heat down to medium. Cook over medium heat for 10–20 minutes, stirring frequently, until the butter turns light brown—be careful not to let it burn. Stir in the chopped shallot and optional garlic and sauté for 1 minute, stirring constantly. Pour browned butter over vegetables, fish, meat or pasta.

Béarnaise Sauce

Béarnaise sauce provides a great package of fat-soluble vitamins, and is fabulous served over rare beef.

Makes about 1½ cups

2 tablespoons white wine vinegar
2 tablespoons dry white wine or vermouth
2 tablespoons finely chopped shallot or the white part of green onion
1 tablespoon finely chopped tarragon leaves, or 1 teaspoon dried tarragon
4 pastured egg yolks
1½ sticks unsalted butter, softened
About 1 teaspoon fresh lemon juice
sea salt and freshly ground pepper to taste

Combine the vinegar, wine or vermouth, shallot and tarragon leaves in a small saucepan. Boil over medium heat until reduced to 1 tablespoon, about 3–5 minutes. Allow to cool slightly and then strain the liquid directly into the top pan of a double boiler. While the water in the lower pan is heating up, add the egg yolks to the reduced vinegar mixture. Whisk until thick and pale, about 2 minutes. As the water in the lower pan begins to simmer, continue to whisk at a reasonable speed, reaching all over the bottom and insides of the pan. The egg yolks should become frothy and increase in volume, then thicken. When the bottom of the pan is visible in the streaks left by the whisk and the egg yolks are thick and smooth, remove from heat.

Add the softened butter by spoonfuls, whisking constantly to incorporate each addition. Continue incorporating the butter until the sauce has thickened to the consistency desired. Add the lemon juice and season with sea salt and freshly ground pepper to taste. Serve immediately.

Better than Mayo

This is so much easier to make than mayonnaise—and more nutritious as well.

Makes 1½ cups

½ cup crème fraîche
2 pastured egg yolks
1 tablespoon extra virgin olive oil
1 tablespoon fresh lemon juice
sea salt and freshly ground pepper to taste

Place all the ingredients into a bowl and whisk together well until thoroughly combined. Use immediately or transfer to a jar and refrigerate.

Ranch Dressing

Store-bought ranch dressing contains vegetable oil, MSG and lots of additives. Better to make your own!

Makes 1⅓ cups

2 cloves garlic, peeled and mashed
½ teaspoon sea salt
1 cup sour cream or crème fraîche

¼–⅓ cup buttermilk or plain, unsweetened full-fat yogurt
2 tablespoons finely chopped parsley
2 tablespoons finely chopped chives
1 green onion, white part only, finely chopped
1 tablespoon white wine vinegar
freshly ground black pepper to taste

Place all the ingredients in a bowl and whisk together until combined. If the dressing is too thick, thin with a little more buttermilk or vinegar. Store in an airtight container in the refrigerator. Use within one week.

Giblet Gravy

Makes 2–4 cups

Reserve the drippings from a chicken or turkey, cooked in a stainless steel or enamel pan
2–4 cups homemade chicken or turkey broth
gizzard from the chicken or turkey, cleaned and cut into pieces
2–4 tablespoons unbleached white flour
sea salt and freshly ground pepper to taste

While the chicken or turkey is cooking, use a small saucepan to simmer the gizzard in the broth. When the gizzard is tender, chop the pieces very fine and set aside.

After your turkey or chicken has finished cooking, remove it (and the rack it was on) from the pan and keep warm in a warm oven. Place the pan over medium heat. Add the flour and stir around until it has completely combined with the poultry fat. (In principle, use 2 tablespoons of flour for a chicken and 4 tablespoons for a turkey, but if there is a lot of fat, use more.) Stir until the fat-flour mixture has lightly browned, being careful not to let it burn. Add the stock slowly, while whisking, and bring to a simmer, whisking constantly to remove any lumps. If the gravy is too thick, thin with a little water; if the gravy is too thin, reduce by gentle boiling. Stir in the reserved chopped gizzard and season to taste with sea salt and freshly ground pepper.

Vegetables

Caesar Salad

Serves 4

For the salad

about ½ cup lard or bacon fat

4 slices sourdough bread, crusts removed and cut into cubes

2 heads romaine lettuce, outer leaves removed, washed and dried

4 ounces Parmigiano-Reggiano cheese, grated or shaved

For the dressing

2 cloves garlic, minced

1 teaspoon sea salt

2 large or 3 medium pastured egg yolks

1½ tablespoons Dijon mustard

4 anchovy filets, cut into ½-inch pieces

juice of 1 small lemon, strained

1 teaspoon fish sauce (preferably Red Boat brand)

3 dashes hot sauce

2 tablespoons red wine vinegar

1 teaspoon freshly ground pepper

⅓–½ cup extra virgin olive oil

½ cup sour cream or crème fraîche (optional)

Melt the bacon fat or lard in a skillet, and sauté the bread cubes until browned. Cut or tear the lettuce into 1-inch pieces. Set the croutons and lettuce aside.

In a large wooden bowl, using a wooden spoon, mash the minced garlic cloves to a fine paste with the salt. Stir in the egg yolks and Dijon mustard. Add the anchovies, and continue to grind into a thick paste. Add the lemon juice, fish sauce, hot sauce and vinegar and season with the pepper. Slowly whisk in the olive oil and optional sour cream or crème fraîche until the dressing is creamy.

Add the lettuce to the bowl, and toss to coat the leaves thoroughly. Divide on 4 plates, sprinkle with the Parmigiano-Reggiano cheese and croutons and enjoy.

Cabbage with Cream

Serves 4

1 cabbage, core removed and sliced thinly

1 cup heavy cream

sea salt and freshly ground pepper to taste

Place the sliced cabbage in a skillet with a close-fitting lid. Pour the cream over the cabbage and sprinkle with the sea salt and freshly ground pepper. Simmer, covered, for 5 minutes over low heat. Remove the lid and bring the liquid to a full boil. Boil gently for about 10 minutes, stirring occasionally, until the liquid has reduced. Serve warm.

Buttered Ginger Carrots

Serves 4

1 pound carrots, peeled and sliced at about 1 inch, on the diagonal

2 tablespoons unsalted butter

2 tablespoons honey

¼ teaspoon powdered ginger

filtered water

Place the carrots, butter, honey and ginger in a medium saucepan and top with filtered water until just covered. Bring to a boil, uncovered, and continue boiling to let the liquid reduce. Use a spoon to skim off any foam that may rise to the surface. As the liquid gets thick, stir constantly to prevent sticking. Carrots will become coated with the butter-honey mixture. Serve warm.

Potato Wedges in Duck Fat

Serves 2–4

4 medium Yukon gold potatoes, peeled, sliced in half lengthwise, with each half cut into 3 sections on an angle

about ½ cup duck fat

sea salt to taste

1 teaspoon finely chopped parsley

Please the potato sections in a colander and rinse with very cold water. Spread on paper towels and pat dry. Meanwhile, place the duck fat in a 9-inch by 13-inch glass baking pan and melt in an oven set at 400 degrees. Add the potatoes to the pan, sprinkle with sea salt and toss to coat in the duck fat. Bake at 400 degrees for about ½ hour until nicely browned, turning once or twice while they are cooking. To serve, sprinkle with parsley.

Twice Fried Potatoes

Serves 8

4 large baking potatoes

1 quart plus 2 tablespoons tallow

sea salt and freshly ground pepper to taste

For best results, use a 1-liter deep fryer.

Peel the potatoes, leaving some skin on the ends. Cut into ⅓-inch slices. Then cut the slices into ⅓-inch sticks. Soak the potatoes in a large bowl of cold water for about 1 hour. Drain in a colander and pat dry with a paper towel to remove excess water.

Heat the tallow in the fryer to 325 degrees. In 4 batches, cook the potatoes in the tallow until light brown, about 5–7 minutes for each batch. Remove the potatoes, shaking off the excess tallow, and allow them to drain on a wire rack. Raise the temperature of the tallow to 350 degrees and cook the potatoes again in 4 batches, about 2 minutes each batch, until golden brown. Shake off the tallow and place the potatoes on paper towels to soak up the excess. Place the potatoes in a bowl and toss with sea salt and freshly ground pepper.

Baked Root Vegetables

Serves 6

2–3 beets, peeled and cut into ½-inch cubes

2 turnips, peeled and cut into ½-inch cubes

2 sweet potatoes, peeled and cut into ½-inch cubes
2 cups baby onions, peeled
1 stick butter
sea salt to taste

While preparing the vegetables, place the butter in a 9-inch by 13-inch glass baking dish and allow it to melt in a 350-degree oven. When butter is melted, place the vegetable cubes (you should have about 10 cups total) in the pan and stir with a wooden spoon to coat the vegetables with the butter. Bake about 1 hour or until tender, stirring occasionally. Toss with sea salt to taste.

Mashed Potatoes

Serves 6

6 large russet potatoes
¼ cup melted butter or lard
1 stick butter, softened
½ cup sour cream or crème fraîche
whole milk, as necessary
sea salt to taste

Cut a small piece off each end of the potatoes and brush with melted butter or lard. Place in a glass baking dish and bake at 350 degrees for 1–1½ hours, or until tender when poked with a fork.

Place the stick of butter in a medium bowl. Cut the potatoes in half lengthwise and scoop out the potato flesh into the bowl. (Reserve the skins for Potato Skins; see recipe below.) Add the sour cream or crème fraîche and mash together. Use a handheld mixer to mix until very smooth. If the mixture is too thick, add a little whole milk to thin. Blend in the sea salt to taste and serve warm.

Potato Skins

Makes 12

12 potato skins as lengthwise halves, baked (see Mashed Potatoes, above)
6 slices bacon, cut into small pieces

3 cups grated Cheddar or Jack cheese
1 cup finely chopped green onions, including green tops
sour cream or crème fraîche for garnish

Cook the bacon in a cast iron skillet until semicrisp and set aside. Place the cooked potato skins in a greased glass baking dish (or dishes, as needed). Place ¼ cup cheese on each skin and top with the bacon pieces and green onions. Broil for several minutes until the cheese is melted. Serve with a dollop of sour cream or crème fraîche.

Seafood

Wild Salmon with Cream Sauce

Serves 4

1½ pounds wild salmon filet, skin on, cut into 4 pieces
2 cups fish stock
½ cup white wine
1 cup sour cream or crème fraîche
1 tablespoon chopped fresh tarragon leaves
sea salt to taste

Place the salmon, skin side down, in a greased glass baking dish—the salmon should fill most of the dish. In a medium bowl, combine the stock and white wine and pour over the salmon—the salmon should be fully covered with the liquid. Bake at 300 degrees for about ½ hour, or until the salmon is flaky, but still slightly underdone in the center. Remove to paper towels and pat dry. Keep warm in a warm oven or warming drawer while making the sauce.

Pour the stock and wine into a large cast iron skillet. Add the sour cream or crème fraîche and boil vigorously until the sauce reduces and thickens. When the sauce coats a wooden spoon, stir in the tarragon leaves and season with sea salt to taste.

To serve, place the salmon pieces into 4 heated bowls and pour the sauce over the fish.

Scallops in Ginger Cream Sauce

Serves 4

1¼ pounds "dry" sea scallops (or 5–6 per serving)
4 tablespoons unsalted butter
½ cup dry white wine or vermouth
1 cup fish stock
1 cup heavy cream

2 cloves garlic, very finely chopped
1 tablespoon grated fresh ginger
3 green onions, including green tops, chopped
1–2 tablespoons fresh lime juice
sea salt to taste
2 tablespoons finely chopped fresh cilantro

Pat the scallops very dry with paper towels. Melt the butter over medium heat in a large cast iron skillet. Sauté the scallops about 5–6 at a time, 4–5 minutes per side, or until just tender. Transfer to a heated platter or dish and keep warm.

Deglaze the skillet with white wine or vermouth. Add fish stock, cream, garlic and ginger and boil vigorously over high heat, skimming any scum that comes to the surface. Continue boiling until the sauce is reduced by at least half and coats a wooden spoon. Stir in the scallions and lime juice, reduce a little more, and season to taste with sea salt. Pour the sauce over the scallops and sprinkle with cilantro. Serve warm.

Note: For best results, choose "dry" sea scallops, which means they have not been soaked in a brine solution.

South-of-the-Border Fish

Serves 4

4 ears fresh corn, husks removed
⅓–½ cup lard
¼ cup chili powder
1 teaspoon sea salt
about 1 ⅓ pounds fresh fish filets, skin on, in 4 pieces
1 jalapeño chile, seeded and diced

Cut the corn off the cob into a medium bowl and set aside. Over medium heat, melt the lard in a cast iron skillet.

Meanwhile, mix the chili powder and sea salt in a shallow dish. Pat the fish very dry with paper towels and dredge in the spice mix. (Set aside any remaining spice mixture.) Sauté the fish on both sides in the hot lard, several minutes on each side, until the fish is cooked through. Transfer to a heated platter and keep warm.

Add the jalapeño chile to the skillet and cook for a few minutes, stirring occasionally. Add the corn and any remaining chili powder–salt mixture. Cook, stirring, for a few minutes until the corn is tender. Serve the corn alongside the cooked fish.

Meats

Italian Meat Loaf

Serves 6–8

1½ cups breadcrumbs, preferably sourdough
½ cup powdered Parmesan cheese
about 1 cup cream
1 pound ground beef
1 pound ground pork
2 whole pastured eggs
1 onion, peeled and minced
2 tablespoons finely chopped parsley
2 teaspoons Italian seasonings
2 teaspoons fish sauce (preferably Red Boat brand)
1 teaspoon pepper
1 teaspoon salt
1 7-ounce jar tomato paste
about ½ cup water

Mix the breadcrumbs and Parmesan cheese together in a small bowl, and add enough cream to completely moisten the mixture, but not so much that it is runny.

Place all the remaining ingredients except the tomato paste in a large bowl, add the breadcrumb mixture, and combine well by hand. Form into a loaf and set into a glass baking dish. Cover the loaf with the tomato paste and fill the bottom of the dish with the water. Bake at 350 degrees for about 1¼ hours, or until cooked through. Leftovers will keep for several days in the refrigerator.

Fried Chicken

Serves 8

2 pastured chickens

1 quart buttermilk or plain unsweetened full-fat yogurt

about 3 cups unbleached flour

½ teaspoon cayenne pepper

2 teaspoons paprika

2 teaspoons salt

1 teaspoon pepper

3–4 cups lard

Cut each chicken into 10 pieces—2 wings, 2 legs, 2 thighs, 2 back pieces and 2 breasts. Place the chicken pieces in a large bowl and mix with the buttermilk or yogurt until thoroughly coated. Cover the bowl and marinate, refrigerated, for 24 hours.

Pour the flour, cayenne pepper, paprika, salt and pepper into a medium-sized paper bag (such as a large lunch bag). Shake to mix the spices thoroughly.

Melt about 1 cup lard in a large cast iron skillet, being careful not to let the fat get too hot. Shake the buttermilk or yogurt off one chicken piece and place it in the paper bag. Shake well to coat the piece with the flour-and-spice mixture. Repeat with 4 additional pieces. Place all 5 pieces in the skillet and fry uncovered at medium-high temperature for 10 minutes. Turn the pieces, lower the heat to medium and continue frying, covered, 10 minutes more, or until cooked through.

Transfer the cooked chicken to a large platter lined with several layers of paper towel and keep warm while completing the remaining batches, adding additional lard to the skillet as needed.

Serve the chicken warm. Can be refrigerated for several days and served cold.

Pulled Pork

Serves 8–10

1 large fatty pork shoulder, about 4 pounds

1 cup fresh lime juice

1 small pig foot or split pig foot

2 teaspoons oregano

3 cloves garlic, peeled and coarsely chopped

sea salt to taste

Cut the pork shoulder into 2-inch chunks. Place the pieces in a large bowl and toss with the lime juice. Cover and marinate in the refrigerator for several hours or overnight.

Place the marinated pork pieces and all remaining ingredients into a slow cooker, adding enough water to cover the pork. Cook on low for about 12 hours, or until the meat is very tender. Turn off the heat and allow to cool. Remove the pork and pig's foot, and reserve the cooking liquid. Chop the meat into small pieces. Remove the meat and skin from pig's foot and chop into small pieces. Mix all the pulled meat with the cooking liquids and season to taste with sea salt. Serve with your favorite sauce, or use pulled pork for tostadas (recipe follows), tacos, burritos or casseroles.

Tostadas

Serves 6

6 corn or flour tortillas, fried until crisp in lard

3 cups pulled pork (recipe above)

3 cups black beans, cooked

6 cups finely sliced Romaine lettuce hearts

3 tomatoes, diced

1 red onion, minced

2 ripe avocados, peeled and diced

3 cups grated Jack cheese

1 cup sour cream

hot sauce

Divide the fried tortillas among 6 heated plates. Top each with pulled pork, warm black beans, Romaine lettuce, tomatoes, onion, avocado, and Jack cheese. Serve with sour cream, and hot sauce as a garnish.

Organ Meats

Chicken Liver and Heart Pâté

Makes about 2 cups

1 pound chicken livers and hearts
3 tablespoons butter or lard
1 onion, peeled and chopped
½ cup brandy
2 cups chicken stock
1 clove garlic, peeled and mashed
1 teaspoon powdered mustard
1 teaspoon dried dill
½ teaspoon powdered rosemary
½ cup butter, softened
sea salt to taste

Trim off any membranes from the livers, and pat hearts and livers dry with paper towels. Melt 3 tablespoons butter or lard in a large cast iron skillet and sauté the chopped onion over medium heat until golden. Add the livers and hearts, raise heat and sauté until they are browned on all sides. Add the brandy to the skillet and bring to a boil. Add the chicken stock, garlic, mustard, dill and rosemary. Boil gently, stirring occasionally, until the liquid is reduced about half, or about 10–15 minutes.

Allow to cool and transfer to a food processor. Add the ½ cup softened butter and process until very smooth. Add additional chicken stock if the pâté is too thick. Add sea salt to taste. Transfer to a 3-cup ramekin or 3 smaller ramekins. Cover well until served. Can be refrigerated or frozen.

Baked Beans with Sausage and Marrow Bones

Serves 8

2 cups dry white beans
1 35-ounce can diced tomatoes
1 cup white wine
2 cloves garlic, peeled and chopped
1 teaspoon sea salt
1 teaspoon peppercorns
2 3-inch marrow bones
1 pound pork sausage, cut into slices
several sprigs fresh rosemary

Soak the beans in 8 cups hot water overnight. Drain through a colander and rinse well. Place the beans and all remaining ingredients into a slow cooker, adding enough water to cover everything. Cook on low heat for about 8 hours, checking occasionally. If the beans seem dry, add more water.

To serve, remove marrow bones from slow cooker. Strip the marrow from the bones and stir into the cooking liquid—the marrow will thicken it nicely. Ladle into bowls and enjoy.

Breaded Marrow Bones

Serves 4

4 4-inch marrow bones, split lengthwise
2 cups breadcrumbs (sourdough if available)
zest of 1 organic lemon
¼ cup parsley, finely chopped
sea salt and freshly ground pepper to taste
¼ cup melted butter

Place the marrow bones in a glass baking dish. In a small bowl, mix the breadcrumbs with the lemon zest, parsley and salt and pepper. Place about ¼ cup of this mixture on each marrow bone and then drizzle the butter over the breadcrumbs. Bake at 350 degrees for about 10 minutes. Place the dish under a broiler for an additional 5 minutes, or until the breadcrumbs are nicely browned. Serve two split bones per plate with small spoons.

Gizzards and Rice

Serves 4

1 pound chicken gizzards
juice of 2 lemons
about 1 cup unbleached white flour
1 teaspoon sea salt
½ teaspoon freshly ground pepper
about ½ cup lard
4 cups cooked rice
4 green onions, including green tops, chopped

Clean the gizzards of any grit or stones and peel away any yellow skin. Cut into small pieces. In a small bowl, mix the gizzards with the lemon juice and marinate for several hours in the refrigerator. Pat dry with paper towels and then dredge in a mixture of the unbleached white flour, sea salt and freshly ground pepper.

Melt the lard in a cast iron skillet over medium high heat. Fry the gizzard pieces in batches, removing with a slotted spoon to paper towels to drain. Serve over hot cooked rice. Garnish with chopped green onion.

Liver Stir-Fry

Serves 2

¾ pound sliced calves liver
¼ cup fresh lemon juice
½ pound bacon, cut into pieces
about 1 cup unbleached white flour
1 teaspoon sea salt
½ teaspoon freshly ground pepper
1 large onion, peeled, quartered and sliced
extra bacon fat, if needed

Cut the liver into strips and toss with the lemon juice in a medium bowl. Marinate, refrigerated, for several hours.

In a large cast iron skillet, cook the bacon pieces over medium heat until the fat is rendered. Meanwhile, pat the liver strips dry with paper towels and dredge in a mixture of unbleached white flour, salt and pepper.

Push the bacon pieces to the edge of the pan and sauté the onion in the rendered fat. When the onion is soft and translucent, push it to the edge of the pan. Raise the heat to high and quickly sauté the liver strips, about 1 minute per side, adding more bacon fat, if needed. The liver should be browned but still pink on the inside. Stir into the bacon and onion and immediately remove to a heated bowl or platter to serve.

Pork and Liver Terrine

Serves 6–8

2 tablespoons butter
1 small onion, peeled and finely chopped
½ pound liver (pork or chicken)
1 pound fatty ground pork
½ pound ground beef or veal
1 clove garlic, peeled and finely chopped
1 teaspoon dried thyme
2 teaspoons sea salt
1 teaspoon black pepper
½ teaspoon nutmeg
⅛ teaspoon allspice
¼ cup cognac or brandy
2 pastured eggs
¼ cup heavy cream
½ cup pistachio nuts
about 12 strips of bacon
sourdough baguette and pickles for serving (optional)

You will need a brick wrapped in aluminum foil or a bacon press (with its wooden handle wrapped in aluminum foil so it doesn't catch fire) to weight the terrine down as it bakes.

Melt the butter in a cast iron skillet and sauté the onion over medium heat until soft. Transfer the onion to a bowl, set aside and let cool.

Pulse the liver in a food processor until smooth. In a large bowl, mix the liver, ground pork, ground beef or veal, cooked onion, garlic, thyme, salt, pepper, nutmeg and allspice. In a separate bowl, whisk together the brandy, eggs and heavy cream. Pour over the meat and stir until completely combined. Stir in the pistachio nuts.

Lay the bacon strips across the bottom of a 5-inch by 9-inch loaf pan, so they completely cover the bottom of the pan without overlapping. Bring the bacon strips up both sides of the pan and let 1–2 inches of bacon overhang the edge. Fill the pan with the meat mixture to create the terrine, taking care not to move the bacon lining the pan. Cover the top of the terrine lengthwise with three strips of bacon then fold the overhang of bacon over the top. Cover the terrine with plastic wrap and refrigerate for 8 hours.

Preheat the oven to 350 degrees. Fill a baking dish with 2 inches hot water, place in the oven and let the water come to a simmer. Remove the terrine from the refrigerator and place a layer of greased parchment paper on top of the bacon and then place the weight on top of the loaf. Place in the simmering hot water bath and bake 1½ hours. Remove from the oven and let cool. Refrigerate for 24 hours with the weight still on top.

To serve, set the loaf pan in a new hot water bath and loosen the sides gently with a knife. Invert terrine onto a platter. Serve with slices of sourdough baguette and pickled gherkins. (Adapted from marksdailyapple.com.)

Desserts

Vanilla Ice Cream

Makes 1 quart

6 pastured egg yolks
⅓–½ cup maple sugar
½ teaspoon vanilla powder or vanilla extract
3 cups cream

In a medium bowl, beat the egg yolks with maple sugar and vanilla powder for about 5 minutes. Beat in the cream. Pour into a home ice cream maker and process according to directions. Store, covered, in the freezer in a shallow glass container. Remove from the freezer and let thaw about 5 minutes before serving.

Almond Spice Cookies

Makes about 18

1½ cups slivered almonds
1½ teaspoons sea salt
1 cup arrowroot powder
½ cup maple sugar
½ teaspoon powdered vanilla
½ teaspoon allspice
½ teaspoon finely ground white pepper
¼ teaspoon powdered cloves
½ cup (1 stick) unsalted butter, softened

Soak the almonds in warm water plus 1 teaspoon sea salt for about 7 hours. Drain in a colander and sprinkle evenly on a baking sheet. Bake at 150 degrees for about 6 hours or until the nuts are completely dry and crisp. This process makes all nuts more digestible.

Place the nuts in a food processor and process until finely ground. Add the arrowroot powder, maple sugar, vanilla, allspice, pepper, cloves, and ½ teaspoon sea salt and process until well mixed. Cut the butter into about 8 pieces and add to the mixture. Process until smooth.

Grease a cookie sheet with butter and lightly coat with unbleached white flour or arrowroot powder. Roll the cookie dough into 1-inch balls and place on the cookie sheet. Flatten each ball with a fork. Bake at 325 degrees for about 20 minutes. Allow to cool before removing to a storage container. Store in the refrigerator for up to 2 weeks.

Cream Cheese Topping

A smooth creamy topping perfect for fruit, pies, tarts, pastries or almond spice cookies.

Makes 1½ cups

8 ounces cream cheese, softened
⅓ cup honey
¼ cup (½ stick) unsalted butter, softened
1 teaspoon vanilla extract

Blend all the ingredients in a blender. Use immediately with your favorite fruit, snack or dessert.

Vanilla Nut Custard

Serves 6

2 cups pecans
1 teaspoon sea salt
4 tablespoons butter
¾ cup maple sugar
1¼ cups heavy cream
1¼ cups whole milk
2 teaspoons vanilla extract
6 large pastured egg yolks

Soak the pecans in warm water and salt for 7 hours. Drain in a colander and sprinkle evenly on a baking sheet. Bake at 150 degrees for about 6 hours or until the nuts are completely dry and crisp. This process makes all nuts more digestible. Finely chop the nuts.

Melt the butter in a cast iron skillet. Add the nuts and ¼ cup maple sugar, and sauté over medium heat until the nuts are lightly browned. Allow to cool and set aside.

Fill a baking pan with about 2 inches water and place in an oven, preheated to 300 degrees. Allow the water to heat while making the custard.

In the top of a double boiler, combine the cream, milk, and vanilla. Heat the mixture over simmering water, stirring frequently. In a medium bowl, whisk the egg yolks with ½ cup maple sugar until light and fluffy. Slowly whisk in the hot milk mixture.

Butter four 6-ounce custard cups and place a tablespoon of the nut mixture at the bottom of each cup. Pour in the hot custard. Place filled custard cups in the hot water bath and bake about 30–40 minutes, or until the custard has set and is no longer liquid in the center. Remove the custard cups from the water, and place on a wire rack to cool. To serve, place another tablespoon of the nut mixture on top. (Any remaining nut mixture can be used in salads or as a topping on fruit or ice cream.) Serve at room temperature or chilled.

Acknowledgments

This book began as a few notes and a hasty table of contents jotted down a dozen years ago, after many conversations with my mentor, Mary G. Enig, PhD. We agreed on the need for a popular book addressing the subject of saturated fats, one that would do more than acknowledge the notion that they "might not be so bad," but explain why they are essential to life. Needless to say, the inspiration for this book, and the basic knowledge on fats and oils, came from her. *Nourishing Fats* is dedicated to the memory of this courageous biochemist, who sacrificed research grants and a prestigious career in order to warn the public about the dangers of *trans* fats.

Then along came Mary Evans, literary agent, who contacted me several years ago about doing the book *Nourishing Broth*. It was her vision and support that has made it possible to finally publish our original ideas, in the form of *Nourishing Fats*.

This book owes a great debt to the ongoing work of Chris Masterjohn, PhD, today's foremost expert in the fat-soluble vitamins, one who has followed in the footsteps of Dr. Weston A. Price in showing the modern scientific validation of his original research.

Nina Teicholz's book, *The Big Fat Surprise,* educated us all about the current science on toxic vegetable oils. Thanks to her persistent sleuthing, we are all a lot wiser about the dangers of processed foods, and I am grateful for her contribution to this effort and for providing key information for this book.

Sylvia Onusic, PhD, helped me track down a great many references, many of them obscure, often making special trips to the University of Pennsylvania library. Her sleuthing skills saved me hours of time and trouble.

What a pleasure it has been to work with Brittany McInerney at Hachette, who helped immensely with her expert editing skills, and with Karen Murgolo, editorial director; many thanks for her confidence in this book.

Mary Woodin's wonderful illustrations greatly enhance the reader's experience in *Nourishing Fats*. No one else has drawn such appealing fatty acid molecules!

Cheesemaker Tess Griebel lived with us the whole year while I worked on the draft, taking over all my farm duties, in the garden, making cheese, and even in the kitchen. I could not have written this book without her.

Finally, much thanks to my patient husband, Geoffrey Morell, whose support and loving presence make possible all the long hours sitting at a desk.

Notes

Chapter 1: The Greatest Villains

1 Pendleton SC. Man's most important food is fat: the use of persuasive techniques in Procter & Gamble's public relations campaign to introduce Crisco, 1911–1913. *Public Relations Quarterly.* Mar 22, 1999.
In footnote: [a] Cotton: Harvest Aid Chemicals, http://ipm.ucanr.edu/PMG/r114800111.html, accessed September 18, 2016.

2 Twain M. *Life on the Mississippi*, 1883, Chap. 39.

3 U.S. Department of Agriculture, U.S. Census Bureau.

4 Visser M. *Much Depends on Dinner: The Extraordinary History and Mythology, Allure and Obsessions, Perils and Taboos of an Ordinary Meal.* New York: Grove Press, 2010, p. 99.

5 *The Baptist Ladies Cook Book: Choice and Tested Recipes Contributed by the Ladies of Monmouth, Ill*, Jan 1, 1895.

6 http://www.second-opinions.co.uk/love-fat.html#.ViEKJrPIoro. Accessed Oct 16, 2015.

7 Cummings RO. *The American and His Food.* Chicago: University of Chicago Press, 1940, p. 235.

8 Parry CH. *An Inquiry into the Symptoms and Causes of the Syncope Anginosa, Commonly Called Angina Pectoris.* Bath, UK: Cruttwell, 1799.

9 Windaus A. Ueber der Gehalt normaler und atheromatoser Aorten an Cholesterol und Cholesterinester. *Zeitschrift Physiol Chemie.* 1910, 67:174.
In footnote: [a] Haas J. Vigantol—Adolf Windaus and the history of vitamin D. *Wurzbg Medizinhist Mitt.* 2007, 26:144–48.

10 Konstantinov IE et al. Nikolai N. Anichkov and his theory of atherosclerosis. *Tex Heart Inst J.* 2006, 33(4):417–23.

11 Connor WE. Dietary cholesterol and the pathogenesis of atherosclerosis. *Geriatrics.* 1961, 16:407.

12 Pardee HEB. An electrocardiographic sign of coronary artery obstruction. *Arch Int Med.* 1920, 26:244–57.

13 http://www.cdc.gov/mmwr/preview/mmwrhtml/figures/m830a1f1.gif. Accessed Dec 13, 2015.
In footnote: [a] https://www.cardiosmart.org/Heart-Basics/CVD-Stats. Accessed Dec. 13, 2015.

14 Gofman JL et al. The role of lipids and lipoproteins in atherosclerosis. *Science.* 1950, 111:166.

15 Enig MG. *Trans Fatty Acids in the Food Supply: A Comprehensive Report Covering 60 Years of Research*, 2d ed. Silver Spring, MD: Enig Associates, Inc., 1995, pp. 4–8.

16 https://tdc.okstate.edu/obesity-epidemic-part-3-sugar. Accessed Dec 13, 2015.

17 Notice of Supelco-AOC Award to Kritchevsky. *Inform.* 1996, 7:315.
In footnote: [a] http://www.nytimes.com/2000/12/16/us/edward-ahrens-cholestrol-researcher-is-dead-at-85.html. Accessed Dec 13, 2015.

18 Teicholz N. *The Big Fat Surprise: Why Butter, Meat and Cheese Belong in a Healthy Diet*. New York: Simon & Schuster, 2014, p. 40.
In footnote: [a] Teicholz N. *The Big Fat Surprise: Why Butter, Meat and Cheese Belong in a Healthy Diet*. New York: Simon & Schuster, 2014, p. 37.

19 Horlick L et al. The effect of a low fat diet on the spontaneously occurring arteriosclerosis of the chicken. *Am Heart J*. Sep 1948, 36(3):472.

20 Stamler J and Shekelle R. Dietary cholesterol and human coronary heart disease: the epidemiologic evidence. *Arch Pathol Lab Med*. Oct 1988, 112(10):1032–40.

21 Stamler J et al. Regional differences in prevalence, incidence and mortality from atherosclerotic coronary heart disease. *Ischaemic Heart Disease*. University Press, 1970, p. 84.

22 http://www.epi.umn.edu/cvdepi/essay/early-prevention-message-your-heart-has-nine-lives-nine-steps-to-heart-health-1963-pocket-books-new-york/. Accessed Dec 13, 2015.

23 Smith RL and Pinckney ER. *The Cholesterol Conspiracy*. Saint Louis: Warren H. Green, Inc., 1991, pp. 125–26.

24 Ibid., p. 128.
In footnote: [a] Taubes G and Couzens C. Big sugar's sweet little lies. http://www.motherjones.com/environment/2012/10/sugar-industry-lies-campaign?page=2. Accessed Dec 15, 2015. [b] Keys A. Sucrose in the diet and coronary heart disease. *Atherosclerosis*. 1971, 14:193–202.

25 Page IH et al. Atherosclerosis and the fat content of the diet. *JAMA*. Aug 31, 1957, 164(18):2048–51.

26 Keys A. Diet and development of coronary heart disease. *J Chron Dis*. Oct 1956, 4(4):364–80.

27 Marvin, HM. *1924–1964: The 40 Year War on Heart Disease*. New York: American Heart Association, 1964.

28 http://www.heart.org/HEARTORG/GettingHealthy/NutritionCenter/HealthyEating/The-American-Heart-Associations-Diet-and-Lifestyle-Recommendations_UCM_305855_Article.jsp#.ViFVZLPIoro. Accessed Oct 16, 2015.

29 Lande KE and Sperry WM. Human atherosclerosis in relation to the cholesterol content of blood serum. *Archives of Pathology*. 1936, 22:301–12.

30 Groom D. Population studies of atherosclerosis. *Annals of Int Med*. Jul 1961, 55(1):51–62; Enos WF et al. Pathogenesis of coronary disease in American soldiers killed in Korea. *JAMA*. 1955, 158:912.

31 Laurie W et al. Atherosclerosis and its cerebral complications in the South African Bantu. *Lancet*. Feb 1958, 231–32.

32 Robertson WB. Atherosclerosis and ischaemic heart disease. *Lancet*. 1959, 1:444.

33 Gordon T. Mortality experience among Japanese in the US, Hawaii and Japan. *Pul Health Rep*, 1957, 51:270. Pollak OJ. Diet and atherosclerosis. *Lancet*. 1959, 1:444.

34 McGill HC et al. General findings of the International Atherosclerosis Project. *Laboratory Investigations*. 1968, 18(5):498.

35 Smith RL and Pinckney ER. *The Cholesterol Conspiracy*. Saint Louis: Warren H. Green, Inc. 1991, p. 125.

36 DeBakey M et al. Serum cholesterol values in patients treated surgically for atherosclerosis. *JAMA*. 1964, 189(9):655–59.

37 General news release issued by the AMA, Oct 12, 1962.

38 Blakeslee A and Stamler J. *Your Heart Has Nine Lives: Nine Steps to Heart Health*. New York: Pocket Books, 1963. Professional edition courtesy of Corn Products Company.

39 Cristakis G et al. Effect of the Anti-Coronary Club program on coronary heart disease: risk-factor status. *JAMA*, Nov 7, 1966, 198(6):597–604.

40 National Diet-Heart Study Research Group. National Diet-Heart Study Final Report. *Circulation*. 1968, 37(Supp. 1).

41 *Dietary Goals for the United States—Supplemental Views*, prepared by the Staff of the Select Committee on Nutrition and Human Needs, United States Senate. Washington DC: Government Printing Office, Nov 1977, pp. 139–40.

42 Food and Nutrition Board, Division of Biology and Agriculture. Council on Foods and Nutrition, American Medical Association. Diet and coronary heart disease. *Preventive Medicine*. 1972, 1:559.

43 Mary G. Enig, personal communication.

44 Proposed Rules. *Federal Register.* Nov 27, 1991, 56(229).

45 http://zerodisease.com/archive/Dietary_Goals_For_The_United_States.pdf. Accessed Oct 16, 2015.

46 Kummerow FA et al. Comparative study of the atherogenecity of dietary trans, saturated and unsaturated fatty acids on swine coronary arteries. *J Nutr Sci Vitaminol* (Tokyo). Apr 1985, 31(2):233–41.

47 Mary G. Enig, personal communication.

48 Rizek RL et al. Fat in today's food supply—level of use and sources. *J Am Oil Chem Soc.* 1974, 51:244.

49 Carroll KK. Experimental evidence of dietary factors and hormone-dependent cancers. *Cancer Res.* Nov 1975, 35(11, Pt. 2):3374–83.

50 Ibid.

51 Fernández NA. Nutrition in Puerto Rico. *Cancer Res.* Nov 1975, 35(11, Pt. 2):3272–91; Martínez I et al. Cancer incidence in the United States and Puerto Rico. *Cancer Res.* Nov 1975, 35(11, Pt. 2):3265–71.

52 Carroll KK. Experimental evidence of dietary factors and hormone-dependent cancers; Gregor O et al. Gastrointestinal cancer and nutrition. *Gut.* Dec 1969, 10(12):1031–34.

53 Correa P. Comments on the epidemiology of large bowel cancer. *Cancer Res.* Nov 1975, 35(11, Pt. 2):3395–97.

54 Phillips RL. Role of life-style and dietary habits in risk of cancer among Seventh-day Adventists. *Cancer Res.* Nov 1975, 35(11, Pt. 2):3513–22.

55 Enig MG et al. Dietary fat and cancer trends—a critique. *Fed Proc.* Jul 1978, 37(9):2215–20.

56 Enig MG. *Trans Fatty Acids in the Food Supply: A Comprehensive Report Covering 60 Years of Research*, 2d ed., Bethesda, MD: Enig Associates, Inc. 1995, p. 135.

57 Smith R and Pinckney ER. *Diet, Blood Cholesterol and Coronary Heart Disease: A Critical Review of the Literature*, vol 2. Sherman Oaks, CA: Vector Enterprises, 1991.

58 Kannel WB. Metabolic risk factors for coronary heart disease in women: perspective from the Framingham Study. *Am Heart J.* Aug 1987, 114(2):413–19.

59 Castelli W. Concerning the possibility of a nut... *Archives of Internal Medicine.* Jul 1992, 152(7):1371–72.

60 Multiple Risk Factor Intervention Trial: Risk factor changes and mortality results. *JAMA.* Sep 24, 1982, 248(12):1465.

61 Mattson FH. Effect of dietary cholesterol on serum cholesterol in men. *Am J Clin Nutr.* 1972, 25:589.

62 Addis P. *Food and Nutrition News.* Mar/Apr 1990, 62(2):7–10.

63 The Lipid Research Clinics Coronary Primary Prevention Trial results. I. Reduction in incidence of coronary heart disease. *JAMA.* 1984, 251:359.

64 Mary G. Enig, personal communication.

65 Anderson KM et al. Cholesterol and mortality: 30 years of follow-up from the Framingham Study. *JAMA.* Apr 24, 1987, 257(16):2176–80.

66 Grundy SM. Cholesterol and coronary heart disease: a new era. *JAMA.* Nov 28, 1986, 256(20):2849–58.

67 Mary G. Enig, personal communication.

68 Samuels SE. Project LEAN: a national campaign to reduce dietary fat consumption. *Am J Health Promot.* Jul–Aug 1990, 4(6):435–40.

69 Smith RL. *Diet, Blood Cholesterol and Coronary Heart Disease: A Critical Review of the Literature.* Santa Monica, CA: Vector Enterprises, Inc. 1988, pp. 9–21.

70 Ibid.

71 Laurie W et al. Atherosclerosis and its cerebral complications in the South African Bantu. *Lancet.* Feb 1958, 231–32.

72 Cohen A. Fats and carbohydrates as factors in atherosclerosis and diabetes in Yemenite Jews. *Heart J*, 1963, 65:291.

73 Malhotra SL. Epidemiology of ischaemic heart disease in India with special reference to causation. *Br Heart J.* Nov 1967, 29(6):895–905; Malhotra SL. Geographical aspects of acute myocardial infarction in India with special reference to patterns of diet and eating. *Br Heart J.* Mar 1967, 29(3):337–44.

74 Kang-Jey H et al. *Archeological Pathology.* 1971, 91:387; Mann GV et al. *Am J Epidemiol.* 1972, 95:26–37.

75 Price WA, *Nutrition and Physical Degeneration*. San Diego, CA: Price-Pottenger Nutrition Foundation, 1945, pp. 59–72.

76 Chen, Junshi. *Diet, Life-Style and Mortality in China: A Study of the Characteristics of 65 Chinese Counties*. Ithaca, NY: Cornell University Press, 1990.

77 Willett WC et al. *Am J Clin Nutr*. Jun 1995, 61(6S):1402S–6S; Perez-Llamas F et al. *J Hum Nutr Diet*. Dec 1996, 9(6):463–71; Alberti-Fidanza A et al. *Eur J Clin Nutr*. Feb 1994, 48(2):85–91.

78 Fernandez NA. *Cancer Res*, 1975, 35:3272; Martines I et al. *Cancer Res*. 1975, 35:3265.

79 Pitskhelauri GZ. *The Long Living of Soviet Georgia*, New York: Human Sciences Press, 1982. *In footnote:* [a] Wilcox B et al. *The Okinawa Program: How the World's Longest-Lived People Achieve Everlasting Health—And How You Can Too*. New York: Clarkson Potter, 2001; Wilcox B et al. *The Okinawa Diet Plan: Get Leaner, Live Longer and Never Feel Hungry*. New York: Clarkson Potter, 2003.

80 Franklyn D. *Health*. Sep 1996, pp. 57–63.

81 Koga Y et al. Recent trends in cardiovascular disease and risk factors in the Seven Countries Study: Japan. In H Toshima et al, eds. *Lessons for Science from the Seven Countries Study*. New York: Springer, 1994, pp. 63–74.

82 Moore TJ. *Lifespan: What Really Affects Human Longevity*. New York: Simon & Schuster, 1990.

83 O'Neill M. *New York Times*. Nov 17, 1991.

84 *European Cardiovascular Disease Statistics*, 2005 ed., http://www.heartstats.org/uploads/documents%5CPDF.pdf. Accessed Oct 13, 2015.

85 HNIS-USDA as compiled by Mary G. Enig.

86 Mary G. Enig, personal communication.

87 Enig, MG. The tragic legacy of CSPI. *Wise Traditions in Food, Farming and the Healing Arts*. Fall 2003.

88 AIN/ASCN Task Force on Trans Fatty Acids. Position paper on trans fatty acids. *Am J Clin Nutr*. 1996, 63:663–70.

89 Lemmon RM et al. The effect of delta-7-cholesterol feeding on the cholesterol and lipoproteins of rabbit serum. *Archives of Biochemistry & Biophysics*. Jul 1954, 51(1):1161–69; Kritchevsky F et al. Effect of cholesterol vehicle in experimental atherosclerosis. *Am J Physiol*. Jul–Sep 1954, 178:30–32.

90 Olson RE. Evolution of ideas about the nutritional value of dietary fat: introduction. *J Nutr*. 1998, 128:421S–25S.

91 http://www.acsh.org/publications.reports/surveysum2001.html. Accessed Oct 13, 2015.

92 http://www.foodnavigator-usa.com/R-D/Low-fat-is-too-simplistic-says-Tufts-professor. Accessed Jan 30, 2016.

93 http://www.sfgate.com/food/article/Eating-by-the-numbers-Getting-real-about-the-2698639.php. Accessed Jan 31, 2016.

94 http://www.nuval.com/. Accessed Jan 30, 2016.

95 http://calorielab.com/news/2008/01/28/food-ranking-system-to-hit-store-shelves/. Accessed Jan 30, 2016.

96 *Nutrition Week*, Aug 25, 2003.

97 *American Journal of Public Health*, Sep 2002.

98 http://tna.europarchive.org/20111116080332/http://www.food.gov.uk/news/pressreleases/2009/feb/launchsatfatcampaign. Accessed Oct 16, 2015.

99 http://www.stuff.co.nz/national/349682/Professor-calls-for-tax-on-poison-butter. Accessed Oct 16, 2015.

100 http://www.telegraph.co.uk/news/health/news/8267876/Statins-the-drug-firms-goldmine.html. Accessed Oct 16, 2015.

101 Diamond DM and Ravnskov U. How statistical deception created the appearance that statins are safe and effective in primary and secondary prevention of cardiovascular disease. *Expert Reviews in Clinical Pharmacology*. Mar 2015, 8(2):201–10.

102 Okuyama H et al. Statins stimulate atherosclerosis and heart failure: pharmacological mechanisms. *Expert Rev Clin Pharmacol*. Mar 2015, 8(2):189–99.

103 Evans D. *Statins Toxic Side Effects: Evidence from 500 Scientific Papers*. Grosvenor House Publishing Limited, 2015.

104 Ridker PM. Rosuvastatin to prevent vascular events in men and women with elevated C-reactive protein. *N Engl J Med.* 2008, 359:2195–207.
In footnote: [a] http://junkfoodscience.blogspot.com/2008/11/when-news-sounds-too-good-statins-new.html. Accessed Oct 13, 2015.

105 http://www.reuters.com/article/us-heart-statins-idUSTRE50C6QO20090113. Accessed Oct 13, 2015.

106 Yeon-Kyun Shin. Cholesterol, statins, and brain function: a hypothesis from a molecular perspective. *IBC.* 2009, 1:1–4.

107 Agalliu I et al. Statin use and risk of prostate cancer: results from a population-based epidemiologic study. *Am J Epidemiol.* Aug 1, 2008, 168(3):250–60.

108 http://www.bmj.com/content/318/7196/1471. Accessed Jan 30, 2016.

109 Nichols M et al. European cardiovascular disease statistics: British Heart Foundation Health Promotion Research Group. *European Heart Network and European Society of Cardiology.* Brussels, 2012.

110 http://www.webmd.com/cholesterol-management/side-effects-of-statin-drugs?page=2. Accessed Jul 10, 2016.

111 Culver AL et al. Statin use and risk of diabetes mellitus in postmenopausal women in the Women's Health Initiative. *Arch Intern Med.* Jan 23, 2012, 172(2):144–52.

112 Preiss D et al. Risk of incident diabetes with intensive-dose compared with moderate-dose statin therapy: a meta-analysis. *JAMA.* Jun 22, 2011, 305(24):2556–64.

113 Sattar N. Statins and risk of incident diabetes: a collaborative meta-analysis of randomised statin trials. *Lancet.* Feb 27, 2010, 375(9716):735–42.

114 http://www.news-medical.net/news/20120110/Statins-may-raise-type-2-diabetes-risk.aspx. Accessed Jan 30, 2016.

115 http://www.diabetes.org/newsroom/press-releases/2012/american-diabetes-association-statement-on-fda-statin-labels-changes.html. Accessed Jan 30, 2016.

Chapter 2: A Short Lesson on the Biochemistry of Fats

1 Kabara JJ. Fatty acids and derivatives as antimicrobial agents—a review. In JJ Kabara, ed. *The Pharmacological Effect of Lipids.* Champaign, IL: American Oil Chemists' Society, 1978; Kabara JJ. Inhibition of staphylococcus aureaus. In JJ Kabara, ed. *The Pharmacological Effect of Lipids II.* Champaign, IL: American Oil Chemists' Society, 1985, pp. 71–75.

2 Mensink RP. Effects of the individual saturated fatty acids on serum lipids and lipoprotein concentrations. *Am J Clin Nutr.* May 1993, 57(5 Suppl):711S–14S.

3 Kabara JJ. Fatty acids and derivatives as antimicrobial agents—a review. In JJ Kabara, ed. *The Pharmacological Effect of Lipids.* Champaign, IL: American Oil Chemists' Society, 1978; Kabara JJ. Inhibition of staphylococcus aureaus. In JJ Kabara, ed. *The Pharmacological Effect of Lipids II.* Champaign, IL: American Oil Chemists' Society, 1985, pp. 71–75.

4 http://www.westonaprice.org/health-topics/the-great-con-ola/. Accessed Jan 30, 2016.

5 http://www.ewg.org/research/ewg-s-dirty-dozen-guide-food-additives/generally-recognized-as-safe-but-is-it. Accessed Jan 30, 2016.

6 Cranton EM and Frackelton JP. Free radical pathology in age-associated diseases: treatment with EDTA chelation, nutrition and antioxidants. *Journal of Holistic Medicine.* Spring/Summer 1984, pp. 6–37.
In footnote: [a]Agarwal V et al. Examination stress: changes in serum cholesterol, triglycerides and total lipids. *Indian J Physiol Pharmacol.* Oct 1997, 41(4):404–8.

7 Engelberg H. Low serum cholesterol and suicide. *Lancet.* Mar 21, 1992, 339:727–28.

8 Kummerow FA. The relationship of oxidized lipids to coronary artery stenosis. *Atherosclerosis.* Mar 2000, 149(1):181–90; Kummerow FA. Changes in the phospholipid composition of the arterial cell can result in severe atherosclerotic lesions. *J Nutr Biochem.* Oct 2001, 12(10):602–7.

9 FD Sauer et al. Additional vitamin E required in milk replacer diets that contain canola oil. *Nutrition Research.* 1997, 17(2):259–69.

10 Trenholm et al. An evaluation of the relationship of dietary fatty acids to incidence of myocardial lesions in male rats. *Canadian Institute of Food Science Technology Journal.* Oct 1979, 12(4):189–93; Kramer JKG et al.

Reduction of myocardial necrosis in male albino rats by manipulation of dietary fatty acid levels. *Lipids.* 1982, 17(5):372–82.

11 O'Keefe S et al. Levels of trans geometrical isomers of essential fatty acids in some unhydrogenated US vegetable oils. *Journal of Food Lipids.* 1994, 1:165–76.

12 Kabara JJ et al. Fatty acids and derivatives as antimicrobial agents. *Antimicrob Agents Chemother.* Jul 1972, 2(1):23–28.

13 http://www.westonaprice.org/health-topics/interesterification/. Accessed Jan 30, 2016.

Chapter 3: Not Guilty as Charged

1 *The Baptist Ladies' Cook Book: Choice and Tested Recipes Contributed by the Ladies of Monmouth, Ill,* Jan 1, 1895.
In footnote: [a] http://www.oysterva.com/oyster-consumption.html, accessed October 20, 2015.

2 Stout C et al. Unusually low incidence of death from myocardial infarction: study of an Italian American community in Pennsylvania. *JAMA.* 1964, 188(10): 845–49.

3 Cassill K. Stress has hit Roseto, Pa., once the town heart disease passed by. *People,* Jun 16, 1980.

4 Egolf B et al. The Roseto Effect: a 50-year comparison of mortality rates. *American Journal of Public Health.* 1992, 82(8):1089–92.

5 Rose GA et al. Corn oil in treatment of ischaemic heart disease. *Br Med J.* Jun 12, 1965, 1(5449):1531–33.

6 http://my.americanheart.org/professional/Sessions/AdditionalMeetings/EmergingScienceSeries/2014-Emerging-Science-Series—July-24-2014_UCM_464850_Article.jsp. Accessed Oct 13, 2015.

7 http://www.health.harvard.edu/blog/the-type-of-fat-you-eat-matters-201509228333. Accessed Oct 16, 2015.

8 Howard BV et al. Low-fat dietary pattern and risk of cardiovascular disease: the Women's Health Initiative Randomized Controlled Dietary Modification Trial. *JAMA.* Feb 8, 2006, 295(6):655–66.

9 http://junkfoodscience.blogspot.com/2007/10/junkfood-science-exclusive-big-one.html. Accessed Oct 16, 2015.

10 Siri-Tarino PW et al. Meta-analysis of prospective cohort studies evaluating the association of saturated fat with cardiovascular disease. *Am J Clin Nutr.* Mar 2010, 91(3):535–46.

11 http://www.wsj.com/articles/SB10001424052748704314904575250570943835414. Accessed Oct 15, 2015.

12 Bonthuis M et al. Dairy consumption and patterns of mortality of Australian adults. *European Journal of Clinical Nutrition.* 2010, 64:569–77.

13 Warensjö E et al. Estimated intake of milk fat is negatively associated with cardiovascular risk factors and does not increase the risk of a first acute myocardial infarction: a prospective case-control study. *Br J Nutr.* Apr 2004, 91(4):635–42.

14 Mozaffarian D et al. Dietary fats, carbohydrate, and progression of coronary atherosclerosis in postmenopausal women. *Am J Clin Nutr.* Nov 2004, 80(5):1175–84.

15 Ransden CE et al. Use of dietary linoleic acid for secondary prevention of coronary heart disease and death: evaluation of recovered data from the Sydney Diet Heart Study and updated meta-analysis. *BMJ.* 2013, 346.

16 Chowdhury R et al. Association of dietary, circulating, and supplement fatty acids with coronary risk: a systematic review and meta-analysis. *Ann Intern Med.* 2014, 160(6):398–406.

17 http://well.blogs.nytimes.com/2014/03/17/study-questions-fat-and-heart-disease-link/?_r=0.

18 https://www.yahoo.com/news/trans-fats-not-saturated-fats-linked-risk-death-231047142.html?ref=gs. Accessed Jul 22, 2016.

19 Saturated fat is not the major issue. *BMJ.* 2013, 347:f6340.

20 http://www.theguardian.com/commentisfree/2013/oct/23/butter-bad-saturated-fat-healthy-eating-industry. Accessed Oct 16, 2015.

21 Siri-Tarino PW et al. Meta-analysis of prospective cohort studies evaluating the association of saturated fat with cardiovascular disease. *Am J Clin Nutr.* Mar 2010, 91(3):535–46.

22 https://www.youtube.com/watch?v=sGIGXfIDaJo. Accessed Oct 15, 2015.

23 https://www.youtube.com/watch?v=X6AkgoY3KEs. Accessed Oct 15, 2015.

24 http://www.sciencenordic.com/low-carb-diets-hold-sway-short-term. Accessed Oct 15, 2015.

25 *American Journal of Cardiology.* 1997, 79:350–54.

26 Agatston A. *The South Beach Diet.* Emmaus, PA: Rodale, 2003.

27 Nicholls SJ et al. Consumption of saturated fat impairs the anti-inflammatory properties of high-density lipoproteins and endothelial function. *J Am Coll Cardiol.* Aug 15, 2006, 48(4):715–20.

28 http://www.nbcnews.com/id/14229538/ns/health-diet_and_nutrition/t/just-one-high-fat-meal-can-be-bad-arteries/#.Vjv_nLPIoro. Accessed Oct 15, 2015.

29 Berstad P et al. Dietary fat and plasma total homocysteine concentrations in 2 adult age groups: the Hordaland Homocysteine Study. *Am J Clin Nutr.* Jun 2007, 85(6):1598–605.

30 Favid MS et al. Dietary linoleic acid and risk of coronary heart disease: a systematic review and meta-analysis of prospective cohort studies. *Circulation.* Oct 28, 2014, 130(18):1568–78.

31 Sinha R et al. Meat intake and mortality: a prospective study of over half a million people. *Arch Intern Med.* Mar 23, 2009, 169(6):562–71.

32 http://www.washingtonpost.com/wp-dyn/content/article/2009/03/23/AR2009032301626.html. Accessed Jan 31, 2016.

33 http://blog.cholesterol-and-health.com/search?q=There+is+absolutely+no+scientific+basis+to+conclude+from+this+study+that+eating+meat+increases+mortality. Accessed Jan 31, 2016.

34 Sacks FM et al. A dietary approach to prevent hypertension: a review of the Dietary Approaches to Stop Hypertension (DASH) Study. *Clin Cardiol.* Jul 1999, 22(7 Suppl):III6-10.

35 http://blood-pressure.emedtv.com/high-blood-pressure/fats-and-high-blood-pressure.html. Accessed Jul 23, 2016.

36 Cutler JA et al. Coronary heart disease and all-causes mortality in the Multiple Risk Factor Intervention Trial: subgroup findings and comparisons with other trials. *Prev Med.* May 1985, 14(3):293–311.

37 http://blog.heart.org/new-heart-disease-and-stroke-prevention-guidelines-released/. Accessed Jan 31, 2016.

38 Fitchett DH et al. Ischemic stroke: a cardiovascular risk equivalent? Lessons learned from the Stroke Prevention by Aggressive Reduction in Cholesterol Levels (SPARCL) trial. *Can J Cardiol.* Sep 24, 2008, 9:705–8.

39 Kazumasa Y and other. Dietary intake of saturated fatty acids and mortality from cardiovascular disease in Japanese: the Japan Collaborative Cohort Study for Evaluation of Cancer Risk (JACC) Study. *Am J Clin Nutr.* Oct 2010, 92(4):759–65.

40 Kagan A et al. Dietary and other risk factors for stroke in Hawaiian Japanese men. *Stroke.* May–Jun 1985, 16(3):390–96.

41 Gillman MW et al. Inverse association of dietary fat with development of ischemic stroke in men. *JAMA.* Dec 24–31, 1997, 278(24):2145–50.

42 http://www.cholesterol-and-health.com/High-Cholesterol-Causes-Stroke.html. Accessed Oct 15, 2015.

43 http://www.diabetes.org/food-and-fitness/food/what-can-i-eat/making-healthy-food-choices/fats-and-diabetes.html. Accessed Oct 15, 2015.

44 Robertson MD et al. Acute effects of meal fatty acid composition on insulin sensitivity in healthy post-menopausal women. *Br J Nutr.* Dec 2002, 88(6):635–40.

45 Ummers LK et al. Substituting dietary saturated fat with polyunsaturated fat changes abdominal fat distribution and improves insulin sensitivity. *Diabetologia.* Mar 2002, 45(3):369–77.

46 Wang LI et al. Plasma fatty acid composition and incidence of diabetes in middle-aged adults: the Atherosclerosis Risk in Communities (ARIC) Study. *Am J Clin Nutr.* Jul 2003, 78(1):91–98.

47 Hu FB et al. Diet lifestyle and the risk of type 2 diabetes mellitus in women. *NEJM.* 2001, 345: 790–97; *A J Clin Nutr.* Jun 2001, 73:1001–2, 1019–20.

48 http://www.webmd.com/diabetes/news/20140916/high-fat-dairy-diabetes. Accessed Jan 4, 2016.

49 http://www.cancer.org/healthy/eathealthygetactive/acsguidelinesonnutritionphysicalactivityforcancerprevention/acs-guidelines-on-nutrition-and-physical-activity-for-cancer-prevention-guidelines. Accessed Jan 4, 2015.

In footnote: [a] http://www.cancer.org/healthy/eathealthygetactive/acsguidelinesonnutritionphysicalactivityforcancerprevention/acs-guidelines-on-nutrition-and-physical-activity-for-cancer-prevention-guidelines. Accessed January 4, 2015.

50 Hope J. Fatty diet link to breast cancer. Dailymail.com, http://www.dailymail.co.uk/health/article-189048/Fatty-diet-link-breast-cancer.html.

51 Holmes MD et al. Meat, fish and egg intake and risk of breast cancer. *Int J Cancer.* Mar 20, 2003, 104(2):221–27.

52 Hunter DJ et al. Cohort studies of fat intake and the risk of breast cancer—a pooled analysis. *N Engl J Med.* Feb 8 1996, 334(6):356–61.

53 Hanf V and Gonder U. Nutrition and primary prevention of breast cancer: foods, nutrients and breast cancer risk. *Eur J Obstet Gynecol Reprod Biol.* Dec 1, 2005, 123(2):139–49; Lof M and Weiderpass E. Impact of diet on breast cancer risk. *Current Opinion in Obstetrics and Gynecology.* 21(1):80–88; Freedman LS et al. Methods of epidemiology: evaluating the fat–breast cancer hypothesis—comparing dietary instruments and other developments. *Cancer Journal.* Mar-Apr 2008, 14(2):69–74.

54 Howard BN et al. Low-fat dietary pattern and risk of cardiovascular disease: the Women's Health Initiative Randomized Controlled Dietary Modification Trial. *JAMA.* 2006, 295(6):655–66.

55 Thiebaut AC et al. Dietary fat and postmenopausal invasive breast cancer in the National Institutes of Health–AARP Diet and Health Study cohort. *J Natl Cancer Inst.* 2007, 99(6):451–62.

56 Wynder EL and Reddy BS. Editorial: Dietary fat and colon cancer. *J Natl Cancer Inst.* Jan 1975, 54(1):7–10.

57 Haenszel W et al. Large-bowel cancer in Hawaiian Japanese. *J Natl Cancer Inst.* Dec 1973, 51(6):1765–79.

58 Willett WC et al. Relation of meat, fat, and fiber intake to the risk of colon cancer in a prospective study among women. *N Engl J Med.* Dec 13, 1990, 323(24):1664–72; Giovannucci E et al. Intake of fat, meat, and fiber in relation to risk of colon cancer in men. *Cancer Res.* May 1, 1994, 54(9):2390–97.

59 Cox BD and Whichelow MJ. Frequent consumption of red meat is not risk factor for cancer. *BMJ.* Oct 18, 1997, 315(7114):1018.

60 Phillips RL. Role of life-style and dietary habits in risk of cancer among Seventh-day Adventists. *Cancer Res.* Nov 1975, 35(11, Pt. 2):3513–22.

61 Harras A, ed. *Cancer Rates and Risks*, 4th ed. National Institutes of Health, National Cancer Institute, 1996.

62 Franceschi S et al. Food groups and risk of colorectal cancer in Italy. *Int J Cancer.* Jul 3, 1997, 72(1):56–61.

63 Graham S et al. Diet in the epidemiology of cancer of the colon and rectum. *J Natl Cancer Inst.* Sep 1978, 61(3):709–14.

64 Merrill AH and Schroeder JJ. Lipid modulation of cell function. *Annu Rev Nutr.* 1993, 13:539–59.

65 Alexander DD et al. A review and meta-analysis of prospective studies of red and processed meat intake and prostate cancer. *Nutr J.* Nov 2, 2010, 9:50.

66 Key TJ. Fruit and vegetables and cancer risk. *Br J Cancer.* Jan 4, 2011, 104(1):6–11.

67 Zhang S et al. Dietary fat and protein in relation to risk of non-Hodgkin's lymphoma among women. *J Natl Cancer Inst.* Oct 20, 1999, 91(20):1751–58.

68 http://cancerres.aacrjournals.org/cgi/content/meeting_abstract/73/8_MeetingAbstracts/148.

69 http://usatoday30.usatoday.com/news/health/2002-11-18-adkins_x.htm. Accessed Jan 4, 2016.

70 *Washington Post*, Oct 29, 2002.

71 The results are posted at http://eatfatlosefat.com/research.php. Accessed Jan 31, 2016.

72 Boden G et al. Effect of a low-carbohydrate diet on appetite, blood glucose levels, and insulin resistance in obese patients with type 2 diabetes. *Ann Intern Med.* Mar 15, 2005, 142(6):403–11.

73 Foster GD et al. Weight and metabolic outcomes after 2 years on a low-carbohydrate versus low-fat diet: a randomized trial. *Ann Intern Med.* 2010, 153(3):147–57.

74 Dhurandhar NV et al. Egg breakfast enhances weight loss. *FASEB Journal.* 2007, 21:538.1.

75 Gardner, CD et al. Comparison of the Atkins, Zone, Ornish, and LEARN diets for change in weight and related risk factors among overweight premenopausal women: the A TO Z Weight Loss Study: a randomized trial. *JAMA.* Mar 7, 2007, 297(9):969–77.

76 http://www.cbsnews.com/news/atkins-study-surprises-doctors/. Accessed Jan 4, 2016.

77 http://www.cbsnews.com/news/atkins-wins-diet-plan-faceoff/; http://www.insidebayarea.com/timesstar/ci_5373373. Accessed Jan 4, 2016.

78 Rosell M et al. Association between dairy food consumption and weight change over 9 y in 19,352 perimenopausal women. *Am J Clin Nutr.* Dec 2006, 84(6):1481–88.

79 Shai I et al. Weight loss with a low-carbohydrate, Mediterranean, or low-fat diet. *N Engl J Med.* 2008, 359:229–41.

80 http://www.reuters.com/article/us-diets-idUSN1642545620080716. Accessed Jan 6, 2016.

81 http://consumer.healthday.com/cardiovascular-and-health-information-20/dieting-to-control-cholesterol-health-news-190/diet-plans-produce-similar-results-617520.html. Accessed Jan 6, 2016.

82 http://www.nytimes.com/2008/07/17/health/nutrition/17diets.html?_r=0. Accessed Jan 6, 2016. *In footnote:* [a] Kavanagh K et al. Trans fat diet induces abdominal obesity and changes in insulin sensitivity in monkeys. *Obesity.* Jul 2007, 15(7):1675–84.

83 McDevitt RM et al. De novo lipogenesis during controlled overfeeding with sucrose or glucose in lean and obese women. *Am J Clin Nutr.* Dec 2001, 74:737–46.

84 Han SN et al. Effect of hydrogenated and saturated, relative to polyunsaturated, fat on immune and inflammatory responses of adults with moderate hypercholesterolemia. *J Lipid Res.* Mar 2002, 43(3):445–52.

85 Wijga AH et al. Association of consumption of products containing milk fat with reduced asthma risk in pre-school children: the PIAMA birth cohort study. *Thorax.* Jul 2003, 58(7):567–72.

86 Zhang SM et al. Dietary fat in relation to risk of multiple sclerosis among two large cohorts of women. *Am J Epidemiol.* Dec 1, 2000, 152(11):1056–64.

87 Magaro M et al. Influence of diet with different lipid composition on neutrophil chemiluminescence and disease activity in patients with rheumatoid arthritis. *Ann Rheum Dis.* Oct 1988, 47(10):793–96.

88 Effects of manipulation of dietary fatty acids on clinical manifestations of rheumatoid arthritis. Kremer JM et al. *Lancet.* Jan 26, 1985, 1(8422):184–87.

89 Young C. New ad links meat-eating and impotence release, Feb 9, 2004, http://forum.lowcarber.org/archive/index.php/t-167095.html.

90 Halkin A et al. HMG-CoA reductase inhibitor-induced impotence. *Ann Pharmacother.* Feb 1996, 30(2):192.

91 http://www.dailymail.co.uk/health/article-2258336/Eating-fatty-diet-reduce-mans-sperm-count-40.html. Accessed Jan 31, 2016.

92 Jensen TK et al. High dietary intake of saturated fat is associated with reduced semen quality among 701 young Danish men from the general population. *Am J Clin Nutr.* Feb 2013, 97(2):411–18.

93 http://www.zoeharcombe.com/2013/01/high-intake-of-saturated-fat-sperm-quality-in-danish-men/. Accessed Jan 31, 2016.

94 Lindqvist A et al. High-fat diet impairs hippocampal neurogenesis in male rats. *Eur J Neurol.* Dec 2006, 13(12):1385–88.

95 http://www.dailymail.co.uk/health/article-434653/Diet-high-cholesterol-trigger-onset-Alzheimers-warn-scientists.html. Accessed Jan 31, 2016.

96 Stewart R et al. Twenty-six-year change in total cholesterol levels and incident dementia: the Honolulu-Asia Aging Study. *Arch Neurol.* Jan 2007, 64(1):103–7.

97 http://www.livescience.com/5635-high-fat-diet-stupid-lazy.html. Accessed Jan 6, 2016.

98 Murray AJ. et al. Deterioration of physical performance and cognitive function in rats with short-term high-fat feeding. *FASEB Journal.* Dec 2009, 23(12):4353–60.

99 http://journals.plos.org/plosone/article?id%3D10.1371/journal.pone.0018604. Accessed Jan 5, 2016.

Chapter 4: The Many Roles of Saturated Fat

1 Elson CE et al. The influence of dietary unsaturated cis and trans and saturated fatty acids on the tissue lipids of swine. *Atherosclerosis.* 1981, 40:115–37.

2 Berg JM, Tymoczko JL, and Stryer L. *Biochemistry.* 5th ed. New York: W. H. Freeman, 2002. http://www.ncbi.nlm.nih.gov/books/NBK22554/#_A3097_.

3 Busconi L and Denker BM. Analysis of the N-terminal binding domain of Go alpha. *Biochem J.* Nov 15, 1997, 328(Pt 1):23–31.

4 Rioux V et al. Dietary myristic acid at physiologically relevant levels increases the tissue content of C20:5 n-3 and C20:3 n-6 in the rat. *Reprod Nutr Dev.* Sep–Oct 2005, 45(5):599–612.

5 http://www.westonaprice.org/know-your-fats/the-importance-of-saturated-fats-for-biological-functions/. Accessed Jul 13, 2016.

6 Nicolosi RJ. Dietary fat saturation effects on low-density-lipoprotein concentrations and metabolism in various animal models. *Am J Clin Nutr.* May 1997, 65(5 Suppl):1617S–27S.

7 http://www.sciencedaily.com/releases/2015/07/150728101220.htm. Accessed Jan 6, 2016.

8 Suárez A et al. Dietary long-chain polyunsaturated fatty acids modify heart, kidney, and lung fatty acid composition in weanling rats. *Lipids.* Mar 1996, 31(3):345–48; Taugbøl O and Saarem K. Fatty acid composition of porcine muscle and adipose tissue lipids as affected by anatomical location and cod liver oil supplementation of the diet. *Acta Vet Scand.* 1995, 36(1):93–101.

9 Gurr M. A fresh look at dietary recommendations. *Inform*, Apr 1996, 7:4:432–35.

10 Stein JH and Rosenson RS. Lipoprotein Lp(a) excess and coronary heart disease. *Arch Intern Med.* Jun 9, 1997, 157(11):1170–76.

11 Marcovina SM et al. Fish intake, independent of apo(a) size, accounts for lower plasma lipoprotein(a) levels in Bantu fishermen of Tanzania: the Lugalawa Study. *Arterioscler Thromb Vasc Biol.* May 1995, 19(5):1250–56.

12 Dahlén GH et al. The importance of serum lipoprotein (a) as an independent risk factor for premature coronary artery disease in middle-aged black and white women from the United States. *J Intern Med.* Nov 1998, 244(5):417–24; Khosla P and Hayes KC. Dietary trans-monounsaturated fatty acids negatively impact plasma lipids in humans: critical review of the evidence. *J Am Coll Nutr.* Aug 1996, 15(4):325–39; Clevidence BA et al. Plasma lipoprotein (a) levels in men and women consuming diets enriched in saturated, cis-, or trans-monounsaturated fatty acids. *Arterioscler Thromb Vasc Biol.* Sep 1997, 17(9):1657–61.

13 Lawson LD and Kummerow FA. Beta-oxidation of the coenzyme A esters of vaccenic, elaidic, and petroselaidic acids by rat heart mitochondria. *Lipids.* May 1979, 14(5):501–3; Garg ML et al. Dietary saturated fat level alters the competition between alpha-linolenic and linoleic acid. *Lipids.* Apr 1989, 24(4):334–39.

14 Felton CV et al. Dietary polyunsaturated fatty acids and composition of human aortic plaques. *Lancet.* Oct 29, 1994, 344(8931):1195–96.

15 Chatterjee TK et al. Pro-inflammatory phenotype of perivascular adipocytes: influence of high-fat feeding. *Circ Res.* Feb 27, 2009, 104(4):541–49.

16 Rudel LL et al. Dietary monounsaturated fatty acids promote aortic atherosclerosis in LDL-receptor-null, human ApoB100-overexpressing transgenic mice. *Arteriosclerosis, Thrombosis and Vascular Biology.* Nov 1998, 18(11):1818–27.

17 http://www.westonaprice.org/know-your-fats/the-importance-of-saturated-fats-for-biological-functions/. Accessed Feb 2, 2016.

18 Watkins BA. Importance of vitamin E in bone formation and in chrondrocyte function. *AOCS Proceedings.* Lafayette, IN: Purdue University, 1996; Watkins BA and Seifert MF. Food lipids and bone health. In RE McDonald and DB Min, eds. *Food Lipids and Health.* New York: Marcel Dekker, Inc., p. 101.

19 Nanji AA et al. *Gastroenterology.* Aug 1995, 109(2):547–54; Cha YS and Sachan, *J Am Coll Nutr*, Aug 1994, 13(4):338–43; Hargrove HL et al. *FASEB Journal.* Meeting Abstracts, Mar 1999, no. 204.1, p. A222.

20 Ronis MJ et al. Dietary saturated fat reduces alcoholic hepatotoxicity in rats by altering fatty acid metabolism and membrane composition. *J Nutr.* Apr 2004, 134(4):904–12.

21 Wang D et al. Saturated fatty acids promote endoplasmic reticulum stress and liver injury in rats with hepatic steatosis. *Endocrinology.* Feb 2006, 147(2):943–51.

22 Kabara JJ, ed. *The Pharmacological Effects of Lipids.* Champaign, IL: The American Oil Chemists' Society, 1978, pp. 1–14; Cohen LA et al. Dietary fat and mammary cancer. II. Modulation of serum and tumor lipid composition and tumor prostaglandins by different dietary fats: association with tumor incidence patterns. *J Natl Cancer Inst.* Jul 1986, 77(1):43–51.

23 Gerster H. Can adults adequately convert alpha-linolenic acid (18:3n-3) to eicosapentaenoic acid (20:5n-3) and docosahexaenoic acid (22:6n-3)? *International Journal of Vitamin and Nutrition Research.* 1998, 68(3):159–73.

24 Garg ML et al. *FASEB Journal.* 1988, 2(4)A852; Oliart Ros RM. Meeting abstracts. *AOCS Proceedings*, Chicago. May 1998, 7.

25 Kabara JJ. Fatty acids and derivatives as antimicrobial agents—a review. In JJ Kabara, ed. *The Pharmacological Effect of Lipids.* Champaign, IL: American Oil Chemists' Society, 1978.

26 Hämäläinen E et al. Diet and serum sex hormones in healthy men. *J Steroid Biochem.* Jan 1984, 20(1): 459–64.

27 Goldin BR et al. The relationship between estrogen levels and diets of Caucasian American and Oriental immigrant women. *Am J Clin Nutr.* Dec 1986, 44(6):945–53.

28 http://www.westonaprice.org/know-your-fats/saturated-fats-and-the-lungs/; Mary G. Enig, personal communication.

29 Von Ehrenstein OS et al. Reduced hay fever and asthma among children of farmers. *Clin Exp Allergy.* 2000, 30:187–93; Von Mutius E et al. Increasing prevalence of hay fever and atopy among children in Leipzig, East Germany. *Lancet.* 1998, 351:862–66; Haby MM et al. Asthma in preschool children: prevalence and risk factors. *Thorax.* 2001, 56:589–95; Bolte G et al. Margarine consumption and allergy in children. *Am J Respir Crit Care Med.* 2001, 163:277–79; Dunder T et al. Diet, serum fatty acids and atopic disease in childhood. *Allergy.* 2001, 56:425–28; Fogarty A and Britton J. The role of diet in the aetiology of asthma. *Clin Exp Allergy.* 2000, 30:615–27; Hodge L et al. Increased consumption of polyunsaturated oil may be a cause of increased prevalence of childhood asthma. *Aust NZ J Med.* 1994, 24:727; Black PN and Sharpe S. Dietary fat and asthma: is there a connection? *Eur Respir J.* Jan 1997, 10(1):6–12.

30 Cranton EM and Frackelton JP. Free radical pathology in age-associated diseases: treatment with EDTA chelation, nutrition and antioxidants. *Journal of Holistic Medicine.* Spring/Summer 1984, pp. 6–37.

31 Alfin-Slater RB and Aftergood. Lipids. In RS Goodhart and ME Shils, eds. *Modern Nutrition in Health and Disease*, 6th ed. Philadelphia: Lea and Febiger, 1980, p. 134.

32 http://www.westonaprice.org/modern-diseases/the-benefits-of-high-cholesterol/. Accessed Feb 2, 2016.

33 Engelberg, H. *Lancet.* Mar 21, 1992, 339:727–28; Wood, WG et al. *Lipids.* Mar 1999, 34(3):225–34.

34 Hamosh M. Digestion in the newborn. *Clin Perinatol.* Jun 1996, 23(2):191–209.

35 http://www.sciencedaily.com/releases/2012/03/120326113713.htm. Accessed Jan 8, 2016.

36 Inbar M and Shinitzky M. Cholesterol as a bioregulator in the development and inhibition of leukemia. *Proc Natl Acad Sci USA.* Oct 1974, 71(10):4229–31.

37 http://www.sciencedaily.com/releases/2005/03/050309144856.htm. Accessed Jan 8, 2016.

38 http://www.westonaprice.org/modern-diseases/the-benefits-of-high-cholesterol/. Accessed Feb 2, 2016.

39 Yackinous C and Guinard JX. Relation between PROP taster status and fat perception, touch, and olfaction. *Physiol Behav.* Feb 2001, 72(3):427–37.

40 http://www.sciencedaily.com/releases/2004/01/040121075702.htm. Accessed Jan 7, 2016; Ajuwon KM and Spurlock ME. Direct regulation of lipolysis by interleukin-15 in primary pig adipocytes. *Am J Physiol Regul Integr Comp Physiol.* Sep 2004, 287(3):R608–11.

Chapter 5: AA and DHA

1 Sears B. *The Zone: A Dietary Road Map.* New York: HarperCollins, 1995.

2 http://www1.cbn.com/700club/understanding-aa-arachidonic-acid-omega-6-%E2%80%93-pro-inflammatory-fat. Accessed Jan 10, 2016.

3 Burr GO and Burr MM. A new deficiency disease produced by the rigid exclusion of fat from the diet. *J Biol Chem.* 1929, 82(2):345–67; Turpeinen O. Further studies on the unsaturated fatty acids essential in nutrition. *J Nutr.* 1938, 15(4):351–66.

4 Newberry RD et al. Cyclooxygenase-2-dependent arachidonic acid metabolites are essential modulators of the intestinal immune response to dietary antigen. *Nat Med.* 1999, 5(8):900–6; D'Arienzo R et al. A deregulated

immune response to gliadin causes a decreased villus height in DQ8 transgenic mice. *Eur J Immunol.* 2009, 39(12):3552–61.

5 Chan MM and Moore AR. Resolution of inflammation in murine autoimmune arthritis is disrupted by cyclooxygenase-2 inhibition and restored by prostaglandin E2-mediated lipoxin A4 production. *J Immunol.* 2010, 184(11):6418–26.

6 http://www.answers.com/Q/Could_you_list_Arachidonic_acid_in_foods; Mann NJ et al. Arachidonic acid content of the Australian diet is lower than previously estimated. *J Nutr.* 1995, 125:2528–35.

7 Borkman et al. The relation between insulin sensitivity and the fatty-acid composition of skeletal-muscle phospholipids. *New Engl J Med.* 1993, 328(4):238–44.

8 Agrawal R and Daniel EE. Control of gap junction formation in canine trachea by arachidonic acid metabolites. *Am J Physiol.* Mar 1986, 250(3, Pt 1):C495–505; Civitelli R et al. Regulation of connexin43 expression and function by prostaglandin E2 (PGE2) and parathyroid hormone (PTH) in osteoblastic cells. *J Cell Biochem.* Jan 1 1998, 68(1):8–21; Blikslager AT et al. Prostaglandins I2 and E2 have a synergistic role in rescuing epithelial barrier function in porcine ileum. *J Clin Invest.* Oct 15, 1997, 100(8):1928–33.

9 du Pre MF and Samson JN. Adaptive T-cell responses regulating oral tolerance to protein antigen. *Allergy.* 2011, 66(4):478–90.

10 Chan MM and Moore AR. Resolution of inflammation in murine autoimmune arthritis is disrupted by cyclooxygenase-2 inhibition and restored by prostaglandin E2-mediated lipoxin A4 production. *J Immunol.* 2010, 184(11):6418–26; Banneberg G and Serhan CN. Specialized pro-resolving lipid mediators in the inflammatory response: an update. *Biochim Biopys Acta.* 2010, 1801(12):1260–73.

11 Crawford MA and Sinclair AJ. Nutritional influences in the evolution of mammalian brain, in *Lipids, Malnutrition & the Developing Brain.* Ciba Foundation symposium. 1971, pp. 267–92.

12 Fukaya T et al. Arachidonic acid preserves hippocampal neuron membrane fluidity in senescent rats. *Neurobiology of Aging.* 2007, 28(8):1179–86.

13 Wang ZJ et al. Neuroprotective effects of arachidonic acid against oxidative stress on rat hippocampal slices. *Chemico-biological interactions.* 2006, 163(3):207–17.

14 Darios F and Davletov B. Omega-3 and omega-6 fatty acids stimulate cell membrane expansion by acting on syntaxin 3. *Nature.* 2006, 440(7085):813–17.

15 Ormes J. Effects of arachidonic acid supplementation on skeletal muscle mass, strength, and power. *NSCA ePoster Gallery.* National Strength and Conditioning Association.

16 Roberts MD et al. Effects of arachidonic acid supplementation on skeletal muscle mass, strength, and power. *Journal of the International Society of Sports Nutrition.* 4:21.
In footnote: [a] http://www.westonaprice.org/health-topics/splendid-specimens-the-history-of-nutrition-in-bodybuilding/. Accessed February 2, 2016.

17 Chowdury R et al. Association of dietary, circulating, and supplement fatty acids with coronary risk: a systematic review and meta-analysis. *Annals of Internal Medicine.* 2014, 160(6):398–406.

18 http://www.westonaprice.org/know-your-fats/precious-yet-perilous/. Accessed Feb 2, 2016.

19 http://www.westonaprice.org/know-your-fats/tripping-lightly-down-the-prostaglandin-pathways/. Accessed Feb 2, 2016.

20 Brenna JT et al. Docosahexaenoic and arachidonic acid concentrations in human breast milk worldwide. *Am J Clin Nutr.* Jun 2007, 85(6):1457–64.

21 Stonehouse W. Does consumption of LC omega-3 PUFA enhance cognitive performance in healthy school-aged children and throughout adulthood? Evidence from clinical trials. *Nutrients.* Jul 22, 2014 6(7):2730–58.

22 Lukiw WJ et al. A role for docosahexaenoic acid-derived neuroprotectin D_1 in neural cell survival and Alzheimer disease. *J Clin Invest.* 2005, 115(10): 2774–83.

23 McNamara RK et al. Selective deficits in the omega-3 fatty acid docosahexaenoic acid in the postmortem orbitofrontal cortex of patients with major depressive disorder. *Biol. Psychiatry.* 2007, 62(1):17; McNamara RK et al. Lower docosahexaenoic acid concentrations in the postmortem prefrontal cortex of adult depressed suicide victims compared with controls without cardiovascular disease. *Journal of Psychiatric Research.* 2013, 47 (9):1187–91.

24 Dietary DHA linked to male fertility. University of Illinois College of Agricultural, Consumer and Environmental Sciences, Jan 18, 2012.

25 http://www.westonaprice.org/know-your-fats/precious-yet-perilous/. Accessed Feb 2, 2016.

26 Serhan CN. Novel omega-3-derived local mediators in anti-inflammation and resolution. *Pharmacol Ther.* Jan 2005, 105(1):7–21.

27 Sanders TA. DHA status of vegetarians. *Prostaglandins Leukot Essent Fatty Acids.* Aug–Sep 2009, 81(2–3):137–41.

28 Gibney MJ and Hunter B. The effects of short- and long-term supplementation with fish oil on the incorporation of n-3 polyunsaturated fatty acids into cells of the immune system in healthy volunteers. *Eur J Clin Nutr.* Apr 1993, 47(4):255–59.

29 Nakamura MT and Nara TY. Structure, function, and dietary regulation of delta6, delta5, and delta9 desaturases. *Annu Rev Nutr.* 2004, 24:345–76.

30 http://www.westonaprice.org/know-your-fats/tripping-lightly-down-the-prostaglandin-pathways/. Accessed Feb 2, 2016.

31 http://in.reuters.com/article/us-health-pufas-epidemiology-idINKBN0P52BN20150625. Accessed Feb 2, 2016.

32 Jones, John. Nutritional Products from Space Research. May 1, 2001. NASA.

33 http://www.cornucopia.org/dha-safety-concerns/. Accessed Feb 2, 2016.

34 http://cornucopia.org/DHA/DHA_QuestionsAnswers.pdf. Accessed Feb 2, 2016.

35 Valenzuela A et al. Tissue accretion and milk content of docosahexaenoic acid in female rats after supplementation with different docosahexaenoic acid sources. *Ann Nutr Metab.* Sep–Oct 2005, 49(5):325–32.

36 http://cornucopia.org/DHA/DHA_QuestionsAnswers.pdf. Accessed Feb 2, 2016.

Chapter 6: Remember the Activators!: The Fat-Soluble Vitamins A, D and K_2

1 Price, WA. *Nutrition and Physical Degeneration.* San Diego, CA: Price-Pottenger Nutrition Foundation, 1945, p. 280.

2 The history outlined here was expertly compiled by G Wolf in: A history of vitamin A and retinoids. *FASEB Journal.* Jul 1996, 10:1102–7.

3 Gerson M, MD. *A Cancer Therapy: Results of Fifty Cases.* Del Mar, CA: Totality Books, 1958.

4 Griffin, GE. *World Without Cancer.* Westlake Village, CA: American Media, 1974, pp. 462–63.

5 Solomons NW and Bulus J. Plant sources of provitamin A and human nutriture. *Nutrition Review.* New York: Springer-Verlag, Jul 1993, 51:1992–94.

6 Jennings IW. *Vitamins in Endocrine Metabolism.* Springfield, IL: Charles C Thomas Publisher, 1970.

7 Dunne LJ. *Nutrition Almanac,* 3d ed. New York: McGraw-Hill Publishing Company, 1990.

8 Olson JA. Absorption, transport, and metabolism of carotenoids in humans. *Pure & Appl. Chem.* 1994, 66(5):1011–16.

9 Crawford M and Marsh D. *Nutrition and Evolution.* New Canaan, CT: Keats Publishing, 1995.
In footnote: [a] http://www.smithsonianmag.com/arts-culture/a-wwii-propaganda-campaign-popularized-the-myth-that-carrots-help-you-see-in-the-dark-28812484/?no-ist.

10 Burri BJ. New clues about carotenes revealed. *Ag Research Magazine.* USDA, Mar 2001.

11 Hickenbottom SJ et al. Variability in conversion of beta-carotene to vitamin A in men as measured by using a double-tracer study design. *Am J Clin Nutr.* May 2002, 75(5):900–7.

12 http://www.sciencedaily.com/releases/2009/11/091118072051.htm. Accessed Jan 11, 2016.

13 Eroglu A et al. Naturally occurring eccentric cleavage products of provitamin A β-carotene function as antagonists of retinoic acid receptors. *J Biol Chem.* May 4, 2012, 287(19):15886–95.

14 The effect of vitamin E and beta carotene on the incidence of lung cancer and other cancers in male smokers: the Alpha-Tocopherol, Beta Carotene Cancer Prevention Study Group. *N Engl J Med.* Apr 14, 1994, 330(15):1029–35.

15 http://researchnews.osu.edu/archive/betacarotene.htm. Accessed Feb 2, 2016.

16 Jayaram M et al. Effect of vitamin A deprivation on the cholesterol side-chain cleavage enzyme activity of testes and ovaries of rats. *Biochem J.* Sep 1973, 136(1); Junekja HS et al. The effect of vitamin A deficiency on the biosynthesis of steroid hormones in rats. *Biochem J.* Apr 1966, 99(1): 138–45.

17 Zadik et al. Vitamin A and iron supplementation is as efficient as hormonal therapy in constitutionally delayed children. *Clin Endocrinol* (Oxford). Jun 2004, 60(6):682–87.

18 Nakano K and Mizutani R. Decreased responsiveness of pituitary-adrenal axis to stress in vitamin A-depleted rats. *J Nutr Sci Vitaminol* (Tokyo). Jun 1983, 29(3):353–63; Marissal-Arvy N et al. Vitamin A regulates hypothalamic-pituitary-adrenal axis status in LOU/C rats. *J Endocrinol.* Sep 6, 2013, 219(1):21–27.

19 Jennings IW. *Vitamins in Endocrine Metabolism*. Springfield, IL: Charles C Thomas Publisher, 1970.

20 Ibid.

21 Meerza D et al. Retinoids have therapeutic action in type 2 diabetes. *Nutrition.* Jul-Aug 2106, 32(7–8):898–903; Iqbal S and Naseem I. Role of vitamin A in type 2 diabetes mellitus biology: effects of intervention therapy in a deficient state. *Nutrition.* Jul–Aug 2015, 31(7–8):901–7.

22 Price, WA. *Nutrition and Physical Degeneration*. San Diego, CA: Price-Pottenger Nutrition Foundation, 1945.

23 Mohanram M et al. Hematological studies in vitamin A deficient children. *Int J Vitam Nutr Res.* 1977, 47(4):389–93.

24 Solomons NW and Bulus J. Plant sources of provitamin A and human nutriture. *Nutrition Review*, New York: Springer-Verlag, Jul 1993, 51:1992–94.

25 Rutstein S. Effects of preceding birth intervals on neonatal, infant and under-five years mortality and nutritional status in developing countries: evidence from the demographic and health surveys. *Int J Gynaecol Obstet.* Apr 2005, 89(Suppl 1):S7-24.

26 Furusho et al. Tissue specific-distribution and metabolism of vitamin A are affected by dietary protein levels in rats. *Int J Vitam Nutr Res.* 1998, 68(5):287–92; Narbonne et al. Protein metabolism in vitamin A deficient rats. II. Protein synthesis in striated muscle. *Ann Nutr Aliment.* 1978, 32(1):59–75.

27 Jennings IW. *Vitamins in Endocrine Metabolism*. Springfield, IL: Charles C Thomas Publisher, 1970.

28 Ruth Rosevear and NW Solomans, personal communication.

29 http://www.westonaprice.org/health-topics/guts-and-grease-the-diet-of-native-americans/.

30 Angler N. Vitamins win support as potent agents of health. *New York Times*, Mar 10, 1992.

31 Brown D. It's cheap and effective, with wonders still being (re)discovered. *Washington Post*, Nov 7, 1994.

32 Vitamin A, retinoids and carotenoids: what's the bottom line? A dialogue between Robert Russell, M.D. and Joel Mason, M.D. Jun 1, 2001. http://www.thedoctorwillseeyounow.com/content/nutrition/art2049.html. Accessed Aug 8, 2016.

33 Rothman, KJ et al. Teratogenicity of high vitamin A intake. *New Engl J Med.* Nov 23, 1995, 333(21):1414–15.

34 Mastroiacovo, P et al. High vitamin A intake in early pregnancy and major malformations: a multicenter prospective controlled study. *Teratology.* Jan 1999, 59(1):1–2.

35 Wiegand UW et al. Safety of vitamin A: recent results. *International Journal of Vitamin and Nutrition Research.* 1998, 68(6):411–16.

36 http://umm.edu/health/medical/reports/articles/vitamins. Accessed Aug 5, 2016.

37 Mann J. Saving young lives with a 2-cent capsule. *Washington Post*, Mar 17, 1999.

38 Semba RD. The role of vitamin A and related retinoids in immune function. *Nutr Rev.* Jan 1998, 56(1, Pt. 2):S38–48.

39 Farber C. A timely firestorm. http://www.ironminds.com. Accessed Oct 18, 2016.

40 Lithgow DM and Politzer WM. Vitamin A in the treatment of menorrhagia. *S Afr Med J.* Feb 12, 1977, 51(7):191–93.

41 Marrakchi S et al.Vitamin A and E blood levels in erythrodermic and pustular psoriasis associated with chronic alcoholism. *Acta Derm Venereol.* Jul 1994, 74(4):298–301.

42 De Keyser J et al. Serum concentrations of vitamins A and E and early outcome after ischaemic stroke. *Lancet*, Jun 1992, 339(8809):1562–65.

43 Kolonel LN et al. Relationship of dietary vitamin A and ascorbic acid intake to the risk for cancers of the lung, bladder, and prostate in Hawaii. *Natl Cancer Inst Monogr.* Dec 1985, 69:137–42.

44 Aschhoff B. Retrospective study of Ukraine treatment in 203 patients with advanced-stage tumors. *Drugs Exp Clin Res.* 2000, 26(5–6):249–52.

45 Findlay GH. History of medicine. Alphonse Loewenthal (1903–1983)—the uncrowned king of dermatology in Africa. *S Afr Med J.* Dec 24, 1983, 64(27):1064–67.

46 Aram H et al. Kyrle's disease: response to high-dose vitamin A. *Cutis.* Dec 1982, 30(6):753–55, 759.

47 Rojas AI and Phillips TJ. Patients with chronic leg ulcers show diminished levels of vitamins A and D, carotenes, and zinc. *Dermatol Surg.* Aug 1999, 25(8):601–4.

48 Layrisse M et al. New property of vitamin A and beta-carotene on human iron absorption: effect on phytate and polyphenols as inhibitors of iron absorption. *Arch Latinoam Nutr.* Sep 2000, 50(3):243–48.

49 Ahmed F et al. Concomitant supplemental vitamin A enhances the response to weekly supplemental iron and folic acid in anemic teenagers in urban Bangladesh. *Am J Clin Nutr.* Jul 2001, 74(1):108–15.

50 Kuzniarz M et al. Use of vitamin supplements and cataract: the Blue Mountains Eye Study. *Am J Ophthalmol.* Jul 2001, 132(1):19–26.

51 Mecocci P et al. Plasma antioxidants and longevity: a study on healthy centenarians. *Free Radic Biol Med.* Apr 2000, 28(8):1243–48.

52 Acin-Perez R et al. Control of oxidative phosphorylation by vitamin A illuminates a fundamental role in mitochondrial energy homoeostasis. *FASEB Journal.* Feb 2010, 24(2):627–36.

53 Sardi B, knowledgeofhealth.com. May 21, 2014. Accessed Oct 15, 2016.

54 Clagett-Dame M and Knutson D. Vitamin A in reproduction and development. *Nutrients.* Apr 2011, 3(4):385–428.

55 http://www.westonaprice.org/our-blogs/cmasterjohn/vitamin-plays-essential-role-setting-circadian-rhythm-allowing-good-sleep/.

56 http://news.bbc.co.uk/2/hi/health/3480053.stm. Accessed Feb 6, 2016.

57 Britons eating too much liver. BBC News. Jan 16, 2004. http://news.bbc.co.uk/2/hi/health/3402891.stm.

58 Michaëlsson K et al. Serum retinol levels and the risk of fracture. *N Engl J Med.* Jan 23, 2003, 348(4):287–94.

59 Kawahara TN et al. Short-term vitamin A supplementation does not affect bone turnover in men. *J Nutr.* Jun 2002, 132(6):1169–72.

60 Barker ME et al. Serum retinoids and beta-carotene as predictors of hip and other fractures in elderly women. *J Bone Miner Res.* Jun 2005, 20(6):913–20.

61 Gabaeff SC. Challenging the pathophysiologic connection between subdural hematoma, retinal hemorrhage and shaken baby syndrome. *West J Emerg Med.* May 2011, 12(2):144–58.

62 Wolf G. The discovery of vitamin D: the contribution of Adolf Windaus. *J Nutr.* 2004, 134(6):1299–302.

63 Milnes GWA and Delander M. *Vitamin D Handbook: Structures, Synonyms, and Properties.* 1st ed. Hoboken, NJ: Wiley InterScience, Nov 9, 2007.

64 Balion C et al. Vitamin D, cognition, and dementia: a systematic review and meta-analysis. *Neurology.* 2012, 79(13): 1397–405.

65 Beard JA et al. Vitamin D and the anti-viral state. *Journal of Clinical Virology.* 2011, 50(3):194–200; Spector SA. Vitamin D and HIV: letting the sun shine in. *Topics in Antiviral Medicine.* 2011, 19(1):6–10; Cannell JJ et al. Epidemic influenza and vitamin D. *Epidemiology and Infection.* 2006, 134 (6):1129–40.

66 Aghajafari F et al. Association between maternal serum 25-hydroxyvitamin D level and pregnancy and neonatal outcomes: systematic review and meta-analysis of observational studies. *BMJ.* 2013, (346):f1169.

67 Dobnig H et al. Independent association of low serum 25-hydroxyvitamin d and 1,25-dihydroxyvitamin d levels with all-cause and cardiovascular mortality. *Arch Intern Med.* Jun 23, 2008, 168(12):1340–49.

68 Zittermann A et al. Low vitamin D status: a contributing factor in the pathogenesis of congestive heart failure? *J Am Coll Cardiol.* Jan 1, 2003, 41(1):105–12.

69 Murphy PK and Wagner CL. Vitamin D and mood disorders among women: an integrative review. *J Midwifery Women's Health.* Sep-Oct 2008, 53(5):440–46.

70 Munger KL et al. Serum 25-hydroxyvitamin D levels and risk of multiple sclerosis. *JAMA*. Dec 20, 2006, 296(23):2832–38.

71 Cheng Y et al. Relation of nutrition to bone lead and blood lead levels in middle-aged to elderly men: the Normative Aging Study. *Am J Epidemiol.* Jun 15, 1998, 147(12):1162–74.

72 Vieth R. The pharmacology of vitamin D, including fortification strategies, in D Feldman et al, eds., *Vitamin D*, 2d ed. Burlington, VT: Elsevier Academic Press, 2005, pp. 995–1015; Heaney RP. The Vitamin D requirement in health and disease. *Journal of Steroid Biochemistry & Molecular Biology.* 2005, 97:13–19.

73 http://www.weegy.com/home.aspx?ConversationId=EE6113FD. Accessed Aug 5, 2016.

74 Bischoff-Ferrari HA. Optimal serum 25-hydroxyvitamin D levels for multiple health outcomes. *Adv Exp Med Biol.* 2008, 624:55–71.
In footnote: [a] http://www.westonaprice.org/health-topics/update-on-vitamins-a-and-d.

75 Prince RL et al. Effects of ergocalciferol added to calcium on the risk of falls in elderly high-risk women. *Arch Intern Med.* Jan 14, 2008, 168(1):103–8.

76 Trang HM et al. Evidence that vitamin D_3 increases serum 25-hydroxyvitamin D more efficiently than does vitamin D_2. *Am J Clin Nutr.* 1998, 68:854–58. Armas LA et al. Vitamin D_2 is much less effective than vitamin D_3 in humans. *J Clin Endocrinol Metab.* 2004, 89(11):5387–91.

77 Brehm W. Potential dangers of viosterol during pregnancy with observations of calcification of placentae. *Ohio State Medical Journal.* 1937, 33(9):989–93.
In footnote: [a] http://www.westonaprice.org/health-topics/cod-liver-oil/vitamin-d-in-cod-liver-oil/.

78 Dionne J et al. Hypertension in infancy: diagnosis, management, and outcome. *Pediatr Nephrol.* 2012, 27:17–32; Vitamin D, *Merck Manual of Diagnosis and Therapy*, professional edition.

79 Better OS et al. Increased incidence of nephrolithiasis in lifeguards in Israel, in Massry et al, eds. *Phosphate and Minerals in Health and Disease.* New York: Plenum Press, 1980.

80 Marshall TG. Vitamin D discovery outpaces FDA decision making. *Bioessays.* Jan 15, 2008, 30(2):173–82.

81 Payne ME et al. Calcium and vitamin D intakes may be positively associated with brain lesions in depressed and non-depressed elders. *Nutr Res.* 2008, 28(5): 285–92.

82 van der Gaag E and Brekhoff L. Effect of food and vitamin D supplements on the serum $25(OH)D_3$ concentration in children during winter months. *Foods.* 2014, 3(4):632–41.
In footnote: [a] Vieth R. Vitamin D supplementation, 25-hydroxyvitamin D concentrations, and safety. *Am J Clin Nutr.* 1999, 69:842–56.

83 Morgan AF et al. A comparison of the hypervitaminoses induced by irradiated ergosterol and fish liver oil concentrates. *Journal of Biological Chemistry.* 1937, 120(1):85–102.

84 Clark I and Bassett CAL. The amelioration of hypervitaminosis D in rats with vitamin A. *J Exp Med.* 1962, 115:147–56; Callari D et al. Retinoic acid action on D_3 hypervitaminosis. *Boll Soc It Biol Sper.* 1986, 62(6): 835–41.

85 Sanchez-Martinez R et al. The retinoid X receptor ligand restores defective signaling by the vitamin D receptor. *EMBO Reports*, 2006.
In footnote: ([a]) (page 114) Aaron J. Studies on the history of rickets I: recognition of rickets as a deficiency disease. *Pharmacy in History.* 1974, 16(3)83–88.

86 Aaron J. Studies on the history of rickets I: Recognition of rickets as a deficiency disease. *Pharmacy in History.* 1974, 16(3)83–88.

87 Galarraga B et al. Cod liver oil (n-3 fatty acids) as a non-steroidal anti-inflammatory drug sparing agent in rheumatoid arthritis. *Rheumatology* (Oxford). May 2008, 47(5):665–69.

88 Vermel AE. Clinical application of omega-3-fatty acids (cod-liver oil). *Klin Med (Mosk).* 2005, 83(10): 51–57.

89 Gruenwald J et al. Effect of cod liver oil on symptoms of rheumatoid arthritis. *Adv Ther.* Mar-Apr 2002, 19(2): 101–17.

90 Macdonald HM et al. Vitamin D status in postmenopausal women living at higher latitudes in the UK in relation to bone health, overweight, sunlight exposure and dietary vitamin D. *Bone.* May 2008, 42(5):996–1003.

91 Barker ME et al. Serum retinoids and beta-carotene as predictors of hip and other fractures in elderly women. *J Bone Miner Res.* Jun 2005, 20(6):913–20.

92 Brustad M et al. Vitamin D status in a rural population of northern Norway with high fish liver consumption. *Public Health Nutr.* Sep 2004, 7(6):783–89.

93 Ceylan-Isik A et al. Cod liver oil supplementation improves cardiovascular and metabolic abnormalities in streptozotocin diabetic rats. *J Pharm Pharmaco.* Dec 2007, 59(12):1629–41.

94 Ohtake T et al. Effects of dietary lipids on daunomycin-induced nephropathy in mice: comparison between cod liver oil and soybean oil. *Lipids.* Apr 2002, 37(4):359–66.

95 Skeie G et al. Cod liver oil, other dietary supplements and survival among cancer patients with solid tumours. *Int J Cancer.* Sep 1, 2009, 125(5):1155–60.

96 Weiner BH et al. Inhibition of atherosclerosis by cod-liver oil in a hyperlipidemic swine model. *N Engl J Med.* Oct 2, 1986, 315(14):841–46.

97 Shimokawa H et al. Effects of dietary supplementation with cod-liver oil on endothelium-dependent responses in porcine coronary arteries. *Circulation.* Oct 1987, 76(4):898–905.

98 Raeder MB et al. Associations between cod liver oil use and symptoms of depression: the Hordaland Health Study. *J Affect Disord.* Aug 2007, 101(1–3):245–49.

99 Olafsdottir AS et al. Relationship between dietary intake of cod liver oil in early pregnancy and birthweight. *BJOG.* Apr 2005, 112(4):424–49.

100 Olafsdottir AS et al. Polyunsaturated fatty acids in the diet and breast milk of lactating Icelandic women with traditional fish and cod liver oil consumption. *Ann Nutr Metab.* 2006, 50(3):270–76.

101 Olafsdottir AS et al. Fat-soluble vitamins in the maternal diet, influence of cod liver oil supplementation and impact of the maternal diet on human milk composition. *Ann Nutr Metab.* 2001, 45(6):265–72.

102 Helland IB et al. Maternal supplementation with very-long-chain n-3 fatty acids during pregnancy and lactation augments children's IQ at 4 years of age. *Pediatrics.* Jan 2003, 111(1):e39–44.

103 Linday LA et al. Effect of daily cod liver oil and a multivitamin-mineral supplement with selenium on upper respiratory tract pediatric visits by young, inner-city, Latino children: randomized pediatric sites. *Ann Otol Rhinol Laryngol.* Nov 2004, 113(11):891–901.

104 Stene LC et al. Use of cod liver oil during the first year of life is associated with lower risk of childhood-onset type 1 diabetes: a large, population-based, case-control study. *Am J Clin Nutr.* Dec 2003, 78(6):1128–34.

105 Linday LA et al. Lemon-flavored cod liver oil and a multivitamin-mineral supplement for the secondary prevention of otitis media in young children: pilot research. *Ann Otol Rhinol Laryngol.* Jul 2002, 111(7, Pt. 1):642–52.

106 Kampman MT et al. Outdoor activities and diet in childhood and adolescence relate to MS risk above the Arctic Circle. *J Neurol.* Apr 2007, 254(4):471–77.

107 Knight JA et al. Vitamin D and reduced risk of breast cancer: a population-based case-control study. *Cancer Epidemiol Biomarkers Prev.* Mar 2007, 16(3):422–29.

108 TheBostonChannel.com, Apr 29, 2010. No longer available.

109 Downes R. Timperley woman celebrates landmark birthday. *Messenger.* Dec 31, 2009.

110 http://www.westonaprice.org/health-topics/abcs-of-nutrition/on-the-trail-of-the-elusive-x-factor-a-sixty-two-year-old-mystery-finally-solved/.

111 Vermeer C and Hamulyak K. Vitamin K: lessons from the past. *J Thromb Haemost.* 2004, 2(12):2115–17.

112 Geleijnse JM et al. Dietary intake of menaquinone is associated with a reduced risk of coronary heart disease: the Rotterdam Study. *J Nutr.* 2004, 134:3100–5.

113 Spronk HMH et al. Tissue-specific utilization of menaquinone-4 results in the prevention of arterial calcification in warfarin-treated rats. *J Vasc Res.* 2003, 40: 531–37.

114 Berkner KL and Runge W. The physiology of vitamin K nutriture and vitamin K-dependent protein function in atherosclerosis. *J Thromb Haemost.* 2004, 2(12):2118–32.

115 Luo G et al. Spontaneous calcification of arteries and cartilage in mice lacking matrix GLA protein. *Nature.* 1997, 386:78–81.

In footnote: [a] Oliva A et al. Effect of retinoic acid on osteocalcin gene expression in human osteoblasts. *Biochem Biophys Res Commun.* 1993, 191(3):908–14; Koshihara Y and Hoshi K. Vitamin K_2 enhances osteocalcin accumulation in the extracellular matrix of human osteoblasts in vitro. *J Bone Miner Res.* 1997, 12(3):431–38; Farzanheh-Far A et al. Transcriptional regulation of matrix gla protein. *Z Kardiol.* 2001, 90(Supp 3): 38–42; Kirfel J et al. Identification of a novel negative retinoic acid responsive element in the promoter of the human matrix Gla protein gene. *Proc Natl Acad Sci USA.* 1997, 94(6):2227–32; Berkner KL and Runge W. The physiology of vitamin K nutriture and vitamin K-dependent protein function in atherosclerosis. *J Thromb Haemost.* 2004, 2(12):2118–32.

116 Price WA. *Nutrition and Physical Degeneration.* San Diego, CA: Price-Pottenger Nutrition Foundation, 1945.

117 Vermeer C et al. Beyond deficiency: potential benefits of increased intakes of vitamin K for bone and vascular health. *Eur J Nutr.* 2004, 43:325–35.

118 Cockayne S et al. Vitamin K and the prevention of fractures. *Arch Intern Med.* 2006, 166:1256–61.

119 Yaegashi Y et al. Association of hip fracture incidence and intake of calcium, magnesium, vitamin D, and vitamin K. *Eur J Epidemiol.* 2008, 23(3):219–25.

120 Johanna M. Geleijnse et al. Dietary intake of menaquinone is associated with a reduced risk of coronary heart disease: the Rotterdam Study. *J. Nutr.* Nov 1, 2004, 134(11):3100–5.

121 Denisova NA and Booth SL. Vitamin K and sphingolipid metabolism: evidence to date. *Nutr Rev.* 2005, 63(4):110–21.

122 Han X et al. Substantial sulfatide deficiency and ceramide elevation in very early Alzheimer's disease: potential role in disease pathogenesis. *J Neurochem.* 2002, 82(4):809–18.

123 Bosio A et al. Functional breakdown of the lipid bilayer of the myelin membrane in central and peripheral nervous system by disrupted galactocerebroside synthesis. *Proc Natl Acad Sci USA.* 1996, 93:13280–85.

124 Sakamoto N et al. Possible effects of one week vitamin K (menaquinone-4) tablets intake on glucose tolerance in healthy young male volunteers with different descarboxy prothrombin levels. *Clin Nutr.* 2000, 19(4): 259–63.

125 Ronden JE et al. Tissue distribution of K-vitamins under different nutritional regimens in the rat. *Biochim Biophys Acta.* 1998, 1379:16–22.

126 Vermeer C et al. Vitamin K and the urogenital tract. *Haemostasis.* 1986, 16: 246–57.

127 Thijssen HHW and Drittij-Reijnders MJ. Vitamin K status in human tissues: tissue-specific accumulation of phylloquinone and menaquionone-4. *Br J Nutr.* 1996, 75:121–27.

128 Vermeer et al. Vitamin K and the urogenital tract. *Haemostasis.* 1986, 16:246–57.

129 Tokita H et al. Vitamin K_2-induced antitumor effects via cell-cycle arrest and apoptosis in gastric cancer cell lines. *Int J Mol Med.* 2006, 17(2):2355–443.

130 Nimptsch K et al. Dietary intake of vitamin K and risk of prostate cancer in the Heidelberg cohort of the European Prospective Investigation into Cancer and Nutrition (EPIC-Heidelberg). *Am J Clin Nutr.* Apr 2008, 87(4):985–92.

131 Nimptsch K et al. Dietary vitamin K intake in relation to cancer incidence and mortality: results from the Heidelberg cohort of the European Prospective Investigation into Cancer and Nutrition (EPIC-Heidelberg). *Am J Clin Nutr.* May 2010, 91(5):1348–58.

132 Gheduzzi D et al. Matrix Gla protein is involved in elastic fiber calcification in the dermis of pseudoxanthoma elasticum patients. *Laboratory Investigation.* 2007, 87: 998–1008.

Chapter 7: The Rancid and the *Trans*

1 http://www.westonaprice.org/know-your-fats/the-tragic-legacy-of-center-for-science-in-the-public-interest-cspi/. Accessed Feb 6, 2016.

2 Enig MG. *Trans Fatty Acids in the Food Supply: A Comprehensive Report Covering 60 Years of Research*, 2d ed. Silver Spring, MD: Enig Associates, Inc., 1995, pp. 67–68.

3 Beare-Rogers JL and Nera EA. Some nutritional aspects of partially hydrogenated oils. *Journal of the American Oil Chemists' Society.* 1976, 53:467A(149).

4 http://www.fda.gov/Food/IngredientsPackagingLabeling/GRAS/SCOGS/ucm260428.htm. Accessed February 6, 2016.

5 Hanis T et al. Effects of dietary trans-fatty acids on reproductive performance of Wistar rats. *Br J Nutr.* May 1989, 61(3):519–29.

6 Alfin-Slater RB and Aftergood L. Nutritional role of hydrogenated fats (in rats). Geometrical and Positional Fatty Acid Isomers, EA Emken and HJ Dutton, eds. Champaign, IL: American Oil Chemists' Society, 1979, pp. 53–74.

7 Teter BB et al. Milk fat depression in C57B1/6J mice consuming partially hydrogenated fat. *Journal of Nutrition.* 1990, 120:818–24; Barnard et al. Dietary trans fatty acids modulate erythrocyte membrane fatty acid composition and insulin binding in monkeys. *Journal of Nutritional Biochemistry.* 1990, 1:190–95.

8 Mary G. Enig, personal communication.

9 Hanis T et al. Effects of dietary trans fatty acids on reproductive performance of Wistar Rats. *Br J Nutr.* May 1989, 61(3):519–29.

10 Koletzko B and Muller J. Cis- and trans-isomeric fatty acids in plasma lipids of newborn infants and their mothers. *Biology of the Neonate.* 1990, 57:172–78.

11 Horrobin D. The regulation of prostaglandin biosynthesis by manipulation of essential fatty acid metabolism. *Reviews in Pure and Applied Pharmacological Sciences.* 1983, 4:339–83.

12 Mann GV. Metabolic consequences of dietary trans fatty acids. *Lancet.* 1994, 343:1268–71.

13 Kohlmeier et al. Stores of trans fatty acids and breast cancer risk. *Am J Clin Nutr.* 1995, 61:896, A25.

14 Mensink RP and Katan M. Effect of dietary trans fatty acids on high-density and low-density lipoprotein cholesterol levels in healthy subjects. *N Eng J Med.* 1990, 323:439–45.

15 Enig MG et al. Isomeric trans fatty acids in the U.S. diet. *J Am Coll Nutr.* 1990, 9:471–86.

16 Willett WC et al. Consumption of trans-fatty acids in relation to risk of coronary heart disease among women. *Society for Epidemiology Research.* Annual Meeting, Jun 1992, Abstract 249.

17 Mary G. Enig, personal communication.

18 Willett WC et al. Intake of trans fatty acids and risk of coronary heart disease among women. *Lancet.* 1993, 341:581–85.

19 http://www.westonaprice.org/know-your-fats/the-oiling-of-america/.

20 Kummerow FA. Nutritional effects of isomeric fats: their possible influence on cell metabolism or cell structure. In EG Perkins and WJ Visek, eds. *Dietary Fats and Health.* Champaign, IL: American Oil Chemists' Society, 1983, pp. 391–402; Kummerow FA. Nutritional aspects of isomeric fats, in Horisberger M and Bracco U, eds. *Lipids in Modern Nutrition.* New York: Nestle Nutrition, Vevey/Raven Press, 1987.

21 Mann GV et al. Atherosclerosis in the Maasai. *Am J Epidemiol*, 1972, 95:26–37.

22 Mann GV, ed. *Coronary Heart Disease, The Dietary Sense and Nonsense.* London: Veritas Society, 1993, p. 1.

23 Enig MG. *Trans Fatty Acids in the Food Supply: A Comprehensive Report Covering 60 Years of Research*, 2d ed., 1995, Silver Spring, MD, Enig Associates, Inc., pp. 93–94.
In footnote: [a] Schiefer HB et al. Long-term effects of partially hydrogenated herring oil on the rat myocardium. *Drug Nutr Interact.* 1982, 1(2):89–102.

24 Enig MG. *Modification of Membrane Lipid Composition and Mixed-Function Oxidases in Mouse Liver Microsomes by Dietary Trans Fatty Acids.* Doctoral dissertation, University of Maryland, 1984.

25 Enig MG et al. Isomeric trans fatty acids in the U.S. diet. *J Am Coll Nutr.* 1990, 9:471–86.

26 Enig, MG. *Trans Fatty Acids in the Food Supply: A Comprehensive Report Covering 60 Years of Research*, 2d ed. Silver Spring, MD: Enig Associates, Inc., 1995, pp. 93–97.
In footnote: [a] Meade CJ and Martin J. Fatty acids and immunity. *Adv Lipid Res.* 1978, 127.

27 Ibid., p. 98.

28 Ibid., p. 101.

29 Willett WC and Ascherio A. Trans fatty acids: are the effects only marginal? *Am J Public Health.* May 1994, 84(5):722–24.

30 Zaloga GP et al. Trans fatty acids and coronary heart disease. *Nutrition in Clinical Practice.* 2006, 21(5):505–12.

31 Mozaffarian D et al. Trans fatty acids and cardiovascular disease. *New Engl J Med.* 2006, 354(15):1601–13.

32 Han SN et al. Effect of hydrogenated and saturated, relative to polyunsaturated, fat on immune and inflammatory responses of adults with moderate hypercholesterolemia. *J Lipid Res.* Mar 2002, 43(3):445–52.

33 Lopez-Garcia E et al. Consumption of trans fatty acids is related to plasma biomarkers of inflammation and endothelial dysfunction. *J Nutr.* Mar 2005, 135(3):562–66.

34 Yanangi S et al. Cumulative Effects of butter, margarine, safflower oil, and dextrin on mammary tumorigenesis in mice and rats. Meeting Abstract 15. *Journal of the American Oil Chemists' Society.* 1988, 65:479–80.

35 Ewertz M and Gill C. Dietary factors and breast-cancer risk in Denmark. *Int J Cancer.* Nov 15, 1990, 46(5):779–84.

36 Van't Veer P et al. Dietary fat and the risk of breast cancer. *Int J Epidemiol.* Mar 1990, 19(1):12–18.

37 Kohlmeier L et al. Stores of trans fatty acids and breast cancer risk. *American Journal of Clinical Nutrition.* 1995, 61:896, A25.

38 Chajès V et al. Association between serum trans-monounsaturated fatty acids and breast cancer risk in the E3N-EPIC Study. *Am J Epidemiol.* Jun 1, 2008, 167(11):1312–20.

39 Chavarro JE et al. A prospective study of trans-fatty acid levels in blood and risk of prostate cancer. *Cancer Epidemiol Biomarkers Prev.* Jan 2008, 17(1):95–101.

40 Kuller LH. Trans fatty acids and dieting (letter). *Lancet.* 1993, 341:1093–94.

41 Kavanagh K et al. Trans fat diet induces abdominal obesity and changes in insulin sensitivity in monkeys. *Obesity.* 2007, 15(7):1675–84.

42 Golomb BA et al. Trans fat consumption and aggression. *PLoS ONE.* 2012, 7(3):e32175.

43 Golomb BA and Bui AK. A fat to forget: trans fat consumption and memory. *PLoS ONE* 2015, 10.

44 Mozaffarian D et al. Trans fatty acids and cardiovascular disease. *New Engl J Med.* 2006, 354(15):1601–13.

45 Enig, MG. *Trans Fatty Acids in the Food Supply: A Comprehensive Report Covering 60 Years of Research*, 2d ed. Silver Spring, MD: Enig Associates, Inc., 1995.

46 http://www.westonaprice.org/health-topics/trans-fats-in-the-food-supply/.

47 Pinckney ER and Pinckney C. *The Cholesterol Controversy.* Los Angeles, CA: Sherbourne Press, 1973.

48 Denham H. Atherosclerosis: possible ill-effects of the use of highly unsaturated fats to lower serum-cholesterol levels (letter). *Lancet*, Nov 30, 1957, 1116–17.

49 Kritchevsky D. *Medical Counterpoint*, Mar 1969.

50 Ohfuji TK and Kaneda K. Characterization of toxic components in thermally oxidized oil. *Lipids.* 1973, 8(6):348–52.

51 Dunder T et al. Diet, serum fatty acids, and atopic diseases in childhood. *Allergy.* May 2001, 56(5):425–28.

52 Haby MM et al. Asthma in preschool children: prevalence and risk factors. *Thorax.* Aug 2001, 56(8):589–95.

53 Takeda M et al. Long-term optional ingestion of corn oil induces excessive caloric intake and obesity in mice. *Nutrition.* Feb 2001, 17(2):117–20.

54 Seddon JM et al. Dietary fat and risk for advanced age-related macular degeneration. *Arch Ophthalmol.* Aug 2001, 119(8):1191–99.

55 Halade GV et al. High fat diet-induced animal model of age-associated obesity and osteoporosis. *J Nutr Biochem.* Dec 2010, 21(12):1162–69.

56 http://www.sciencedaily.com/releases/2009/12/091231163503.htm. Accessed Jan 17, 2016.

57 http://www.sciencedaily.com/releases/2010/02/100209124352.htm. Accessed Jan 17, 2016.

58 Lasserre M et al. Effects of different dietary intake of essential fatty acids on C20:3 omega 6 and C20:4 omega 6 serum levels in human adults. *Lipids.* Apr 1985, 20(4):227–33.

59 Tang J et al. Isolation and identification of volatile compounds from fried chicken. *Journal of Agricultural and Food Chemistry.* 1983, 31(6):12.

60 World Health Organization, International Agency for Research on Cancer (IARC). Household use of solid fuels and high-temperature frying. IARC Monographs on the Evaluation of Carcinogenic Risks to Humans. 2006, 95:392.

61 Esterbauer H et al. Chemistry and biochemistry of 4-hydroxynonenal, malonaldehyde and related aldehydes. *Free Radic Biol Med.* 1991, 11(1):81–128.

62 Tong Z et al. Age-related formaldehyde interferes with DNA methyltransferase function, causing memory loss in Alzheimer's disease. *Neurobiol Aging.* Jan 2015, 36(1):100–10; Benedetti E et al. Involvement of peroxisome proliferator-activated receptor β/δ (PPAR β/δ) in BDNF signaling during aging and in Alzheimer disease: possible role of 4-hydroxynonenal (4-HNE). *Cell Cycle.* 2014, 13(8):1335–44.

63 Conklin DJ et al. Acrolein-induced dyslipidemia and acute-phase response are independent of HMG-CoA reductase. *Mol Nutr Food Res.* Sep 2011, 55(9):1411–22.

64 Sundram K et al. Stearic acid-rich interesterified fat and trans-rich fat raise the LDL/HDL ratio and plasma glucose relative to palm olein in humans. *Nutr Metab (Lond).* Jan 15, 2007, 4:3.

Chapter 8: Remember the Little Ones: Why Children Need Animal Fats

1 Luo T et al. Dräger UC. Retinoids, eye development, and maturation of visual function. *J Neurobiol.* 2006, 66(7):677–86; Rawson NE and LaMantia AS. Once and again: retinoic acid signaling in the developing and regenerating olfactory pathway. *J Neurobiol.* 2006, 66(7):653–76.

2 http://www.sciencedaily.com/releases/2010/03/100317091301.htm. Accessed Jan 18, 2016.

3 Zile MH. Function of vitamin A in vertebrate embryonic development. *J Nutr.* Mar 2001, 131(3):705–8.

4 Price WA. *Nutrition and Physical Degeneration*, 6th ed. La Mesa, CA: Price-Pottenger Nutrition Foundation, 2004, pp. 334–49.

5 Gilbert T. Vitamin A and kidney development. *Nephrol Dial Transplant.* 2002, 17(Supp 9):78–80.

6 Biesalski HK and Bohr D. Importance of vitamin-A for lung function and development. *Mol Aspects Med.* 2003, 24:431–40.

7 Checkley W et al. Maternal vitamin A supplementation and lung function in offspring. *N Engl J Med.* 2010, 362:1784–94.
In footnote: [a] Checkley W et al. Maternal vitamin A supplementation and lung function in offspring. *N Engl J Med.* 2010, 362:1784–94.

8 Biesalski HK and Bohr D. Importance of vitamin-A for lung function and development. *Mol Aspects Med.* 2003, 24:431–40.

9 http://www.news-medical.net/news/2005/05/11/9979.aspx#sthash.ZqXFSRvc.dpuf. Accessed Feb 7, 2016.

10 Chen F et al. Prenatal retinoid deficiency leads to airway hyperresponsiveness in adult mice. *J Clin Invest.* Feb 2014, 124(2):801–11.

11 Strobel M et al. The importance of beta-carotene as a source of vitamin A with special regard to pregnant and breastfeeding women. *Eur J Nutr.* Jul 2007, 46(supp 1):11–20.

12 Devereux G. Early life events in asthma—diet. *Pediatr Pulmonol.* 2007, 42(8):663–73.

13 Hoogenboezem T et al. Vitamin D metabolism in breast-fed infants and their mothers. *Pediatric Research.* 1989, 25:623–28; Ala-Houhala M et al. Maternal compared with infant vitamin D supplementation. *Archives of Disease in Childhood.* 1986, 61:1159–63.

14 Maiya S et al. Hypocalcaemia and vitamin D deficiency: an important, but preventable, cause of life-threatening infant heart failure. *Heart.* May 2008, 94(5):581–84; Soliman A. Clinical, biochemical, and radiological manifestations of vitamin D deficiency in newborns presented with hypocalcemia. *Indian J Endocrinol Metab.* Jul 2003, 17(4):697–703; Mehrotra P et al. Hypovitaminosis D and hypocalcemic seizures in infancy. *Indian Pediatrics.* Jul 17, 2010, 47: 581–86; Lee JY et al. A review on vitamin D deficiency treatment in pediatric patients. *J Pediatr Pharmocol Ther.* Oct–Dec 2013, 18(4):277–91.

15 Bishop N. Perinatal vitamin D actions. In Feldman D et al, eds. *Vitamin D*, 2d ed. Burlington, VT: Elsevier Academic Press, 2005, 803–10.

16 Stene LC et al. Use of cod liver oil during the first year of life is associated with lower risk of childhood-onset type 1 diabetes: a large, population-based, case-control study. *Am J Clin Nutr.* Dec 2003, 78(6): 1128–34.

17 Berkner KL. The vitamin K-dependent carboxylase. *Annu Rev Nutr.* 2005, 25:127–49.

18 Howe AM et al. Severe cervical dysplasia and nasal cartilage calcification following prenatal warfarin exposure. *Am J Med Genet.* 1997, 71(4):391–96.

19 Innis SM. Dietary (n-3) fatty acids and brain development. *J Nutr.* 2007, 137:855–59.

20 Hibbeln J. Seafood consumption, the DHA content of mothers' milk and prevalence rates of postpartum depression: a cross-national, ecological analysis. *Journal of Affective Disorders.* 2002, 69:15–29.

21 Cheruku SR et al. Higher maternal plasma docosahexaenoic acid during pregnancy is associated with more mature neonatal sleep-state patterning. *Am J Clin Nutr.* Sep 2002, 76(3):608–13.

22 Zeisel, SH. The fetal origins of memory: the role of dietary choline in optimal brain development. *J Pediatr.* 2006, 149:S131–36.

23 Oberlander TF. Prenatal exposure to maternal depression, neonatal methylation of human glucocorticoid receptor gene (NR3C1) and infant cortisol stress responses. *Epigenetics.* Mar-Apr 2008, 3(2):97–106.

24 Jiang X et al. Maternal choline intake alters the epigenetic state of fetal cortisol-regulating genes in humans. *FASEB Journal.* Aug 2012, 26(8):3563–74.

25 Olafsdottir AS et al. Fat-soluble vitamins in the maternal diet, influence of cod liver oil supplementation and impact of the maternal diet on human milk composition. *Ann Nutr Metab.* 2001, 45(6):265–72.

26 Gordon CM et al. Prevalence of vitamin D deficiency among healthy infants and toddlers. *Arch Pediatr Adolesc Med.* Jun 2008, 162(6):505–12.

27 Stoltzfus RJ and Underwood BA. Breast-milk vitamin A as an indicator of the vitamin A status of women and infants. *Bull World Health Organ.* 1995, 73(5):703–11.

28 Alm B et al. Vitamin A and sudden infant death syndrome in Scandinavia 1992–1995. *Acta Paediatr.* 2003, 92(2):162–64.

29 Fischer LM et al. Choline intake and genetic polymorphisms influence choline metabolite concentrations in human breast milk and plasma. *Am J Clin Nutr.* 2010, 92:336–46.

30 Anderson NK et al. Dietary fat type influences total milk fat content in lean women. *J Nutr.* 2005, 135:416–21.

31 Teter BB et al. Milk fat depression in C57Bl/6J mice consuming partially hydrogenated fat. *J Nutr.* 1990, 120:818–24.

32 Anderson NK et al. Dietary fat type influences total milk fat content in lean women. *J Nutr.* 2005, 135:416–21.

33 Hamosh M. Digestion in the newborn. *Clin Perinatol.* Jun 1996, 23(2):191–209.

34 Koletzko B et al. Long chain polyunsaturated fatty acids (LC-PUFA) and perinatal development. *Acta Paediatr.* Apr 2001, 90(4):460–64.

35 Chen ZY. Breast milk fatty acid composition: a comparative study between Hong Kong and Chongqing Chinese. *Lipids.* 1997, 32(10):1061–67.

36 Birch, EE et al. A randomized controlled trial of early dietary supply of long-chain polyunsaturated fatty acids and mental development in term infants. *Developmental Medicine & Child Neurology.* 2007, 42(3):174.

37 Reddy S et al. The influence of maternal vegetarian diet on essential fatty acid status of the newborn. *European Journal of Clinical Nutrition.* May 1994, 48(5)358–68.

38 Garg ML et al. *FASEB Journal.* 1988, 2(4):A852; Oliart-Ros RM et al. Meeting Abstracts. *AOCS Proceedings.* Chicago, May 1998, 7.

39 Jensen RG. Lipids in human milk. *Lipids.* Dec 1999, 34(12):1243–71.

40 German JB and Dillard CJ. Saturated fats: a perspective from lactation and milk composition. *Lipids.* 2010, 45(10):915–23.

41 Bilbo SD and Tsang V. Enduring consequences of maternal obesity for brain inflammation and behavior of offspring. *FASEB Journal.* 2010, 24:2104–15.

42 Smedts HP et al. Maternal intake of fat, riboflavin and nicotinamide and the risk of having offspring with congenital heart defects. *Eur J Nutr.* 2008, 47:357–65.

43 Aaltonen J et al. Impact of maternal diet during pregnancy and breastfeeding on infant metabolic programming: a prospective randomized controlled study. *Eur J Clin Nutr.* 2011, 65:10–19.

44 Khoury J et al. Effect of a cholesterol-lowering diet on maternal, cord, and neonatal lipids, and pregnancy outcome: a randomized clinical trial. *Am J Obstet Gynecol.* 2005, 193(4):1292–301.

45 Khoury J et al. Effects of an antiatherogenic diet during pregnancy on markers of maternal and fetal endothelial activation and inflammation: the CARRDIP study. *BJOG.* 2007, 114(3):279–88; Khoury J et al. Effect of a cholesterol-lowering diet during pregnancy on maternal and fetal Doppler velocimetry: the CARRDIP study. *Am J Obstet Gynecol.* 2007, 196(6):549.e1-7.

46 Chavarro JE et al. A prospective study of dairy foods intake and anovulatory infertility. *Hum Reprod.* May 2007, 22(5):1340–47.

47 McCollum EV. *The Newer Knowledge of Nutrition.* New York: Macmillan, 1921, p. 58.

48 http://www.second-opinions.co.uk/cholesterol_myth_1.html#.Vp1a-73I0r1. Accessed Jan 19, 2016.

49 McGill HC et al. Origin of atherosclerosis in childhood and adolescence. *Am J Clin Nutr.* Nov 2000, 72(5 Suppl.):1307S–15S.

50 Questions surround treatment of children with high cholesterol. *JAMA.* 1970, 214(10):1783–94.

51 *Cornell Magazine*, May–Jun 1999.
In footnote: [a] http://www.westonaprice.org/book-reviews/the-china-study-by-t-colin-campbell/.

52 *Gerson Healing Newsletter*, 2000, 15(1).

53 American Academy of Pediatrics Committee on Nutrition. Prudent life-style for children: dietary fat and cholesterol. *Pediatrics.* Sep 1986, 78(3):521–25.

54 Lifshitz F and Moses N. Growth failure: a complication of dietary treatment of hypercholesterolemia. *Am J Dis Child.* May 1989, 143(5):537–42.

55 Dagnelie PC et al. Stunting and nutrient deficiencies in children on alternative diets. *Acta Paediatr Scand Suppl.* 1991, 374:111–18.

56 Dagnelie PC et al. High prevalence of rickets in infants on macrobiotic diets. *Am J Clin Nutr.* Feb 1990, 51(2):202–8.

57 Samuel SG et al. Dietary recommendations for children and adolescents: a guide for practitioners. Consensus statement from the American Heart Association. Endorsed by the American Academy of Pediatrics. *Circulation.* 2005, 112:2061–75.

58 American Academy of Pediatrics. Committee on Nutrition. Cholesterol in childhood. American Academy of Pediatrics. Committee on Nutrition. *Pediatrics.* Jan 1998, 101(1, Pt. 1):141–47.

59 Steinberg D et al. Evidence mandating earlier and more aggressive treatment of hypercholesterolemia. *Circulation.* Aug 5, 2008, 118(6):672–77.

60 http://www.washingtonpost.com/wp-dyn/content/article/2007/10/26/AR2007102602504.html.

61 Ward EM. *MyPlate for Moms, How to Feed Yourself & Your Family Better.* Reading, MA: Loughlin Press, 2011, p. 99.

62 World Health Organization. *Preterm Birth.* Fact Sheet No. 363. Geneva: WHO, 2014.

63 Grieger JA et al. Preconception dietary patterns in human pregnancies are associated with preterm delivery. *J Nutr.* Jul 2014, 144(7):1075–80.

64 Blanchard LT et al. Emotional, developmental, and behavioral health of American children and their families: a report from the 2003 National Survey of Children's Health. *Pediatrics.* 2006, 117(6):e1202–12.

65 Kogan MD et al. A national profile of the health care experiences and family impact of autism spectrum disorder among children in the United States, 2005–2006. *Pediatrics.* Dec 2008, 122(6):e1149–58.

66 http://www.nytimes.com/learning/students/pop/articles/Gross2.html. Accessed Feb 7, 2016.

67 http://usatoday30.usatoday.com/news/health/2006-06-26-recess-bans_x.htm. Accessed Feb 7, 2016.

68 http://sci.rutgers.edu/forum/showthread.php?30240-U-S-Counts-One-in-12-Children-As-Disabled. Accessed Feb 7, 2016.

69 Wijga AH et al. Association of consumption of products containing milk fat with reduced asthma risk in pre-school children: the PIAMA birth cohort study. *Thorax.* Jul 2003, 58(7):567–72.

70 http://www.upi.com/Science_News/2003/03/01/High-fat-diet-protects-brain-cells/23771046514393/. Accessed Feb 7, 2016.

71 Helland IB et al. Maternal supplementation with very-long-chain n-3 fatty acids during pregnancy and lactation augments children's IQ at 4 years of age. *Pediatrics.* Jan 2003, 111(1):e39–44.

72 Judith G. Hall, OC, MD, reviewing Edison RJ and Muenke M. Statins and low cholesterol may be bad news for human embryos and fetuses. *Am J Med Genet.* Dec 15, 2004.

73 http://www.foxnews.com/story/2010/01/28/couple-accused-starving-baby-so-doesnt-get-fat.html. Accessed Feb 7, 2016.

74 http://abcnews.go.com/GMA/fat-babies-parents-put-fat-babies-diet/story?id=12216642. Accessed Feb 7, 2016.

75 Moon RJ et al. Maternal plasma polyunsaturated fatty acid status in late pregnancy is associated with offspring body composition in childhood. *J Clin Endocrinol Metab.* Jan 2013, 98(1):299–307.

76 http://sciencenordic.com/vegetable-oils-promote-obesity. Accessed Feb 7, 2016.

77 Garemo M et al. Metabolic markers in relation to nutrition and growth in healthy 4-y-old children in Sweden. *Am J Clin Nutr.* Nov 2006, 84(5):1021–26.

78 Scharf RJ et al. Longitudinal evaluation of milk type consumed and weight status in preschoolers. *Arch Dis Child.* May 2013, 98(5)335–40.

79 Dorgan JF et al. Diet and sex hormones in girls: findings from a randomized controlled clinical trial. *J Natl Cancer Inst.* Jan 15, 2003, 95(2):132–41.

80 http://www.theguardian.com/science/2005/mar/03/1. Accessed Feb 7, 2016.

81 Hulett JL et al. Animal source foods have a positive impact on the primary school test scores of Kenyan schoolchildren in a cluster-randomised, controlled feeding intervention trial. *Br J Nutr.* Mar 14, 2014, 111(5):875–86.

82 Michael A. Woodley et al. Were the Victorians cleverer than us? The decline in general intelligence estimated from a meta-analysis of the slowing of simple reaction time *Intelligence.* 2013, 41(6):843–50.

83 http://www.huffingtonpost.com/2013/05/22/people-getting-dumber-human-intelligence-victoria-era_n_3293846.html. Accessed Feb 7, 2016.

84 http://www.thestar.com/news/canada/2012/09/24/hold_the_pablum_give_that_baby_some_meat_new_canadian_guidelines_advise.html. Accessed Feb 7, 2016.

85 Lozoff B et al. Preschool-aged children with iron deficiency anemia show altered affect and behavior. *J Nutr.* Mar 2007, 137(3):683–89.

86 Jamil KM et al. Micronutrients and anaemia. *Journal of Health, Population, and Nutrition.* Sep 2008, 26(3):340–55.

87 Linday LA et al. Lemon-flavored cod liver oil and a multivitamin-mineral supplement for the secondary prevention of otitis media in young children: pilot research. *Ann Otol Rhinol Laryngol.* Jul 2002, 111(7, Pt. 1):642–52.

88 http://www.nytimes.com/2012/03/06/health/rise-in-preschool-cavities-prompts-anesthesia-use.html?_r=0. Accessed Feb 7, 2016.

89 http://www.westonaprice.org/health-topics/the-arrest-of-dental-caries-in-childhood/. Accessed Feb 7, 2016.

90 Tanaka K et al. Dairy products and calcium intake during pregnancy and dental caries in children. *Nutr J.* May 17 2012, 11:33.

91 http://usatoday30.usatoday.com/news/health/2009-12-02-schoollunch02_st_N.htm. Accessed Feb 7, 2016.

92 Reedy J and Krebs-Smith SM. Dietary sources of energy, solid fats, and added sugars among children and adolescents in the United States. *J Am Diet Assoc.* Oct 2010, 110(10):1477–84.

93 http://dailycaller.com/2013/08/27/kentucky-students-to-first-lady-michelle-obama-your-food-tastes-like-vomit/. Accessed Feb 7, 2016.

94 http://blogs.naturalnews.com/kentucky-school-district-opts-federal-lunch-program-provides-healthy-school-lunches/. Accessed Feb 7, 2016.

95 http://www.foodnavigator-usa.com/Suppliers2/Consumer-psychology-could-be-used-to-eat-healthy-says-USDA. Accessed Feb 7, 2016.

96 http://www.fns.usda.gov/wic/background-revisions-wic-food-package. Accessed Feb 7, 2016.

97 http://www.azed.gov/health-nutrition/files/2011/06/cn017-11-nutrition-requirements-for-fluid-milk-and-fluid-milk-substitutions-in-the-cacfp-051311-cnr-2010-revised.pdf. Accessed Feb 7, 2016.

98 http://www.nytimes.com/2008/07/07/health/07cholesterol.html?pagewanted=print. Accessed Aug 8, 2016.

99 http://well.blogs.nytimes.com/2008/07/07/cholesterol-drugs-for-kids/?_r=0. Accessed Feb 7, 2016.

100 http://www.sfgate.com/business/article/EU-body-OKs-chewable-Lipitor-for-older-children-3259492.php. Accessed Feb 7, 2016.

101 Edison RJ and Muenke M. Mechanistic and epidemiologic considerations in the evaluation of adverse birth outcomes following gestational exposure to statins. *American Journal of Medical Genetics.* 2004, 131A:287–98.

102 Girardi G. Role of tissue factor in the maternal immunological attack of the embryo in the antiphospholipid syndrome. *Clin Rev Allergy Immunol.* Dec 2010, 39(3):160–65.

103 Merialdi M and Murray JC. The changing face of preterm birth. *Pediatrics.* Nov 2007, 120(5):1133–34.

104 Troisi A. Low cholesterol is a risk factor for attentional impulsivity in patients with mood symptoms. *Psychiatry Research.* Jun 30, 2011, 188(1):83–87.

105 http://www.westonaprice.org/childrens-health/healthy-baby-photo-gallery/.

Chapter 9: Animal Fats for the Mind

1 http://www.greatplainslaboratory.com/cholesterol/web/. Accessed Jan 23, 2016.

2 Mutka AL and Ikonen E. Genetics and molecular biology: brain cholesterol balance—not such a closed circuit after all. *Curr Opin Lipidol.* Feb 2010, 21(1):93–94.

3 Mary G. Enig. Unpublished study, personal communication.

4 Leutwyler K. Glia cells help neurons build synapses. *Scientific American*, Jan 29, 2001.

5 Mauch DH et al. CNS synaptogenesis promoted by glia-derived cholesterol. *Science.* Nov 9, 2001, 294(5545):1354–57.

6 Yu W et al. Segregation of Nogo66 receptors into lipid rafts in rat brain and inhibition of Nogo66 signaling by cholesterol depletion. *FEBS Letters.* Nov 5, 2004, 577(1–2):87–92.

7 http://www.nytimes.com/2000/01/04/science/a-decade-of-discovery-yields-a-shock-about-the-brain.html. Accessed Feb 8, 2016.

8 Mielke MM et al. High total cholesterol levels in late life associated with a reduced risk of dementia. *Neurology.* May 24, 2005, 64(10):1689–95.

9 West R et al. Better memory functioning associated with higher total and low-density lipoprotein cholesterol levels in very elderly subjects without the apolipoprotein e4 allele. *Am J Geriatr Psychiatry.* Sep 2008, 16(9):781–85.

10 http://www.lifeclinic.com/fullpage.aspx?prid=525859&type=1. Accessed Feb 8. 2016.

11 Elias PK et al. Serum cholesterol and cognitive performance in the Framingham Heart Study. *Psychosom Med.* Jan–Feb 2005, 67(1):24–30.

12 http://cbsn.ws/1RHsY4m; http://huff.to/1Pw4CnJ; http://carbwars.blogspot.com/2009/10/fat-improves -performance-for-pilots.html. Accessed Feb 8, 2016.

13 http://megson.com/readings/MedicalHypothesis.pdf. Accessed Feb 8, 2016.

14 Misner DL et al. Vitamin A deprivation results in reversible loss of hippocampal long-term synaptic plasticity. *Proc Natl Acad Sci USA.* Sep 25, 2001, 98(20):11714–19.

15 Stoney PN and McCaffery P. A vitamin on the mind: new discoveries on control of the brain by vitamin A. *World Rev Nutr Diet.* 2016, 115:98–108.

16 Latimer CS et al. Vitamin D prevents cognitive decline and enhances hippocampal synaptic function in aging rats. *Proc Natl Acad Sci USA.* Oct 14, 2014, 111(41):E4359–66.

17 Schlögl M and Holick MF. Vitamin D and neurocognitive function. *Clin Interv Aging.* Apr 2, 2014, 9:559–68; Zhang Y et al. The association of serum 25-hydroxyvitamin D levels with multiple sclerosis severity and progression in a case-control study from China. *J Neuroimmunol.* Aug 15, 2016, 297:127–31; Chiang M et al. Vitamin D in schizophrenia: a clinical review. *Evid Based Ment Health.* Feb 2016, 19(1):6–9; Holló A et al. Correction of vitamin D deficiency improves seizure control in epilepsy: a pilot study. *Epilepsy and Behavior.* Apr 11, 2012.

18 Mizwicki MT et al. 1α,25-dihydroxyvitamin D_3 and resolvin D_1 retune the balance between amyloid-β phagocytosis and inflammation in Alzheimer's disease patients. *J Alzheimers Dis.* 2013, 34(1):155–70.

19 Nagel G et al. Serum vitamin D concentrations and cognitive function in a population-based study among older adults in South Germany. *J Alzheimers Dis.* 2015, 45(4):1119–26.

20 Soni M et al. Vitamin D and cognitive function. *Scand J Clin Lab Invest Suppl.* 2012, 243:79–82.

21 Pilz S et al. Low vitamin D levels predict stroke in patients referred to coronary angiography. *Stroke.* Sep 2008, 39(9):2611–13.

22 Llewellyn DJ et al. Vitamin D and risk of cognitive decline in elderly persons. *Arch Intern Med.* Jul 12, 2010, 170(13):1135–41; Slinin Y et al. 25-Hydroxyvitamin D levels and cognitive performance and decline in elderly men. *Neurology.* Jan 5, 2010, 74(1):33–41.

23 Schneider AL et al.Vitamin D and cognitive function and dementia risk in a biracial cohort: the ARIC Brain MRI Study. *Eur J Neurol.* Sep 2014, 21(9):1211–8, e69–70; Michos ED et al. Vitamin D and subclinical cerebrovascular disease: the Atherosclerosis Risk in Communities Brain Magnetic Resonance Imaging Study. *JAMA Neurol.* Jul 1, 2014, 71(7):863–71.

24 Littlejohns TJ et al. Vitamin D and the risk of dementia and Alzheimer disease. *Neurology.* Sep 2, 2014, 83(10):920–28.

25 Maden M. Retinoids have differing efficacies on alveolar regeneration in a dexamethasone-treated mouse. *Am J Respir Cell Mol Biol.* 2006, 35(2):260–67.

26 Welsh et al. Night blindness precipitated by isotretinoin in the setting of hypovitaminosis A. *Australas J Dermatol.* 1999, 40(4):208–10.

27 Sieving PA et al. Inhibition of the visual cycle in vivo by 13-cis retinoic acid protects from light damage and provides a mechanism for night blindness in isotretinoin therapy. *Proc Natl Acad Sci USA.* 2001, 98(4):1835–40.

28 Danby FW. Oral isotretinoin, neuropathy and hypovitaminosis A. *Clin Exp Dermatol.* 2008, 33(2):190.

29 Bousvaros et al. Vitamins A and E serum levels in children and young adults with inflammatory bowel disease: effect of disease activity. *J Pediatr Gastroenterol Nutr.* 1998, 26(2):129–35; Mizuno et al. Serum vitamin A concentrations in asthmatic children in Japan. *Pediatrics International.* 2006, 48: 261–64; Arora et al. Vitamin A status in children with asthma. *Pediatr Allergy Immunol.* 2002, 13: 223–26. 897.

30 Bremner JD and McCaffery P. The neurobiology of retinoic acid in affective disorders. *Prog Neuropsychopharmacol Biol Psychiatry.* 2008, 32(2):315–31; O'Reilly K et al. Retinoid-mediated regulation of mood: possible cellular mechanisms. *Exp Biol Med.* 2008, 233:251–58.

31 Landy D. Pibloktoq (hysteria) and Inuit nutrition: possible implication of hypervitaminosis A. *Soc Sci Med.* 1985, 21(2):173–85.

32 Denisova NA and Booth SL. Vitamin K and sphingolipid metabolism: evidence to date. *Nutr Rev.* 2005, 63(4):110–21.

33 Han X et al. Substantial sulfatide deficiency and ceramide elevation in very early Alzheimer's disease: potential role in disease pathogenesis. *J Neurochem.* 2002, 82(4):809–18.

34 Bosio A et al. Functional breakdown of the lipid bilayer of the myelin membrane in central and peripheral nervous system by disrupted galactocerebroside synthesis. *Proc Natl Acad Sci USA.* 1996, 93:13280–85.

35 http://www.sciencedaily.com/releases/1998/04/980409080807.htm; Pyapali GK et al. Prenatal dietary choline supplementation decreases the threshold for induction of long-term potentiation in young adult rats. *J Neurophysiol.* Apr 1998, 79(4):1790–96.

36 Kuratko CN, et al. Relationship of docosahexaenoic acid (DHA) with learning and behavior in healthy children: a review. *Nutrients.* Jul 2013, 5(7):2777–810.

37 Horrocks LA and Yeo YK. Health benefits of docosahexaenoic acid (DHA). *Pharmacol Res.* Sep 1999, 40(3):211–25.

38 Matthew M et al. Serum phospholipid docosahexaenonic acid is associated with cognitive functioning during middle adulthood. *Journal of Nutrition.* 2010, 140(4):848–53.

39 Lukiw WJ et al. A role for docosahexaenoic acid-derived neuroprotectin D_1 in neural cell survival and Alzheimer disease. *J Clin Invest.* 2005, 115(10):2774–83.

40 McNamara RK et al. Selective deficits in the omega-3 fatty acid docosahexaenoic acid in the postmortem orbitofrontal cortex of patients with major depressive disorder. *Biol. Psychiatry.* 2007, 62(1):17–24; McNamara RK et al. Lower docosahexaenoic acid concentrations in the postmortem prefrontal cortex of adult depressed suicide victims compared with controls without cardiovascular disease. *Journal of Psychiatric Research.* 2013, 47(9):1187–91.

41 Rapoport SI. Arachidonic acid and the brain. *Journal of Nutrition.* 2008, 138(12):2515–20.

42 http://www.westonaprice.org/health-topics/the-pursuit-of-happiness/.
In footnote: [a] http://www.naturalchoice.net/blogs/Art13_Gut_Flora_Probiotics_Affect_Mood.html. Accessed Feb 7, 2016.

43 http://adh.fr.yuku.com/topic/470#.VqaRQL3rwUE. Accessed Feb 9, 2016.

44 http://cocaine.org/cart/cart.html. Accessed Feb 8, 2016.
In footnote: [a] is http://www.westonaprice.org/health-topics/the-pursuit-of-happiness/.

45 Patel S et al. Endocannabinoid signaling negatively modulates stress-induced activation of the hypothalamic-pituitary-adrenal axis. *Endocrinology.* 2004, 145:5431–38.

46 Kathuria S et al. Modulation of anxiety through blockade of anandamide hydrolysis. *Nature Med.* 2003, 9(1):76–81.

47 Placzek EA et al. Mechanisms for recycling biosynthesis and of endogenous anandamide and 2-arachidonylglycerol. *J Neurochem.* 2008, 107(4):987–1000.
In footnote: [a] Weaver CM and Heaney RP. Calcium. In Shils et al., eds. *Modern Nutrition in Health and Disease,* 10th ed. Baltimore, MD: Lippincott Williams & Wilkins, 2006, pp. 194–210.

48 Patrick RP and Ames BN. Vitamin D and the omega-3 fatty acids control serotonin synthesis and action, part 2: relevance for ADHD, bipolar disorder, schizophrenia, and impulsive behavior. *FASEB Journal.* Jun 2015, 29(6):2207–22.

49 Basky G. Suicide linked to serotonin gene. *CMAJ.* 2000, 162(9):1343.

50 Lesch KP et al. Association of anxiety-related traits with a polymorphism in the serotonin transporter gene regulatory region. *Science.* 1996, 274(5292):1527–31.

51 Alenina N et al. Growth retardation and altered autonomic control in mice lacking brain serotonin. *Proc Natl Acad Sci USA.* 2009, 106(25):10332–37.

52 Badawy A. Serotonin: the stuff of romance. *The Biochemist.* 2000, 15–17.

53 Frost M et al. Levels of serotonin, sclerostin, bone turnover markers as well as bone density and microarchitecture in patients with high bone mass phenotype due to a mutation in Lrp5. *J Bone Miner Res.* 2011, 26(8):1721–28.

54 http://www.webmd.com/depression/features/serotonin. Accessed Aug 11, 2016.

55 Badawy A. Serotonin: the stuff of romance. *The Biochemist*: 2000, 15–17.

56 http://www.mayoclinic.org/diseases-conditions/depression/in-depth/ssris/art-20044825. Accessed Aug 11, 2016.

57 Engelberg H. Low serum cholesterol and suicide. *Lancet.* Mar 21, 1992, 339:727–28.

58 Cocchetto DM et al. Behavioral perturbations in the vitamin K-deficient rat. *Physiology & Behavior.* 1985, 34(5):727–34.

59 Bremner JD and McCaffery P. The neurobiology of retinoic acid in affective disorders. *Prog Neuropsychopharmacol Biol Psychiatry.* 2008, 32(2):315–31.

60 Sink KS. *CB1 Inverse Agonists and Antagonists as Obesity Therapies: Effects on Food Motivation and Emotion.* PhD thesis. University of Connecticut, 2008.

61 http://psychcentral.com/lib/the-dopamine-connection-between-schizophrenia-and-creativity/. Accessed Aug 11, 2016.

62 http://medlicker.com/789-low-dopamine-causes-symptoms-diagnosis-and-treatment-options. Accessed Aug 11, 2016.

63 Salamone JD et al. Nucleus accumbens dopamine and the regulation of effort in food-seeking behavior: implications for studies of natural motivation, psychiatry, and drug abuse. *J Pharmacol Exp Ther.* 2001, 305(1):1–8.

64 Sink KS. *CB1 Inverse Agonists and Antagonists as Obesity Therapies: Effects on Food Motivation and Emotion.* PhD thesis. University of Connecticut, 2008.

65 http://www.westonaprice.org/health-topics/the-pursuit-of-happiness/.

66 Brunstein JC. Personal goals and subjective well-being: a longitudinal study. *Journal of Personality and Social Psychology.* 1993, 65(5):1061–70; Elliott AJ et al. Avoidance personal goals and the personality-illness relationship. *Journal of Personality and Social Psychology.* 1998, 75(5):1282–99; Sheldon KM et al. Pursuing personal goals: skills enable progress but not all progress is beneficial (PDF). *Personality and Social Psychology Bulletin* 1998, 24(12):1319–31.

67 Kessler RC et al. Lifetime prevalence and age-of-onset distributions of DSM-IV disorders in the National Comorbidity Survey Replication. *Arch Gen Psychiatry.* 2005, 62:593–602.

Chapter 10: The Queen of Fats: Why Butter Is Better

1 Chowdhury R et al. Association of dietary, circulating, and supplement fatty acids with coronary risk: a systematic review and meta-analysis. *Ann Intern Med.* Mar 18, 2014, 160(6):398–406.

2 Siri-Tarino PW et al. Meta-analysis of prospective cohort studies evaluating the association of saturated fat with cardiovascular disease. *Am J Clin Nutr.* Mar 2010, 91(3):535–46.

3 *Nutrition Week.* Mar 22, 1991, 21(12)2–3.

4 Gillman MW et al. Margarine intake and subsequent coronary heart disease in men. *Epidemiology.* Mar 1997, 8(2):144–49.

5 http://www.slideshare.net/rocomara/functional-foods-weekly-vol-4-no-36, #9. Accessed Feb 8, 2016.
In footnote: [a] http://www.westonaprice.org/health-topics/toxins-on-your-toast/.

6 Holmberg S et al. Food choices and coronary heart disease: a population based cohort study of rural Swedish men with 12 years of follow-up. *Int J Environ Res Public Health.* Oct 2009, 6(10):2626–38.
In footnote: [a] Pala V et al. Meat, eggs, dairy products, and risk of breast cancer in the European Prospective Investigation into Cancer and Nutrition (EPIC) cohort. *Am J Clin Nutr.* Sep 2009, 90(3):602–12.

7 de Oliveira Otto MC et al. Biomarkers of dairy fatty acids and risk of cardiovascular disease in the Multi-ethnic Study of Atherosclerosis. *J Am Heart Assoc.* Jul 18, 2013, 2(4):e000092.

8 Holmberg S and Thelin A. High dairy fat intake related to less central obesity: a male cohort study with 12 years' follow-up. *Scand J Prim Health Care.* Jun 2013, 31(2):89–94.

9 Kratz M et al. The relationship between high-fat dairy consumption and obesity, cardiovascular, and metabolic disease. *Eur J Nutr.* Feb 2013, 52(1):1–24.

10 Li Y et al. Saturated Fats Compared With Unsaturated Fats and Sources of Carbohydrates in Relation to Risk of Coronary Heart Disease: A Prospective Cohort Study. *J Am Coll Cardiol.* Oct 6, 2015, 66(14):1538–48.

11 http://www.hsph.harvard.edu/news/press-releases/butter-is-not-back-limiting-saturated-fat-still-best-for-heart-health/. Accessed Jan 25, 2016.

12 http://www.zoeharcombe.com/2015/10/butter-or-margarine/. Accessed Jan 25, 2016.

13 Enig MG. Health and Nutritional Benefits from Coconut Oil. *Price-Pottenger Nutrition Foundation Health Journal.* 1998, 20:1:1–6.

14 Nishii Y. n-Butyrate enhances induction of thyroid hormone-responsive nuclear proteins. *Endocrine Journal.* Oct 1993, 40(5):515–21.

15 Prasad KN. Butyric acid: a small fatty acid with diverse biological functions. *Life Sci.* Oct 13, 1980, 27(15):1351–58; Gershon H and Shanks L. In JJ Kabara, ed. *Symposium on the Pharmacological Effect of Lipids.* American Oil Chemists' Society, Champaign, IL, 1978, 51–62.

16 Belury MA. Conjugated dienoic linoleate: a polyunsaturated fatty acid with unique chemoprotective properties. *Nutr Rev.* Apr 1995, 53(4, Pt. 1):83–89; Kelly ML et al. Effect of intake of pasture on concentrations of conjugated linoleic acid in milk of lactating cows. *J Dairy Sci.* Jun 1998, 81(6):1630–36.

17 Rainer L et al. Conjugated linoleic acid: health implications and effects on body composition. *J Am Diet Assoc* (review). 2004, 104(6):963–68.

18 Onakpoya IJ et al. The efficacy of long-term conjugated linoleic acid (CLA) supplementation on body composition in overweight and obese individuals: a systematic review and meta-analysis of randomized clinical trials. *Eur J Nutr* (systematic review). 2012, 51(2):127–34.

19 Carta G et al. Metabolic interactions between vitamin A and conjugated linoleic acid. *Nutrients.* Mar 24, 2014, 6(3):1262–72.

20 Connor AB. The relation of the spectro vitamin A and carotene content of butter to its vitamin A potency measured by biological methods. *Texas Agricultural Experiment Station.* Bulletin 560, Feb 1938.

21 Price WA. *Nutrition and Physical Degeneration*, 6th ed. La Mesa, CA: Price-Pottenger Nutrition Foundation, 2004, p. 424.

22 Jennings IW. *Vitamins in Endocrine Metabolism.* Springfield, IL: Charles C Thomas Publisher, 1970.

23 http://www.westonaprice.org/wp-content/uploads/TheFatSolubleActivators.pdf.

24 Jetter A et al. Calcidiol form of vitamin D is better: pharmacokinetics of oral vitamin D(3) and calcifediol. *Bone.* Feb 2014, 59:14–19.

25 Wall CR et al. Vitamin D activity of breast milk in women randomly assigned to vitamin D_3 supplementation during pregnancy. *Am J Clin Nutr.* Feb 2016, 103(2):382–88.
In footnote: (§) [a] Murray MT. *Encyclopedia of Nutritional Supplements: The Essential Guide for Improving Your Health Naturally.* New York: Three Rivers Press. 1996.
In footnote: (*) (page 177) [a] Koopman JS et al. *AJPH,* 1984, 74(12)1371–73.

26 http://www.westonaprice.org/health-topics/dioxins-in-animal-foods-a-case-for-vegetarianism/.

27 Stohs et al. Effects of BHA, d-alpha-tocopherol and retinol acetate on TCDD-mediated changes in lipid peroxidation, glutathione peroxidase activity and survival. *Xenobiotica.* 1984, 14(7):533–37.

28 Chavarro JE et al. A prospective study of dairy foods intake and anovulatory infertility. *Hum Reprod.* May 2007, 22(5):1340–47.

29 Mercer JM. An experiment in milk pasteurization. *Nature's Path.* Mar 1941. In CP Bryant. *The Truth About Pasteurization.* Seattle, WA: National Nutrition League, 1943.

30 Price WA. *Nutrition and Physical Degeneration*: 6th ed. La Mesa, CA: Price-Pottenger Nutrition Foundation, 2004.

31 van Wagtendonk WJ and Wulzen R. *Arch Biochemistry.* New York: Academic Press, Inc., 1943, 1:373–77.

32 Hogg JA. Steroids, the steroid community, and Upjohn in perspective: a profile of innovation. *Steroids.* 1992, 57(12):593–616.

33 http://www.countrycrock.com/product/detail/91770/original. Accessed Feb 8, 2016.

34 http://www.icantbelieveitsnotbutter.com/product/detail/129799/i-can-t-believe-it-s-not-butter-original-spread. Accessed Feb 8, 2016.

35 http://www.statista.com/statistics/188760/top-margarine-spread-butter-blend-brands-in-the-united-states/. Accessed Feb 8, 2016.

36 http://www.poweredbyosteons.org/2012/01/lead-poisoning-in-rome-skeletal.html.

Index

Page numbers in italics refer to charts, and illustrations in the text.